Antithrombotic Drugs in Thrombosis Models

Author

Josef Hladovec

Senior Scientist
Laboratory of Thrombosis
4th Department of Medicine
Charles University
Prague, Czechoslovakia

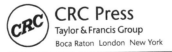

CRC Press
Taylor & Francis Group
Boca Raton London New York

CRC Press is an imprint of the
Taylor & Francis Group, an **informa** business

T0174917

CRC Press
Taylor & Francis Group
6000 Broken Sound Parkway NW, Suite 300
Boca Raton, FL 33487-2742

© 1989 by Taylor & Francis Group, LLC
CRC Press is an imprint of Taylor & Francis Group, an Informa business

First issued in paperback 2019

No claim to original U.S. Government works

ISBN 13: 978-0-367-45098-4 (pbk)
ISBN 13: 978-0-8493-5162-4 (hbk)

Visit the Taylor & Francis Web site at
http://www.taylorandfrancis.com

and the CRC Press Web site at
http://www.crcpress.com

Library of Congress Cataloging-in-Publication Data

Hladovec, Josef.
  Antithrombotic drugs in thrombosis models / Josef Hladovec.
    p. cm.
  Includes bibliographies and index.
  ISBN 0-8493-5162-6
  1. Thrombosis--Animal Models. 2. Fibrinolytic agents--Testing.
3. Thrombosis--Chemotherapy--Testing. I. Title.
  [DNLM: 1. Disease Models, Animal. 2. Fibrinolytic Agents-
-therapeutic use. 3. Thrombosis--drug therapy. QV 190 H677a]
RC694.3.H57 1989
616.1'35061--dc19
DNLM/DLC
for Library of Congress   88-38833
                                                                        CIP

Library of Congress Card Number 88-38833

PREFACE

This book is intended to serve as information about thrombosis models to all those interested, and particularly as a guide to those who are actively working on drug research. It is not a handbook and does not uncritically accumulate a host of data about as many thrombosis models as possible. Instead it attempts to bring a relatively new and integrated look to the problem with a sort of philosophy of thrombosis models and subjects the models described to a critical survey from this new viewpoint. This is why only a single author was necessary.

Meanwhile, the author was not alone in his task and is indebted to many people for help. Thus, he is indebted for the invaluable assistance to Mrs. Polyxeny Theodoru. His thanks are also due to the personnel of the Information Service of the Institute for the most helpful cooperation and particularly to Mr. Prahl for his linguistic assistance. Furthermore, he acknowledges the beneficial support of the head of the Experimental Department of the Institute, Dr. M. Vrána.

Josef Hladovec

THE AUTHOR

Josef Hladovec, M.D., Ph.D., is chief of the Laboratory of Thrombosis, 4th Department of Medicine, Charles University, in Praha, Czechoslovakia.

Dr. Hladovec graduated in 1950 from the medical faculty at Charles University in Praha, and in 1961 obtained a Ph.D. degree from the Czechoslovak Academy of Sciences.

Dr. Hladovec is a member of the Association of the Czechoslovak Medical Societies J. E. Purkyně (Cardiological Society, Physiological Society, and Haematological Society), the International Society on Thrombosis and Haemostasis, Serotonin Club, and is one of the editors of Thrombosis Research.

Dr. Hladovec has published over 200 scientific papers, almost all of them in international journals and in English. His main interest was always thrombosis research and particularly the pharmacology of thrombosis prophylaxis.

TABLE OF CONTENTS

Chapter 1
Introduction... 1

Chapter 2
The Rational Basis of Thrombosis Models 3
  I.   The Thrombosis Triad.. 3
  II.   Thrombosis Factors.. 4
         A.   Humoral Factors 4
              1.   Blood Clotting System 4
              2.   Fibrinolytic System.. 6
              3.   Platelets 7
         B.   Blood Flow Factors 8
         C.   Vascular Lesion 9
  III.   Multifactorial Pathogenesis 15
  IV.   What is a Model? 19
  V.   Classification of Thrombosis Models.................................... 20
         A.   Localization... 20
         B.   Type of Provocation 23
         C.   Experimental Animals 25
         D.   Method of Indication... 26
         E.   Time Span of the Experiment...................................... 26
         F.   Comprehensiveness of the Viewpoint 27
         G.   Number of Provoking Factors..................................... 27
         H.   Research Objectives 28
  VI.   Conclusions from the Survey.. 28
References.. 30

Chapter 3
Basic Methods 39
  I.   Model of Vascular Lesion... 39
  II.   Arterial Thrombosis Model.. 55
  III.   Venous Thrombosis Model 67
  IV.   Possible Additional Models 71
  V.   The Use of New Models in the Drug Screening............................ 71
References.. 72

Chapter 4
Effects of Antithrombotics and Results of Drug Screening 75
  I.   Acetylsalicylic Acid (ASA) 75
         A.   Activation... 76
         B.   Adhesion... 76
         C.   Aggregation.. 77
         D.   Release 78
  II.   Dipyridamole... 87
  III.   Sulfinpyrazone 94
  IV.   Heparin..101
  V.   Pentoxifylline...111

VI. Ticlopidine 113
VII. Nafazatrom 115
VIII. Suloctidil 118
IX. Drugs Interacting with the Eicosanoid System 121
X. Adrenolytics 124
XI. Calcium Channel Blocking Agents 130
XII. Ketanserin 135
XIII. Bioflavonoids 141
XIV. Clofibrate 149
XV. Anagrelide 151
XVI. Dextran 152
XVII. Oral Anticoagulants 153
XVIII. Other Agents 156
XIX. Conclusions 159
References 161

Chapter 5
Drug Combinations 189
I. Introduction 189
II. Combinations of ASA with Dipyridamole 189
III. Other Drug Combinations 191
IV. Conclusions of the Combination Section 218
References 220

Chapter 6
General Conclusions 225

Index 227

Chapter 1

INTRODUCTION

Ever since the recognition of the pathogenetic role of thrombosis, that is since the mid-19th century, many authors have attempted to find effective ways to dispose of this killer number one. First, it was necessary to know more about the mechanism of thrombus development.

One line of research followed the humoral changes which would predispose to or even cause thrombosis. This line leaned heavily on biochemical methods and scored tremendous successes particularly in our times. Another line represented a predominantly experimental approach which, in distinction to the first one, attempted to see thrombosis as a whole in model situations induced in experimental animals. This line has been present since the start of thrombosis research and has been never completely abandoned. Nevertheless, it was very often, and not to the benefit of our knowledge, eclipsed by the successes of the biochemical line of research. The third line is a clinical and pathological one. It supplies us with new and alarming data about the deadly character of thrombosis, leads to attempts to recognize this process in time and to offer more or less effective prevention and even treatment.

It is necessary to state straightly that the problem of effective prevention and treatment remains, in general, unsolved. Nevertheless, an impression is present all the time that more effective ways are feasible and waiting behind the door for discovery. One way to discover them is to pursue the first successful biochemical line; accumulation of further and more detailed information about new systems and factors which would once more appear as the most important and ultimately decisive ones. A probably more useful way would be to proceed along the second experimental line which alone can mediate healthy relations with the clinic and serve also as a corrective of the excesses of sometimes exaggerated self-assurance of the first research line.

Chapter 2

THE RATIONAL BASIS OF THROMBOSIS MODELS

I. THE THROMBOSIS TRIAD

In this chapter thrombosis will be dealt with as a general problem even though differences undoubtedly exist between thrombosis on the arterial and venous side, and even more so, between both and the disseminated intravascular coagulation. This general view allows us to pay particular attention to the traits and mechanisms common to thrombosis in all localizations and then point out differences if necessary.

Essentially, thrombosis is a multifactorial process, just as almost all serious and still incompletely understood and controlled circulatory derangements of our days are. The simple ones have already been solved. It is generally handed down that the multifactorial character of thrombosis was discovered by Virchow[1] who formulated his triad as a combination of stasis, inflammatory changes in the vessel wall, and changes in the properties of blood. It would be only fitting to mention that all three factors were recognized some time before Virchow by the Viennese pathologist of Czech origin, Rokitansky, in his "Krasenlehre".[2] He pointed out in a quite up-to-date way the role of systemic humoral changes, whereas Virchow emphasized in his somewhat polemic studies mostly local conditions of thrombus development. On the other hand, credit is due to Virchow for using an experimental approach and for having been the first to formulate the concept of embolism. Virchow mentioned that he introduced the term thrombosis, even though the term thrombus is of a much older date and was used, e.g., by Galenus. Rokitansky distinguished thrombi developing on the basis of vessel-wall inflammation combined with stasis and assigned an important role to the liberation of materials from the vascular wall in the process ("Exudate"). This reminds us of the modern knowledge about the secretory function of the endothelium. He also distinguished inflammation which was secondary to the development of thrombus, but in his eyes thrombus may be the result of inflammatory processes in other areas of circulation outside the site of thrombosis or may be a consequence of "einer aus einem inneren Momente (Blutkrankheit) hervorgegangener Blutgerinnung". He knew well the differences between arterial and venous thrombi and recognized thrombolysis as a "feine Zertheilung" or "Auflösung" of thrombi. A close relation existed in his concept between a vascular inflammatory reaction, blood clotting, and thrombus development on one side and atherosclerotic processes on the other. He also described "die Prozesse von Stase und Blutgerinnung in den verschiedensten Abschnitten des Capillargefässsystems" that came to be known much later as disseminated intravascular coagulation. All that may be summarized in the statement that Rokitanski's views of thrombogenesis were characterized by unusual dynamism and anticipation. As his ideas were published in advance of Virchow's it would probably be just to call Rokitanski the father not only of modern atherosclerosis theories, but also of current concepts of thrombosis. This is not meant to diminish the credit due to Virchow in the field of our knowledge about thrombosis. He has, for example, introduced the term fibrinogen and stimulated the studies of A. Schmidt who laid the ground to our present knowledge about the coagulation system.

If the thrombogenesis triad is approximated to the present state of the problem, the three factors have now rather the form of three groups of related factors (Table 1). All these factors contribute to the production of a special state of the organism, mostly existing for a limited period of time and confined particularly to a circumscribed site of the vascular system to result in thrombus formation. Meanwhile, thrombosis may be defined as local adhesion to the vascular wall of more or less structured masses accumulating locally from

TABLE 1
Thrombosis Triad and its
Contemporary Correlates

Originally	Presently
Humoral factor ("crasis")	Blood clotting
	Fibrinolysis
	Platelets
Stasis	Hemodynamic factors
	Hemorheologic factors
Vascular lesion	Vascular lesion

constituents of flowing blood as a consequence of a deviation of hemostatic mechanism and leading to a partial or complete obstruction of blood flow.

II. THROMBOSIS FACTORS

A. HUMORAL FACTORS
1. Blood Clotting System

Sometimes a primary role in the development of thrombosis is ascribed to changes in the blood clotting system. The meaning of the designation "primary", however, is not very clear. If it is accepted that thrombosis is a multifactorial process, the primary contribution is meant to be made by such factors which would produce thrombosis alone, without the preliminary assistance of other factors implicated in the process only as secondary consequences. However, this is not the case even in hereditary blood clotting defects connected with a predisposition to thrombosis because they exist mostly for a lifetime whereas thrombosis develops only in case of favorable coincidence with other contributing factors. Nevertheless, it is possible to admit their important influence.

If the clinical experience is taken into account in only a portion of thrombosis patients, between 10 and 20%, a hereditary defect of a known blood clotting factor or inhibitor may be of such an important influence, or may have substantially contributed to the development of thrombosis.[3-6] Antithrombin III deficiency, caused either by the lack of or a qualitative defect in the molecule, was found in about 2% of thrombosis cases. Deficiency of protein S was estimated in 10% of cases up to 40 years of age. The frequency of factor C defects is still difficult to assess. Other hereditary defects such as dysfibrinogenemias, factor XII deficiency, and sickle cell anemia are infrequently connected with the occurrence of thrombosis. Another portion of thrombosis patients may have inherited defects of the fibrinolytic system such as deficient or defective plasminogen, deficient tissue plasminogen activator (tPA) synthesis or release, as well as increased plasminogen activator inhibitor (PAI). This particularly concerns patients with recurrent attacks of deep vein thrombosis. Of course, not all possibly important factors and their hereditary defects have been properly identified as yet. Some factors inhibiting endothelial synthesis, accumulation or release of blood clotting or fibrinolytic factors or endothelial viability may exist as well, such as in homocysteinemia.[7,8] A special kind of a hereditary predisposition in thrombosis patients is suggested by the high freqency of some HLA antigens (Cw 4)[9] and the prevalence of blood group A.[10-14]

As mentioned above, in patients with hereditary predispositions relatively weak additional provocation is needed for thrombosis development and it is in this subgroup of thrombosis patients that humoral factors may play an important role. However, even under such conditions the process of thrombosis is still multifactorial.

A rather different situation exists in the case of acquired humoral defects. They may be manifested as hypercoagulable states, if defined on the basis of laboratory tests, or as

TABLE 2
Laboratory Tests for Hypercoagulability

From the side of the coagulation system	APTT
	Factor VII level
	Factor VIII level
	Fibrinogen
	FP-A and other fibrinogen split products
	AT III and its complexes with serine proteases
	Proteins C and S
From the side of the fibrinolytic system	Basal PA level
	PA level after
	Exercise
	DDAVP
	Venostasis
	PAI

thrombophilia, if related simply to an increased frequency of thrombotic episodes.[4,15-17] Numerous tests have been suggested for the detection of hypercoagulable state, to name but the most important or most discussed ones (Table 2).[18-20] They were looked for particularly in the hope of finding better prediction indicators so that radical antithrombotic treatment, or rather prophylaxis, might be reserved predominantly for detected high risk patients. On the other hand, there is no universal agreement as to their value due to the inherent weakness of the definition and concept of hypercoagulability or prethrombotic state. Positivity in such tests appears to be generally of a secondary character, their proponents having been to some extent, misled by the easiness of obtaining blood and simplicity of their performance. The fact that it may occur often in advance of manifest thrombosis does not prove any causal relationship. Despite some recent improvements, these tests if carried out in well-selected batteries, are more useful for population studies than for individual diagnosis. Moreover, we do not know which of them are really representative of the supposed thrombosis-prone state, and above all, they are not yet sufficiently standardized to be comparable from laboratory to laboratory. Some of them, as FP-A, are so sensitive that they may be positive even under normal conditions.

Another problematic aspect is the difficulty to distinguish between a tendency to thrombosis, developing thrombosis, and existing latent or fully manifest thrombosis. Of course, in the diagnosis of existing thrombosis, laboratory tests may have only supporting value for instrumental diagnosis, which is in general preferred. In addition, it is almost impossible to recognize what is primary or predominant in the pathogenesis of thrombosis and what is of secondary compensatory or reactive nature. All these difficulties are not surprising if the dynamic character of thrombosis is taken into account. A stabilized cut-and-dried state almost never exists. The picture is further complicated by the concept of a continuous dynamic equilibrium between thrombus formation and thrombolysis.[21,22] Even though this concept of continuous latent clotting is not generally accepted, the formation of small transitory non-occluding thrombi is probably much more frequent than generally supposed, e.g., after prolonged immobilization during travel in leg veins, after inflammatory and reparatory processes, etc.

Another objection to the concept of hypercoagulability is the fact that most of these acquired defects are, in all probability, the consequence of a vascular lesion. This is particularly evident if the typical pathological states are considered in which hypercoagulability is most often observed (Table 3). In some conditions the contribution of a vascular lesion may be less conspicuous, as for example with artificial prostheses and other foreign surfaces inserted in the circulation. The same is observed with hereditary humoral defects, nephrotic

TABLE 3
The Relation of Hypercoagulability to the
Presence of a Vascular Lesion

Hypercoagulability states with evident primary role of vascular lesion	Postoperative states
	Posttraumatic states
	Malignancies
	Inflammatory conditions
	Myocardial infarction and other ischemias
	Smoking
Hypercoagulable states with probable primary role of vascular lesion	Cardiac insufficiency
	Prolonged stasis
	Diabetes mellitus
	Atherosclerosis
	Cardiomyopathy
	Hepatic insufficiency
	Bürger's disease
	Behcet's disease
	Immunology reactions
	Homocystinuria
	Oral contraceptive use
	Lupus erythematodes, etc.

syndrome (probably caused by AT III deficiency) and after administration of coagulation factor concentrates. Exceptionally it was described after EACA, during rebound after oral anticoagulants, heparin-induced thrombocytopenia, and AT III decrease.

It is evidently exceptional to show that an acquired hypercoagulable state could start without vascular lesion, and the other way around, with every vascular lesion or even functional perturbation anywhere in the vascular tree, blood clotting and platelet activation resulting in a local or disseminated thrombosis even at distant sites should be expected as a possible consequence. In fact, most hypercoagulability tests represent an indirect indication of the presence or recent presence of vascular lesion somewhere in the circulatory bed.

All this should not mean that humoral factors are not necessary in the process. Acquired deficiencies of anticoagulant inhibitors may result from their consumption during thrombotic or excessive hemostatic processes. Such deficiencies or excessive release of some factors may contribute to the positive feedback leading to thrombosis. In arterial thrombosis, a contributing factor may be the release of serotonin from platelets into the systemic circulation leading to the potentiation of platelet aggregation by usual mediators in an avalanche-like way. In both venous and arterial thrombosis, a mild vascular lesion might produce a defective function of the endothelium, and possibly, also a systemic humoral change which cannot be specified as yet (tissue factor release?). Under special conditions, predisposing humoral changes may originate from some dietary influences such as hyperlipidemia after consumption of saturated fats or cholesterol,[23-26] from stressful situations, etc.

2. Fibrinolytic System

Reviews on the fibrinolytic system may be found elsewhere.[27-29] Only those aspects will be dealt with in this book which concern its integration into the process of thrombosis as a whole. In fact, fibrinolysis steps into the process probably later than other humoral factors and represents predominantly a defense against an already forming or formed thrombus. It might be argued that according to the theory of the continuous dynamic equilibrium between thrombus formation and thrombolysis, the participation of the latter should be shifted already to the beginning of the process. This assumption is supported, to some extent, by the fact that hereditary defects of the fibrinolytic system, such as defects in tPA synthesis or release as well as the presence of excess PAI, may be connected with an increased frequency of clinical thrombosis. On the other hand, this may be explained on the basis of a very frequent occurrence of latent, short-lived, and small thrombi that get rapidly dissolved under normal conditions. Administration of antifibrinolytics such as epsilonaminocaproic acid or aprotinin may serve, particularly EACA, as hemostatic agents. Their administration is not, with rare exceptions, associated with local thrombosis,[30,31] even though they may contribute to the development of disseminated intravascular thrombosis and local thrombosis in some models.[32] This contribution is probably based on the stabilization of microthrombi which would be quickly dissolved under normal conditions. In general, fibrinolysis represents only a secondary modifying factor and is probably not closely connected with the early stages of thrombus development.

3. Platelets

Platelets play an even more important role in the earliest stages of thrombosis than the blood clotting system which is, from the phylogenetic point of view, a later development. They contribute decisively to arterial thrombosis and may participate largely even in a portion of clinical venous thrombosis cases. At the same time, the descriptions of platelet derangements involve almost invariably ''minus'' defects leading to hemorrhagic diathesis. It is somewhat surprising to find that inherited ''plus'' defects are practically unknown, but it is possible that they have only remained undetected as yet. A hereditary condition with hypersensitive platelets to aggregating agents complicated by cerebral infarction at a relatively low age has been described.[4] Primary acquired ''plus'' defects of platelet function are infrequent. Thrombocythemias, whether of myeloproliferative, postsplenectomic, e.g., for hemolytic anemia, or reactive etiology (thrombocytosis), are more often connected with bleeding than thrombosis which prevails only in thrombocythemia accompanying polycythemia vera.[34,35] Of course, in that condition other factors may also contribute such as high blood viscosity and slowing of blood flow. In other types of thrombocythemia, the occurrence of thrombosis is not high enough to justify their classification as thrombophilias. Knizley and Noyes[36] linked iron deficiency thrombocytosis with the development of thrombosis. Some cases of ulcerative colitis are connected with thrombocytosis and thrombosis.[37] Thrombosis after heparin administration exists even though this claim may sound odd.[38]

There are two types of postheparin thrombocytopenias of the consumption type. The first one may be called a heparin-induced thrombotic thrombocytopenia. It is a serious condition probably of immune origin. The other type connected with an acute transitory decrease of platelet counts after heparin administration is dependent on the origin and probably the purity of preparations. The mechanism of its development is still not well understood. The classical thrombotic thrombocytopenic purpura is probably an immune disorder. It may be a disease of the vessel wall rather than of platelets themselves associated, according to some authors, with a deficient prostacyclin production or with circulating polymers of von Willebrand's factor.[39,40]

A large group of secondary platelet activation states as indicated by hypersensitivity to various aggregating agents, or more appropriately, the release of platelet factors and constituents as in complicated atherosclerosis,[41,42] diabetes mellitus,[43-45] smoking,[46,47] advanced age,[48,49] and perhaps even in hypertension[50] and emotional stress,[51] is characterized by a previous vascular lesion. Nevertheless, some studies were negative.[52,53] Platelets and the vascular wall have very close functional relations and platelet activation may be considered one of the most sensitive indicators of endothelial dysfunction. A large number of tests have been devised to detect platelet activation (Table 4).

Here, the contribution of other formed elements of blood may be mentioned. Leukocytes play an important role in the pathology of microcirculation due to their size and high reactivity. They have a very important function in the further history of already formed thrombi and may contribute significantly to thrombolysis. Their role in the early phases of thrombus formation is very little known but they might participate already in the development

TABLE 4
Tests for Platelet Activation

Beta-thromboglobulin release (β—TG)
Platelet antiheparin factor (PF—4)
Thromboxane A_2 (TXA$_2$) metabolite, TXB$_2$
Platelet turnover (suitable for group studies only)
Circulating platelet aggregates (still disputed)

of a vascular lesion due to their high content of potential mediators, e.g., proteolytic enzymes, components of the immune and complement system, kinin system, their capability to produce constituents of the prostaglandin and leukotriene system,[54,55] interleukins,[56] as well as the ability of polymorphonuclear leukocytes to exhibit the "oxygen burst" connected with the production of potentially very harmful oxygen free radical species.[57] Of importance may be the procoagulant activity in monocytes and other mononuclear leukocytes.[58,59] On the other hand, the ability of leukocytes to remove or destroy some procoagulant mediators should be kept in mind. Leukocytes may be also actively attracted by the already damaged vascular wall, and their enhancing effect on the local vascular spasm could contribute to thrombotic occlusion. The thrombogenic potential of leukocytes is illustrated by the existence, even if in a minority of cases, of a marked thrombotic tendency in leukemia.[34]

The contribution of erythrocytes should not be underestimated if only in view of their large quantity. They influence, particularly if their number is increased above the normal range, (e.g., in polycythemia vera) and with some pathological qualitative changes, the rheological properties of blood increasing the interaction of platelets with the vessel wall, increasing stasis, and producing a "sludge". Their influence could be also of a chemical character as they release (or unmask) thromboplastic material in hemolysis,[32,60] contribute to the ADP production,[61] and even their passive inclusion into the bulk of the thrombus may be of significance. The marked thrombotic tendency in sickle cell anemia may serve as an example of erythrocyte contribution.[62]

B. BLOOD FLOW FACTORS

Thrombosis factors related to blood flow may be divided into rheological (flow properties of blood) and hemodynamic (flow conditions of blood), the latter dependent on the properties of the vascular bed such as size, smoothness of surface, etc. Rheological factors are much more important in microcirculation than in large vessels and more so in arteries than in veins. Of course, they may indirectly influence venous return and in this way the stagnation in large veins. From the rheological point of view a particular importance may acquire an increased viscosity of whole blood at low shear rates mainly connected with increased erythrocyte aggregation either reversible, or more often irreversible (sludge). It is also often associated with an increased hematocrit and/or fibrinogen level. Another important predisposing derangement may be decreased erythrocyte deformability which is often a consequence of ischemia. Under special conditions some influence may be attributed to a greatly increased plasma viscosity such as that often seen in myeloma or even to much increased leukocyte and platelet counts. Increased fibrinogen is often observed in connection with an acute phase reaction as well as in some degenerative and chronic inflammatory conditions.

Hemodynamic changes are particularly important for thrombosis in large vessels such as stasis resulting from a decreased venous tonus, decreased pumping activity of the heart on the venous side, or various defects in flow-laminarity in large arteries caused mostly by stenotic atherosclerotic changes. These defects occurring in most cases at particularly exposed predisposing sites result in a disturbed flow with the development of turbulences, vortex formation, etc., and are connected with an increased frequency of platelet impacts on the vessel wall. Local predisposition to thrombosis in arteries may also be related to sites of boundary layer separation with stasis, local hypoxia of endothelial lining, and silting off formed elements, particularly platelets and leukocytes.

The effect of stasis is more complex than evident at first sight. It includes changes in endothelial function amounting to a secondary vascular lesion as manifested by the appearance of interendothelial gaps and increased permeability.[63,64] This induces, in turn, further increases in stasis. Another consequence of stasis is decreased removal of activated blood clotting factors by the reticuloendothelial system leading to their local accumulation sufficient to overwhelm the local defense system and start on an avalanche-like process.

On the arterial side, a more or less systemic role may be ascribed to a vascular lesion brought about by an increased shear stress in hypertension. A local influence is exerted by stenosis and unevenness of the vascular surface, or even changes in its adhesive properties as a consequence of a vascular lesion of various degree, or at least, functional perturbations. It should be kept in mind that even spastic stenosis may produce an acute flow disturbance in muscular arteries to start a thrombosis.[65]

Of the various tests available for the estimation of the rheologic properties of blood, it is necessary to name hematocrit, fibrinogen estimation, and to some extent, even the sedimentation rate. A more objective method is viscosity estimation at various shear rates. Rotation viscosimeters are generally used for this purpose. Erythrocyte deformability may be determined by various methods such as the filtration rate or viscosity measurement at relatively higher shear rates with whole blood and plasma. None of these deformability methods is adequately standardized.

In conclusion, blood flow factors have the main localizing function in both venous and arterial thrombosis.

C. VASCULAR LESION

A vascular lesion often plays a primary role in thrombosis in the sense that a major lesion may take along both blood clotting and platelet activation. In most other situations, a vascular lesion has a central or predominant position in the sense that it decides about the localization in both arterial and venous thrombosis, or timing in venous thrombosis, and that all relevant processes converge on the vessel wall, e.g., platelet-vessel wall interactions, blood-clotting activation and fibrin formation, thrombolysis, vascular tonus regulation, etc.

What is, in fact, a vascular lesion? The term vascular covers all constituents of the vessel wall, but in most situations, the key role is played by the endothelium forming a barrier between tissues and circulation. To define lesion is much more difficult and it may be useful to distinguish four categories of lesions:

1. It is most probable that already such changes may be of importance which are still purely functional, such as those resulting from stimulation or perturbation. Such changes may still be completely reversible and it is questionable whether morphological methods could be of any value in their detection, ultramicroscopic methods not excepted. After such stimulation, some of the many endothelial functions may be enhanced, others inhibited, and the delicate balance between prothrombotic and antithrombotic functions may be disturbed. This category may include adaptive processes leading to structural reconstruction of cells with subsequent functional changes. Agents may be released from or unmasked in the surface layer of the endothelium, surface coat or glycocalyx, or even actively secreted by the cytoplasm. Exhaustion of some defensive functions may take place after prolonged stimulation.

2. The next category includes changes that already have some morphological correlates such as demonstrable changes in the thickness of glycocalyx,[66] increased formation of vacuoles, blebs and other projections,[67] mitochondrial swelling,[68] nuclear bulging,[67] shape alterations,[69] etc. Such changes should be evaluated with utmost care because of the danger of methodological artifacts. It is appropriate to mention here the story

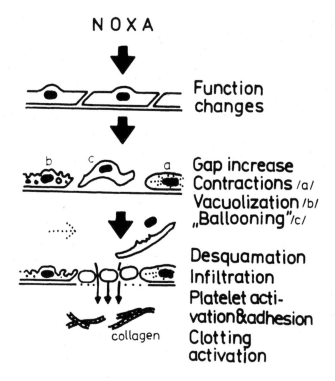

FIGURE 1.   Morphological changes characteristic of endothelial lesions.

of interendothelial bridges,[70,71] the disputed existence of endothelial contractility,[72,73] or the controversy over the existence of glycocalyx, once called endothelial cement,[74-76] whose existence was denied for a long time by electron microscopists to be accepted at last after methodological improvements.

3.   The third category includes defects in continuity of the endothelial lining. They are connected at first with the appearance of gaps and holes in the region of intercellular junctions or craters in the cell body.[67,69] In the following stage, ballooning of cells may eventually result in their partial detachement from the subendothelium, or even in complete desquamation and washing away with blood flow.[77] Such losses may involve single cells or whole groups (Figure 1). Large scale denudations are most often connected with the next stage of lesions.

4.   The last category concerns subendothelial structures and may include lesions of media and adventitia. The processes activated by such deep lesions may be very different from those characteristic for mild lesions with some of them stressed (prothrombotic, hemostatic) and others inhibited.

Meanwhile, it is important to realize that vascular lesion does not need to be present particularly at the site of developing thrombosis, and may be more or less of a systemic character. An example is deep vein thrombosis which was in former German terminology called "Fernthrombose", i.e., thrombosis taking place at another site than the activation of the humoral factor. An analogous situation may be present in arterial thrombosis as well.

In general, using morphological criteria, the presence of a vascular lesion may be confirmed but never excluded. It is important to accept the fact that endothelium can no longer be looked upon in an over-simplified way as a passive lining of a pipe with an adaptable diameter, but that it represents a tissue very much alive and active, having a high metabolic rate based on aerobic glycolysis, and due to its content of many enzymatic systems, capable of exerting various functions some of which play a key role in maintaining blood fluidity. It synthesizes many matrix and glycocalyx constituents including glycoproteins, some of them closely related to those of platelets, glycosaminoglycans such as heparan monosulfate, and proteins such as collagen III, IV, and V, fibronectin, elastin, laminin, etc.[78-81]

Various enzymes are present such as ATPase, ADPase, 5-nucleotidase, carboanhydrase (particularly in the lung), angiotensine-converting enzyme and lipoprotein lipase.[79] Many mediators such as adenosine, some of autacoid character such as prostacyclin and EDRF, are produced contributing to the regulation of vascular tonus. Other products are involved in the regulation of blood fluidity such as tissue factor, factor VIII, von Willebrand's factor, factor V, PAF (platelet activating factor), PAI (plasminogen activator inhibitor) on the one hand and tissue plasminogen activator (tPA), antithrombin III, heparinlike materials, thrombomodulin, etc.,[80] on the other hand. The endothelium possesses probably a very complex system for the regulation of its own multiplication as well as that of cells in the subendothelial layers (contact inhibition, EDGF).[82,83] Permeability changes lead, in addition, to an infiltration of platelet-derived growth factor (PDGF).[84] Endothelium metabolizes many circulating mediators such as biogenic amines by monoaminooxidase (particularly in the lung) and bradykinin by kininases.[85] A high adenylate metabolism is present particularly in the coronary circulation.[79] Furthermore, endothelium possesses receptors for acetylcholine, noradrenaline, and other catecholamines, angiotensin II, histamine, serotonin, bradykinin, thrombin, ATP, ADP, adenosine, substance P, etc.[78]

Some authors have pointed out differences between the functions of the endothelium in different organs and in various portions of the vascular bed.[86,78] On the other hand, the basic reactions to various kinds of vascular injury are very stereotyped due to a very similar fixation of cells to the subendothelial matrix and to each other, presence of a surface coat and its main constituents (glycosaminoglycans), the contribution of calcium ions to its properties, as well as the response to various desquamating agents. All that is very similar not only in the endothelium from various regions but even in corneal endothelium, mesothelium of the peritoneal cavity, and possibly in some epithelial linings such as stomach mucosa. All these cellular linings have certain functional and morphological characteristics in common. It is true that the enzymatic and receptor equipment may be very different, for example, the presence of particularly high levels of ATP and xanthin dehydrogenase in coronary arteries or carboanhydrase in lung vessels. Nevertheless, all these differences may represent only adaptations to local requirements based on the particular development of inherent potentials present in all endothelial cells. Sometimes such differences may result from a methodology of cell cultivation. Of course, in special situations such differences should be kept in mind.

The importance of the role of endothelium in maintaining blood fluidity stands out after consulting several numbers. The total endothelial surface is about 200 m^2 in man at rest. This area may be increased by opening further portions of the microcirculation about three times. On the average, 1 ml of blood is distributed at rest as a thin film over a surface area of 30 $\times$ 30 cm and this surface is formed by very active cells. Of the value of 200 m^2 about 56% come from capillaries and 98% from the whole microcirculation including arterioles and venules. Meanwhile, one endothelial cell has a surface area of about 600 μm^2. It may be accepted that under normal conditions and in most organs, with the notable exception of lungs, this surface is relatively smooth but it may increase markedly by the pathological formation of blebs and other projections. The total number of endothelial cells in man is about 4 $\times$ 10^{11}. They have a variable half-life *in situ* of about 12 months and the value may decrease many times under special conditions.[87,88] This means that under normal conditions about 55 elements must appear in 1 ml of blood per 1 min as it is supposed that cells that have lost their viability are desquamated. Their replacement at the abandoned site is probably a matter of minutes, particularly if they are probably pushed out by neighboring

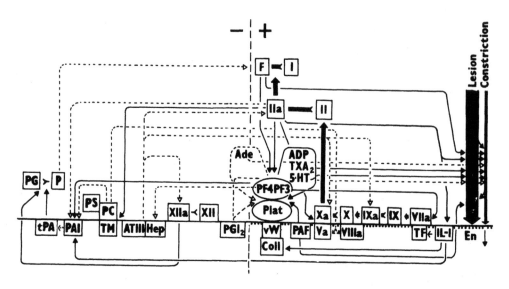

FIGURE 2.   Pro- and antithrombotic functions of endothelium. Full horizontal line: endothelial lining with the right half damaged. Broken line divides pro- and antithrombotic factors produced or associated with endothelium. Inhibition — — — →; passing into⟩——— ; enhancing effect ———→; PG: plasminogen; P: plasmin; TM: thrombomodulin; vW: von Willebrand's factor; PS: protein S; IIa: thrombin; Aden: adenosine; F: fibrin; I: fibrinogen; En: endothelium.

cells.[77] Temporary accumulation of platelets on the subendothelium may be accomplished in seconds and some active subendothelial surface must be unmasked continually. Under pathological conditions platelets may be probably attached even to seemingly "intact" (possibly degenerated) endothelial cells. This is still the object of discussions.[77,89]

Figure 2 shows schematically some more important prothrombotic and antithrombotic factors active at the endothelial surface and their mutual interactions. Of course, the figure cannot show all interrelations and despite all simplifications it is still quite complicated. The relations of thrombus formation and vascular lesions are emphasized. Prothrombotic activity is exerted by some fibrinogen and fibrin degradation products (early stage products), thrombin, thromboxane A_2, serotonin, as well as interleukin-1 which is synthesized not only by leukocytes but also by endothelial cells. Interleukin-1 (IL-1) not only increases the synthesis of various matrix components, but also of plasminogen activator inhibitor (PAI) and tissue factor (tissue thromboplastin).[55,56,90] Factor XIIa appears in the diagram on the inhibitory side as thrombotic complications prevail in its deficiency at least partially due to its enhancing effect on the activation of the fibrinolytic system. Thrombin (IIa) exerts many influences on both sides which are (1) enhancement of PAI decay; (2) activation of the protein C (PC) system on one side; (3) platelet activation; (4) factor V and VIII activation; and (5) stimulation of interleukin-1 synthesis on the other. PAI decay is also activated by protein C. Platelets likewise contribute to both the inhibitory (adenosine and prostacycline release) and enhancing side (ADP, TXA_2, serotonin, PF 4 and PF 3). The serine-esterase inhibiting system of the AT III-heparan complex inhibits not only thrombin, but also XIIa, Xa, and IXa. The endothelium produces both tissue plasminogen activator (tPA) and PAI, thrombomodulin (TM), AT III and heparin-like mucopolysaccharides (hep), collagen and von Willebrand's factor (vW), factor VIII, tissue factor, and IL-1. It manifests also the factor V activity. All the above effects do not necessarily step into action simultaneously and some need not join at all. It depends on the degree and character of a vascular lesion, as well as on the stage of the process with some portions entering the action at the start and others at the end of the whole process. This is illustrated by the production from fibrinogen and fibrin of split products which at first increase a vascular lesion (early split products), activate platelets and blood clotting to be later replaced by products activating fibrinolysis and stimulating repair.[91-94]

There exists a very finely tuned equilibrium between both prothrombotic and antithrombotic functions. Nawroth rightfully points out the discrepancy between laboratory findings concerning the blood-clotting system and clinical observations.[95,96] All important processes of thrombogenesis are taking place on the endothelial surface and are also strongly modified by this close association. To study only blood removed from the vessel cannot correctly indicate the actual situation in the organism as the sample has broken loose from a complex dynamic equilibrium with the vessel wall, seeking a new artificial end-stage. Nevertheless, some endothelial functions might be reflected to some extent by changes in blood levels of agents and their metabolites (factor VIII, tPA, PGI_2 metabolites). In this context, the old question of why blood does not clot in vessels under normal conditions might at last be answered.

From the etiological aspect of the vascular lesion various agents may be involved (Table 5). The ability to regulate blood fluidity is not the only deranged function of the damaged endothelium. Beside changes in permeability with the resulting rheologic defects (dehydration, increased hematocrit), it is also the deficient regulation of vascular tonus possibly bringing about a vascular spasm. Of course, a prolonged spasm may produce a flow disturbance and even stasis. In this way it may represent an additional factor in the final thrombotic occlusion of the vascular lumen.[97] The primary and particularly the secondary spasm, i.e., secondary to the already existing thrombus, may be related to the release of platelet constituents or products such as serotonin and thrombin (stimulating TXA_2 production), as well as a deficient production of EDRF (endothelium-derived relaxing factor) in the damaged endothelium with the resulting inability of adenosine derivatives to produce relaxation.[98,99] Simultaneously the damaged endothelium loses its ability to metabolize biogenic amines by monoaminooxidase and all mediators can readily enter the vessel wall due to the loss of the barrier function. It is possible that other products of thrombus formation may play an additional role such as some fibrinogen (fibrinopeptide B) and fibrin split products.

The degree and character of the vascular lesion may lead to a characteristic dissociation of prothrombotic and antithrombotic endothelial function. This dissociation is more probable with lesions of low or intermediate degree, whereas with severe lesions uncovering the deeper structures such as collagen, the hemostatic function would probably prevail and thrombogenesis may be even inhibited. With very mild lesions defensive functions could be supported; thus, even thrombin in very low concentrations would support the anticoagulant activity of protein C at the endothelial surface.

On the other hand, it is easy to imagine special kinds of even mild endothelial lesions which would result in an unfavorable disproportion of procoagulant and anticoagulant endothelial functions. Such lesions might depend on the particular properties of noxious agents. The number of possible challenges is almost unlimited and the stereotyped equipment of the endothelium cannot cope with all of them. It is possible to imagine, for example, damage concerning predominantly the glycocalyx critically decreasing the activity of inhibitory systems (AT III-heparan) without seriously diminishing the prothrombotic potential. Of critical significance may also be a repeated or prolonged mild injury exhausting the defensive capacity particularly if there is not time enough for the replacement of inhibitors, and of course for adaptive processes. Unfortunately not much is known about all these possibilities. If we define a disease as a manifestation of an overburdening with possible exhaustion and collapse of the regulatory systems, it is easy to see thrombosis as such exhaustion of a correspondingly very limited portion of the regulatory system. To some extent this is prevented in the organism on the basis of the "multiline" principle. Most defensive regulations have multiple safety checks against failure, just as in a space shuttle, and if one defense

TABLE 5
Noxious Influences Leading to Endothelial Lesion

Physical
  Heat
  Radiation
  Electric current
  Osmotic changes
Mechanical
  Mechanical trauma
  Rheologic effects (hyperviscosity)
  Hemodynamic effects (hypertension)
Ischemia
  Vascular occlusions, embolism (lactate, pH)
  Stasis
  Shock
  Bleeding
Inflammation
  Infections (particularly viral)
  Endotoxins
  Complement system
  Immune reactions and diseases (particularly immune complexes)
Myeloproliferative and malignant diseases
Metabolic defects
Blood lipids (particularly low density lipoproteins)
  Cholesterol
  Fatty acids and their oxidative products
  Bile acids
  Homocysteine and homocystine
  Diabetes?
Thrombocytopenia, activated leukocytes
Fibrin- and fibrinogen degradation products
Mediator release
  Catecholamines
  Histamine
  Serotonin
  TXA_2
Toxic and iatrogenic influences
  Nicotin
  Oral contraceptives
  Animal toxins (snake venoms)
  Proteolytic enzymes
  Various drugs (e.g., many antibiotics)
  Oxygen-free radicals
Inhibition of detoxifying capacity
  Dysfunction of the reticuloendothelial system
  Dysfunction of the liver
  Dysfunction of the kidneys

line is blocked another may serve as a substitute. With the current body of our knowledge, this is more evident in the hemostatic than in the antithrombotic function, e.g., several independent aggregation mediators. For a primitive organism engaged in the daily struggle for life hemostasis is naturally more important.

From all that has been said about the importance of the endothelium in the process of thrombogenesis it is evident that suitable tests indicating the presence of an endothelial lesion might be very useful. As morphological methods are of no use in the clinical diagnosis, various factors known to be released by the endothelium readily stand out as possible candidates. The factors are factor VIII, angiotensin II, tPA, and PGI_2 metabolites.[100] Unfortunately all such tests lack specificity, the factors could often be produced elsewhere and

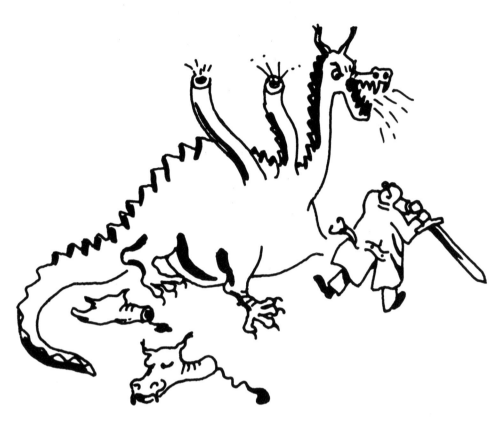

FIGURE 3. Challenging a multifactorial disease.

their change in blood after the induction of a vascular lesion is not very marked. Above all, it may be expected that after a mild injury they could increase to be easily exhausted increasing no longer after a prolonged damaging influence. To some extent, various tests for the early phases of platelet and blood-clotting activation might serve as a kind of indicator: increased platelet sensitivity to aggregating agents or even spontaneous aggregation, release of beta-TG and PF 4. From the side of activated blood clotting particularly FPA release may be mentioned. All these methods are, of course, very indirect indicators.

The only method which would show directly the presence of a lesion is to count circulating desquamated endothelial cells in blood. The method may be applicable also under clinical conditions. While the details of the method will be given later in this book, it could be mentioned here that it is based on the presence of a functional lesion which, in only a small fraction of injured cells, results in desquamation. Some basal levels are demonstrable even under normal resting conditions reflecting endothelial turnover. A particularly sensitive modification suitable for clinical use is the function test using oral methionine as a challenge. This modification may even discover latent lesions or increased vulnerability of the endothelium.

III. MULTIFACTORIAL PATHOGENESIS

What does it actually mean to claim that thrombogenesis has a multifactorial character (Figure 3)? For a better understanding of the term, an attempt was undertaken to build a suitable mental construction, provided that some license is granted for speculation. All three factors (or three or more groups of factors) can be imagined as cone-shaped forms situated side by side so that they overlap to a variable degree (Figure 4). This overlapping illustrates the interdependence of factors, i.e., interrelations of a mostly positive feedback character.

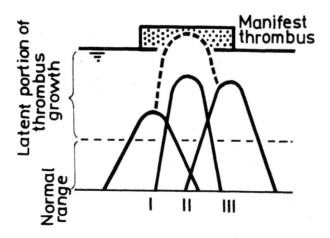

FIGURE 4.   The interrelation of three groups of factors; I, humoral; II, blood flow; III, vascular lesion, and the emergence of a manifest thrombus.

For example, activation of platelets leads to a secondary blood-clotting activation by way of PF 3 release and blood-clotting activation causes thrombin production with subsequent activation of platelets. Of course, we are unable to sufficiently offer exact data not only concerning the relevance of each group of factors, but also the importance of their interrelations. The distance between the highest limit of still normal factor levels and the level of clinical perception, the penetration of which is connected with the appearance of the phenomenon of thrombosis, probably involves two closely interrelated positions.

1.   The latent period of thrombus formation showing a ''supersaturation'' of at least one factor. In such situations, an accidental additional increase of another factor may trigger thrombus formation.
2.   The latent period of thrombus detection dependent on the sensitivity of the diagnostic method used.

As suggested by the ''false-positive'' results of the fibrinogen uptake test, even incipient mural thrombus formation can still be compensated by an increased activity of defensive processes. Experimental studies have shown that a 50% occlusion does not necessarily produce a serious decrease in blood flow with resulting organ ischemia. Such consequences are seen only after attaining a decrease of about 90% of the cross-sectional area. Clinical experience shows that about 50% of thromboses remain clinically silent. In such situations, an increase in the turnover of some factors (fibrinogen) and the appearance of FP-A or platelet-released factors may be observed in blood. However, such changes are not yet recognized as signs of a definite thrombus.

Only three groups of factors are taken into account in our diagrams even though the number of factors changing relatively independently of each other may be larger.

Figure 4 shows a combined intermediate increase in all three factors, e.g., simultaneous presence of vascular lesion (possibly at some other site), blood-clotting activation, and stasis in venous thrombosis and this may be probably the most common combination. The combination of two increased factors may also be common. Another situation is depicted in Figure 5: a massive increase in one factor alone, e.g., a severe vascular damage leading to a secondary activation of all the remaining factors and by the action of all of them in concert, thrombosis comes into appearance. Is the situation shown in Figure 6 possible? It is not. Even with maximum activation no factor is able to produce thrombosis alone, i.e., without the assistance of additional factors. Thrombosis is unthinkable, e.g., in complete absence

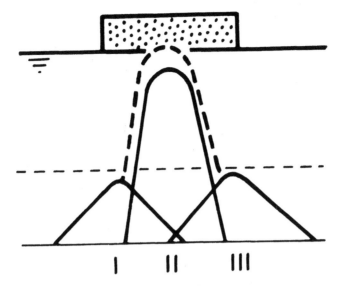

FIGURE 5. The situation characterized by one group of factors only above normal range.

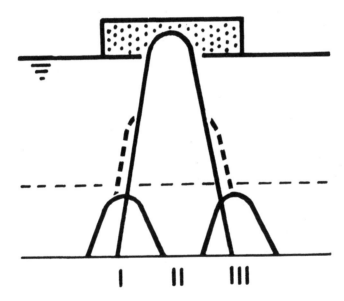

FIGURE 6. Extreme increase in one factor group does not lead to thrombosis without the assistance of remaining groups.

of humoral factors as evident already from its definition. For all factors, there evidently exist certain levels which represent an excess or "supersaturation" and further increases do not change anything. Even a very massive vascular trauma does not necessarily and invariably lead to thrombosis. Similarly, complete activation of blood clotting as following an intravenous injection of thrombin may produce defibrination with consumption of coagulation factors and total blood unclottability. It does not produce, in general, a local thrombosis. Very extensive and prolonged stasis as that occurring in immobilized patients does not necessarily lead to thrombosis even though its frequency may increase.

The situation shown in Figure 4 may be quite frequent in "idiopathic" venous thrombosis. On the other hand, typical postoperative venous thrombosis is better illustrated in

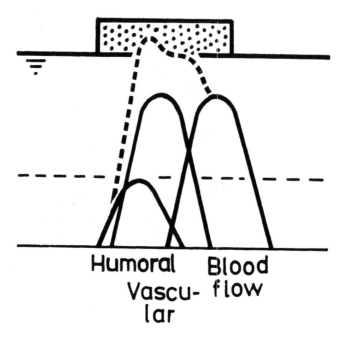

Humoral   Blood
Vascu-   flow
lar

FIGURE 7.   Combination of factors frequently encountered in postoperative venous thrombosis.

Figure 7: a massive vascular lesion resulting from a surgical intervention at some other site in combination with postoperative immobilization produces thrombosis despite the originally normal levels of humoral factors. With a sufficiently intensive derangement of both factors, the frequency of venous thrombosis may attain more than 50% after hip reconstructions. It is easy to imagine many other situations resulting from various combinations of factors activated to various degrees, particularly if more factors are involved.

The interaction of factors could also be expressed as a direct or indirect relationship with thrombosis as the endpoint (T):

$$T = \frac{\text{blood viscosity}}{\text{blood flow}} \times \frac{\text{endothelial lesion}}{\text{fibrinolytic activation}} \times \frac{\text{platelet activation}}{\text{platelet inhibition}} \times \frac{\text{clotting activation}}{\text{clotting inhibition}}$$

Nevertheless, various weights should be given to the relative contribution made by single factors. The mechanism of this contribution has been already discussed with each factor. Even though it depends on the individual situation, on a very general level the factors are not equivalent and the importance of their contribution may be very different. They are all involved in the production (or prevention) of a state existing for a limited period of time and consummated by the appearance of a thrombus. Here again, if a very schematic representation is allowed, the relative interrelations of all three main factors or factor groups may be imagined as three rings corresponding to the overlapping bases of the three-dimensional truncated cones shown in the frontal view in previous diagrams (Figure 8). The relations between a vascular lesion and the other factors are almost one-sided. While a vascular lesion heavily influences the activity of the blood-clotting system, platelets and fibrinolytic system, on the contrary, it is affected little by these factors. Some notable exceptions include effects of mediators released from platelets (serotonin, TXA_2, and PAF) as well as of thrombin and fibrinogen- or fibrin-split products, the consequences of the close

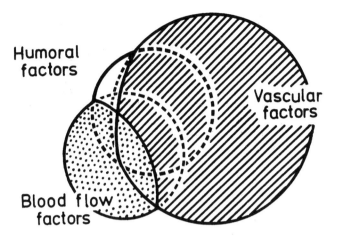

FIGURE 8. Another schematic diagram of all three groups of factors according to their supposed relative importance.

relation of the fibrinolytic system with the kallikrein and complement systems, and the untold influence of an already present thrombus on the nutrition of the vascular wall. The effect of a vascular lesion on the flow conditions may be seen in chronic atherosclerotic changes, while on the contrary, high shear rates are known to produce endothelial lesions. Nevertheless, high shear rates are due mostly to an already existing atherosclerotic lesion, with the exception of hypertension. The relation between humoral and flow factors is again almost one-sided: pathologic flow conditions such as stasis, turbulence, vortex formation, etc., may have a profound influence on the activity of the blood-clotting system and platelets, but there is not much hard evidence for an inverse influence. One possible exception may be the effect of increased fibrinogen levels and platelet aggregation on viscosity. In general, vascular factor appears as the relatively most independent and all-influencing factor, whereas humoral factors are the most dependent. This, of course, does not mean that they are not necessary.

The schematic representation of the multifactorial thrombotic pathogenesis presented here should serve to illustrate an important principle for model design. If it is intended to study drug effects on thrombosis it is not recommended to use any factor in excess because this would preclude the detection of any external influence on the factor concerned. There exists an analogy with the experience in the field of blood clotting: such factors whose effects are the object of investigation should never be added to the reaction mixture in excess. It is surprising to see that this simple rule has been ignored in most thrombosis models to date. Logically, it should be possible to design several models with an excess of another factor in each so that each factor could be investigated under the conditions of a relatively tight supply. However, a probably better alternative would be a model with all three factors as low-dosed as possible.

IV. WHAT IS A MODEL?

In general a model may be understood to represent a reproduction of the main characteristics of one object or system in another object or system, both being connected by homomorphic relations. In our case we are dealing with a biomodel, which is a living organism the behavior of which may allow us to infer by analogy as well as on the basis of more or less close phylogenetic relations on the behavior of another organism which is the object of our main interest, i.e., man. Thus a biomodel is a biological experiment of a special kind in which the response to a challenge possesses a global character proceeding

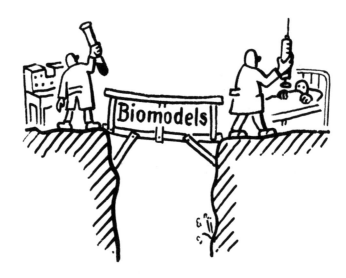

FIGURE 9.   Biomodels bridging the gap between laboratory and clinical experience.

after the initiation in a series of successive mutually linked-up processes according to its own still not completely understood inner program. Mostly, we are not looking for agents inducing a standard response, as usual in pharmacological experiments, but on the contrary, for a response produced by a standard challenge. The sensitivity to this challenge and the possibility of the modification of this sensitivity by drugs are of particular interest.

Biomodels are sometimes used only as a final experimental proof of results obtained by screening methods of analytical and often *in vitro* character. This is probably not a very reasonable approach as biomodels should stand at the start as well as at the conclusion of the search for new drugs (Figure 9). They should bridge the gap between the clinical practice and laboratory research. Meanwhile, analytical methods should serve to the elucidation of the mechanism of drug action, otherwise the outlook is unacceptably narrowed and accidental or circumstantial observations may simulate a causal relationship. In addition, important findings may be easily missed. The recent trend to eliminate biomodels on ethical grounds is extremely dangerous for further progress. Meanwhile, all models used in the author's laboratory are carried out on animals (rats) under deep general anethesia.

V. CLASSIFICATION OF THROMBOSIS MODELS

Thrombosis models have been surveyed in detail by several authors including Henry,[101] Deutsch,[102] Didisheim,[103] Dodds,[104] Day,[105] and Philp.[106] The number of methods described until now is very large, between 300 and 350. Although it is not possible to mention every one of them, the methods have been classified into different groups and, in general, "core citations" are only referred to around which other papers are clustered.

Classification of thrombosis models can be carried out along various lines, according to the sought-after answers (Table 6).

A. LOCALIZATION

According to the *localization*, it is possible to distinguish thrombosis in arteries, veins, and microcirculation. This survey will be concerned mainly with thrombosis models in large vessels. As mentioned previously, the main pathomechanisms of arterial and venous thrombosis are considered to be closely related and may be treated jointly. In fact, some transitions and overlappings can be observed. Arterial thrombi forming at the site of stasis after complete

TABLE 6
Classification of Thrombosis Models from Various Viewpoints

According to the localization	Arterial
	Venous
	Microcirculatory (DIC)
	Artificial surfaces
According to the type of provocation	Physical
	Chemical
	Physico-chemical
	Biological
According to the experimental animals used	Single species
	Several species
According to the indication method	Qualitative (including morphologic)
	Quantitative
	One estimation (end-point)
	Continuous
According to the time span	Acute
	Chronic
According to the comprehensiveness of the viewpoint	Global
	Analytical
According to the number of provoking factors	Unifactorial
	Plurifactorial
According to the research objectives	Pathogenetic
	Diagnostic
	Therapeutic and prophylactic

obstruction are not much different from vein thrombi and those forming in saphenous vein grafts in aorto-coronary bypass surgery are almost identical with arterial thrombi. The differences lie mostly in the quantitative representation of factors and their entering the process under different disguises. Nevertheless, differences do exist and should be kept in mind for special opportunities. As will be shown later, some drug combinations may very differently affect venous and arterial thrombosis models. That is why two separate models were necessary. The main difference is in the relatively more important role of the localizing influence of a vascular lesion and in a different kind of flow influence in arterial thrombosis. The high-flow rate is probably the main factor leading to increased involvement of platelets. This does not imply that platelets do not contribute to venous thrombosis. Steele has shown that two kinds of idiopathic venous thromboses exist according to the relative participation of platelets. It may be noted that even in the early but invaluable survey on thrombosis models by Henry, the venous and arterial models were treated jointly and very often the methods used in one type of vessel were used similarly in the other with some minor modifications.

Some arterial models deal with coronary arteries. They are often concerned not so much with problems of thrombogenesis but with its consequence, myocardial infarction. Of course, it is possible to stress the differences in the equipment of coronary endothelium in comparison with other arteries, e.g., the strong representation of the adenosine system, in order to justify the much more complicated and cumbersome work with coronaries, particularly in small animals. However, if myocardial infarction is accepted as the end-point indicator, the effectiveness of a drug in similar models may be caused by other mechanisms besides the antithrombotic one, such as antiarrhythmic, metabolic, spasmolytic, etc. It is true that most antiplatelet drugs find their use to be chiefly in the prevention of coronary thrombosis. On the other hand, results of clinical trials do not show any marked tendency to distinguish coronary arteries from those of other regions, e.g., carotid arteries as the main source of TIA.

We are not concerned here in particular with models of disseminated thrombosis in the microcirculation, not because of their minor importance, but because of differences in the pathomechanisms, and particularly in the design of the models.[32,33,107,108] The scope of this topic has grown to such proportions that it would deserve a special monograph. The terminology itself; disseminated intravascular coagulation (DIC), generalized intravascular coagulation, consumption coagulopathy, microembolism syndrome, thrombotic microangiopathy, etc., demonstrates the many sided and pluricausal character of the condition. This complex pathogenetic character is by no means completely clarified and in this section the main differences only to local thrombosis in large vessels will be pointed out. Above all, it is simply the relative lack, or on the contrary, systemic excess of those factors which provide the localizing influence, i.e., local hemodynamic factors and local vascular lesions. Moreover, the process of activation of platelets and blood clotting in DIC is often rapidly followed by consumption and reactive phenomena, particularly hyperfibrinolysis, which preclude any local thrombus formation. In general, local thrombus formation requires relatively mild systemic changes which would not go beyond a certain maximum level lest the localizing factors should be obscured and could have their own way. Therefore, release of tissue materials with only incomplete thromboplastic activity or merely foreign body character are under suitable conditions connected with local thrombosis more often than the release or administration of fully active thromboplastic materials or even thrombin, capable of coagulating fibrinogen directly and without delay. In fact, intravenously administered thrombin may be experimentally shown to have antithrombotic properties, i.e., it may prevent the formation of local thrombosis. In most situations connected with DIC, both clinical and experimental, the vascular lesion is generalized and often severe, with platelet and blood-clotting activation greatly increased. In addition, strong contribution of leukocytes may be present. The fibrinolytic activity, if in abundance, may enhance the hemostatic defect, or organ lesion, if in shortage (e.g., after antifibrinolytics). A modifying influence is exerted also by the reticuloendothelial system. All these changes take place against the background of a generalized hemodynamic crisis, manifested as hypocirculation, ischemia of vital organs, and shock. The interaction of all these powerful factors may be very intricate under clinical conditions and experimental simplifications mostly show only one aspect of the process.

A problem deserving special attention arises from the fact that many models applied in the investigation of antithrombotic effects use vessels in or very close to the microcirculatory bed. They include the use of mesenteric, mesorchial, hamster cheek pouch, and brain surface microvessels. Of course, such methods have many advantages: a number of experiments can be carried out in a single animal, one animal may serve as its own control, it is possible to use modern imaging methods with computer quantification, there is an easy administration of drugs by external ways, and an easy direct observation of the process under the microscope. On the other hand, thrombosis factors are not represented in such areas in the same way as in large vessels. In arterial thrombosis the hemodynamic factors are very different and probably so is the endothelial equipment with constituents of the prothrombotic and antithrombotic, in particular fibrinolytic, system. As a result there may be significant differences in the contribution of humoral factors. That is why the otherwise satisfactory method of venous thrombosis using the mesenterium of rats was replaced as part of a routine set of models in our laboratory.

In conclusion, this kind of method has a decreased value as thrombosis models of global character and should be classified as models of a more or less analytical type (see further in the chapter about the comprehensiveness of models) suitable for the investigation of single relatively isolated problems of thrombogenesis. Application of results obtained with such models particularly in testing drugs for clinical use is more indirect and requires special cautiousness. On the other hand, these kinds of models contributed so much to our present knowledge about thrombosis that the discussion of some of them is inevitable in this survey.

Thrombosis on artificial surfaces is, like DIC, not the object of the present treatise. The number of methods in this field is rapidly expanding with the use of various kinds of shunts, catheters, small extracorporeal loops, and prostheses. Many of them are very specialized to the study of antithrombotic properties of particular kinds of prostheses and plastic materials. In general, in these kinds of models the lesion of the endothelial surface does not play a localizing role, with the possible exception of endothelium-seeded prostheses. Nevertheless, the endothelium may exert a "distant" effect mediated by humoral activation. It should be kept in mind that the prosthesis is never inserted in a completely atraumatic way and the transition between prosthesis and normal vascular tissue is probably the source of many derangements in normal function of the blood-fluidity maintaining system. It is very probable that according to the character of the artificial surface the relative contribution of various mechanisms may be very different, and consequently, so may be the effect of drugs. A particularly conspicuous example is a relatively good antithrombotic effect of dipyridamole on artificial surfaces in comparison with an almost nonexistent effect in clinical arterial thrombosis if given alone. This could mean that adenosine derivatives may be relatively more important in thrombosis on artificial prostheses. However that may be, it is again not possible to ignore completely some models of this kind particularly if the borderline between thrombosis models produced by a mechanical vascular lesion and models based on the presence of foreign bodies in the circulation is not well defined.

B. TYPE OF PROVOCATION

According to the *type of provocation*, most models, particularly earlier ones, have been based on physical challenges. A review of about 300 models shows that approximately 60% were based on a deliberate vascular lesion by physical means and the majority of the remaining models is not free of an unintentional lesion of variable degree. The definition of *physical means* has a very broad meaning, and as generally noted with attempts at classification, there are no clear-cut borders between various categories. Mechanical induction may imply the direct or indirect trauma inflicted to the vessel wall and/or nearby tissue by an instrument, e.g., hammer,[109] on the one hand, and fluid-mechanical effects based on acute or chronic changes in flow rate caused by various mechanical flow-restricting devices, on the other hand.[110-112] Many models based on the introduction into the circulation of foreign materials, i.e., catheters, files, etc., may be effective less on account of their material properties than of producing a mechanical trauma to the vessel wall or disturbing the blood flow. Similarly, clamps and ligatures produce a mechanical trauma combined with the impediment to the blood flow. Therefore, most such methods are, in principle, at least two-factorial, only the relative contribution of both factors is, in general, not well defined. An additional influence may come from the particular character of the foreign surface, e.g., the obligatory treatment of the alloy file in Friedman's model with $ZnCl_2$.[113] This latter influence may be direct (influence on blood properties) or again indirect (affecting the vascular wall).

Direct mechanical trauma includes various kinds of crushing,[114-117] contusion,[118,120] stretching,[121-123] stripping and scraping,[116,124-126] using scalpels, clamps, forcepses,[121,122] as well as highly specialized instruments and devices such as dental broaches,[127] dental excavators,[128] and dental ultrasonic devices.[129,130] The lesions may be inflicted from the outside, from the luminal side or from both, such as incisions and sutures.[131-133] Into the vessel may be introduced catheters,[134] balloon catheters,[135-137] threads, and files.[112,113,138,139] Special surgical procedures may result, for example, in an inversion of an arterial branch.[140] All these methods have serious inherent drawbacks: not only is the local vascular lesion poorly quantified, but most importantly, the lesion is almost invariably in excess, i.e., the endothelium is destroyed and the deep layers of the vessel wall are as a rule more or less involved. This situation leads to the detrimental failure to realize the fact that many existing or potential antithrombotics may also affect (or even predominantly affect) the endothelial function. It is a similar misconception, as if the postoperative deep vein thrombosis was modeled in the operation field and myocardial infarction was always supposed to precede the thrombotic occlusion of the coronary (the latter theory was given extensive publicity about 10 years ago). It ought to be kept in mind that the authors of the models were forced to use an excessive lesion to obtain thrombosis in at least a majority of animals. Less severe trauma was ineffective and the results not well reproducible showed a variable latency period. Occasionally, it was necessary to repeat the lesion several times. Only exceptionally was the minimum necessary degree of trauma investigated in detail but quantification was difficult and thresholds depended on too many variables. In some studies a relatively mild but poorly reproducible trauma was used.[141-143] In general, local trauma was used with systemic trauma (e.g., by endotoxin) reserved for the study of DIC. Assumptions of a direct relationship between the degree of the local damage inflicted and the ease of inducing thrombosis may be rather unsubstantiated here. Very different mechanisms may come into play with a severe and deep trauma when a rapid hemostasis serves to provide an entirely purposeful defense and a mild and possibly extensive trauma which while leaving many functions intact may bring about only a disequilibrium between the prothrombotic and antithrombotic functions of the endothelium. This lack of discrimination led to a scepticism about the necessity of a vascular lesion in venous thrombosis.[144] A severe local vascular lesion produces something very different from clinical thrombosis where it is never in excess.

More interesting are the attempts to use some well quantifiable physical effects to produce a vascular lesion. This includes the use of electric current,[145-151] laser beams,[152-156] thermic lesions (burning and scalding),[157,158] UV-irradiation,[159-160] freezing, and "chilling".[161-164] The dosage is, in general, well reproducible and simple to apply. Of course, there is the need for a special device. Nevertheless, these methods share the main disadvantage with the previous group: to obtain reproducible thrombosis it is necessary to inflict an excessive vascular damage. The attempts of some authors to look for a physiological background for the use of electric current in electric potential differences across the vascular wall were not sufficiently substantiated particularly if the electrical stimuli necessary to produce thrombosis were much stronger.[165] The electrochemical lesion produced by polarization phenomena may be more important than potential differences. In the case of laser the interpretation is complicated by the very artificial thermic influence on formed blood elements and dependence on an exact vessel wall geometry. The "chilling" ($-15°C$) experiments evidently gave excellent results.[161] They are well reproducible and the model is highly sensitive to the effects of drugs. Of course, the vessel is probably damaged also by the extensive dissection and manipulation. The vascular wall lesion is again not very well defined and is probably deep and extensive. The arterial modification is combined with the use of a clip and should be classified as a two-factorial model. It is important to emphasize that in almost all models induced by physical means the vascular lesion is combined with stasis in veins or a blood flow disturbance in arteries. This is often achieved already by the intervention designed to produce a lesion. Very often stasis is produced independently by ligation. In fact, stasis is accepted, since Wessler's studies, as necessary in venous models just as some derangement in flow rate and laminarity in arterial models, as localizing factors. Meanwhile, is the slow development of the obstruction in arterial models necessary? Probably not, as it would mimic more the result of atherosclerosis rather than the starting precondition of thrombosis. Clinical stenosis alone, if not joined by other factors, can exist for a life without causing thrombosis. There is, of course, always the problem of the vascular lesion inflicted by the flow restriction and the necessary manipulation. This can never be completely eliminated but should be kept as small and constant as possible.

Models induced by the administration of chemical substances either parenterally, perivascularly, or even intraosseously[166] differ mainly by the vast range of materials administered. Most earlier models used the intravenous route of administration of very highly effective prothrombotic agents, such as thrombin and thromboplastin,[166-171] trypsin and other proteases,[172-175] Russel's viper venom,[101,176] ADP,[122] endotoxin,[177] combined as a rule with a local stasis. Under such conditions the process did not differ very much from the clotting of blood in the test tube. Without stasis, such agents tended to produce rather a DIC. More interesting was perhaps the use of less effective agents, such as ellagic acid,[139,178] serum and serum derivatives,[179] activated contact factor,[180] hemolysates,[60] kaolin,[181] collagen covered threads,[182] etc. These agents often produced a hypercoagulable state whereas the more active materials caused a more or less hypocoagulable state by the abrupt consumption processes. The combination of stasis with serum or serum products is the basis of the famous Wessler's model[183,184] used in various modifications for more than 3 decades. All such materials cut short the way from the vascular lesion to blood-clotting activation. Such changes may be the cause of many postoperative clinical thromboses, but it might be asked whether this shortcutting was necessary as it neglected the activation phase in which many drugs may be effective.

The other group of agents was not effective in the coagulation system directly, but more or less indirectly by a local vascular lesion. Various sclerosing agents,[185-190] fixatives,[138,191] silver nitrate,[192-195] or even sulfuric acid[171,196] were used for this purpose, mostly in combination with local stasis. The agents were often administered perivascularly[197] and combined with other agents, even with thrombin and thromboplastin. More logical was the combination with antifibrinolytics such as EACA.[139] In most such models the local vascular lesion was likewise excessive. On the other hand, there was a bit of good reasoning: the vascular lesion is capable of activating blood clotting and platelets, being more likely to occur at the start of clinical thrombosis than, for example, the appearance in blood of Russel's viper venom or high concentrations of thrombin.

Among the physico-chemical influences the effect of hypertonic[198] or hypotonic[199] saline, changes in pH[171,196] just as fatty acid infusions[200,201] might be interesting. In our opinion the systemic administration of hypotonic saline is one of the best reproducible mildly damaging effects on the endothelium despite the impossibility to completely exclude some effect on formed blood elements.

Biological inducing agents include infections like bacterial endocarditis,[202] parasitic infestations such as dirofilariasis and angiostrongylosis.[104] This group also covers the inductions by some neoplastic processes and immune reactions.[104,203] They do not all depend solely on the dose of the inducing agent, but also on the responsiveness of animals. For routine purposes, an unsatisfactory quantification and reproducibility has to be expected.

Another subgroup of biological influences is dietary means of thrombus induction.[23,204-206] A relatively large number of such models served a special purpose: the investigation of the pathogenetic role of various lipid and other dietary constituents. Such models are, in general, time consuming and may be influenced not only by species differences in thrombogenic mechanisms but also in fat metabolism.

The last subgroup of biological models includes the relatively infrequent cases of spontaneous thrombosis in wild, household, and experimental animals.[104,207-211] Unfortunately, no hereditary disease characterized by a high frequency of thrombosis has been described in animals. Veterinary medicine knows thrombosis in connection with strongylosis in horses and racehorses may suffer thrombosis of leg veins even without this background. All these models are probably more interesting from the viewpoint of pathogenetic studies than the testing of drugs.

C. EXPERIMENTAL ANIMALS

According to the *experimental animals* used, it was possible to induce thrombosis in numerous animal species, mostly in rats, mice, rabbits, hamsters, guinea pigs, and dogs, but also in cats,[213-214] sheep,[215,216] goats, calves,[104,217] pigs,[137,164] rhesuses,[218] baboons,[219] and even bats,[220] if we omit frogs used in the stone-age of thrombosis models. Some studies were carried out in chickens[222] and human volunteers.[127] This illustrates that experimental thrombosis can be induced in practically all mammals and probably even in many other vertebrates. Two main strategies may be distinguished in the use of experimental animals. Species differences do exist and are undisputable. The first strategy, therefore, used a battery of several models, each in a different animal species. The extrapolation to man is hoped to be a little easier than from one model in one species only. This solution has serious disadvantages: the models are not comparable between each other and can be compared less with the situation in man. Research is poorly coordinated, and consequently, very superficial.

Another strategy is to rely on one commonly used animal species, e.g., the rat which is rather inexpensive and represents a relatively homogeneous population. It is necessary to use the same sex and age and to devise in this animal a battery of tests as mutually compatible as possible in order to increase the comparability of results. This strategy has been used in a rudimentary form in some studies applying the same induction method in rats for arteries and veins and acquired relatively clear outlines in the studies of Seuter and Meng[161] who used chilling in both arteries and veins in rats. It is important to work as systematically as possible and accumulate as much experience as possible to increase the predicting value of a similar system of models. The argument generally used against such strategy is the relatively distant phylogenetic relation between the species used in models and in man. There could be, for example, important differences in the drug pharmacokinetics based on differences in metabolism. On the other hand, the hemostatic function is so important for survival that it is probably following the convergence rule: the same function to be efficient is probably brought to effect by the same general mechanism in all mammalian species, in spite of minor differences in detail. This is also why the global type of models is more suitable than an analytical one. In our experience, large species differences observed while comparing many drug effects in man and experimental animals are due more often to an unsuitable model design than to species differences. Very practical disadvantages in using, e.g., primate models are hardly justified by the questionable advantage in the closer relation to man which may be misleading. Serious differences may exist even inside the species of man, e.g., relative resistance of Eskimos.

D. METHOD OF INDICATION

According to the *method of indication* it is possible to distinguish between methods expensive and simple, cumbersome and easy, methods based on qualitative characteristics (like most morphological methods) or on semiquantitative and qualitative parameters. It is probably of advantage to use a method as simple as possible, based on principal physical quantitative parameters such as weight, pressure, time, and temperature. A continuous registration of the process of thrombus formation or direct visualization of the process, while having many advantages from the point of view of a theoretical investigation, may be too time-consuming, does not allow several animals to be used in the experiment at the same time, and in the case of direct visualization, a subjective factor may be brought into play. The models should be suitable for routine study in a large number of animals and sufficiently quantitative to be easily accessible to statistical analysis.

E. TIME SPAN OF THE EXPERIMENT

According to the *time span of the experiment* it is possible to distinguish models of acute, subacute, and even chronic character. Of course, many clinical thrombotic processes may have a chronic character or at least development of the predisposition to thrombosis may be of such a character. Subacute development of vascular obstruction was modeled, for example, by placing swelling sleeves[111,112] around arteries and chronic development of predisposition to thrombosis is illustrated by dietary means. On the other hand, it is mostly acute arterial occlusion or acute venous thromboembolism which we are dealing with in the clinical practice and the process of thrombus development may be very rapid in man. For special purposes, chronic models can be helpful, but in general, an acute experiment is acceptable in thrombosis research even though it may be out of place, e.g., in atherosclerosis research. In clinical practice thrombosis is the result of a shift in a dynamic balance between processes of its development and growth on the one hand and those of its prevention and thrombolysis on the other. Thrombus may develop quickly, get stabilized, disappear, or resume growth repeatedly often giving the impression of a chronic process. All this depends on a favorable or unfavorable combination of predisposing factors such as systemic depression of the endothelial function, release of tissue factors, temporary stasis, e.g., during a prolonged travel, dietary influences, etc.

F. COMPREHENSIVENESS OF THE VIEWPOINT

The distinction according to the *comprehensiveness of the viewpoint* is very important. It has been stressed repeatedly that two types of models, analytical and global, can be used. Whereas global models attempt to represent the processes in their integrity, analytical ones emphasize one aspect only, e.g., the effect of ADP. It is impossible to deny the value of analytical models for the study of particular pathomechanical, narrowly formulated questions. Nevertheless, they do not allow any synthetic view on the whole process as well as an adequate appreciation of the relative contribution of various factors and their integration in the process. Thus, if a global test has shown some drug to be effective, a series of analytical tests may help solve the question of its mechanism of action. The reverse direction of investigation cannot be recommended and the tendency to use analytical tests (which may often be very simple, particularly if carried out *in vitro*) for screening purposes may easily lead expensive efforts into a blind alley. The only useful screening possible is one employing a well-selected system of global methods.

G. NUMBER OF PROVOKING FACTORS

According to the *number of provoking factors*: with thrombosis being a multifactorial process, its model should necessarily be multifactorial as well. Many models are covertly multifactorial even though seemingly one inducing factor is used, as excessive activation of one factor takes along a secondary activation of other Virchow's factors in the process. However, the factors should be dosed independently and just sufficient doses of challenges should be used in the model. A notable example is the Wessler's model combining humoral activation and venous stasis in the venous thrombosis model. Only in this way can sensitivity to the influence of agents capable of affecting one particular factor be preserved. A hypothesis has been offered in the literature suggesting that an ideal model should not be overly sensitive because too many drugs could be more or less effective in the system lacking a meaningful specificity.[106] This does not look like a reasonable approach. In view of the convergence rule it is recommended from the start to have a model not only comparable in its patho-mechanism to the real situation in man, but also showing a similar sensitivity to drugs. The differences between drugs could be preserved even at a lower dose level and it might also be possible to recognize the negative effects which would otherwise be easily overlooked. According to this view it is just the high sensitivity that should be looked for. The objections on the part of pharmacokinetics are of no concern here. Pharmacokinetics serve to explain observations difficult to understand by other ways, but cannot be used in advance to assess the appropriateness of the model. We know too little about the mechanisms of action of most drugs, at least in the field of antithrombotics. In fact, one of the main targets is endothelium, the first tissue besides blood with which the drug comes into contact if given parenterally. We still know very little about the time necessary for the drug to reach and occupy its targets, the duration of this occupation, the quantity of the drug necessary, the character and relevance of receptors, etc.

H. RESEARCH OBJECTIVES

If we look for classification according to *research objectives*, the main area for use of thrombosis models described in this book is experimental therapy, or more correctly, experimental prevention of thrombosis. This does not mean that similar models cannot be used to solve questions of pathogenetic character. Already the design of adequate models must be based on sound understanding of the pathogenesis of thrombosis and vice versa, the results of drug studies must provide useful material for such understanding. Another open field is the study of the possible coagulation or biochemical changes in blood and tissues which would be characteristic for the development of thrombosis and could even serve as predictive or diagnostic indicators.

One question may easily arise: why is it necessary to develop thrombosis models if it is possible to simply use tests for hemostasis which can be, in addition, used in man. Almost all components participating in thrombosis are also involved in hemostasis including the endothelium and other portions of the vascular wall which have suffered a more or less severe trauma, mostly of a mechanical nature. There is an evident contribution of humoral factors, platelets, blood clotting, and fibrinolysis. It is only the hemodynamic factors that are obviously different. Whereas in arterial thrombosis blood flow supports thrombosis; in the venous one an opposite situation is present. In hemostasis it is again necessary to distinguish venous, arterial, and capillary bleeding. In bleedings from large vessels, hemostasis is often of minor importance for the organism, with an ability to compensate for and replace the heavy blood losses being more important. In bleeding from capillaries, endothelial function is probably less important than the involvement of deeper portions of the vessel wall and other tissues. The relative contribution of various humoral factors is probably quite different as compared with thrombosis. Clinical experience shows that almost all antithrombotics also produce a defect in hemostasis. Nevertheless, this defect often remains latent (clinically silent). Ideally, the desired antithrombotic treatment should exert no marked effect on hemostasis or possibly no effect at all. This claim is based on the possible differences in the pathomechanisms of thrombosis and hemostasis. If we use tests for hemostasis to detect antithrombotics we would probably end up with drugs in our hands that would readily produce severe bleeding without affecting thrombogenesis. In other words, we cannot use hemostatic tests in the search for new antithrombotics because we are looking for drugs with a low antihemostatic effect. This does not mean that hemostatic tests should not be used altogether, but only as part of looking for undesirable side effects of drugs and in pathogenetic studies. We will often probably be forced to put up with some degree of undesirable side effects anyway.

VI. CONCLUSIONS FROM THE SURVEY

As far as the general recommendations for a suitable system of models are concerned, it is possible to draw the following conclusions:

1. It is advisable to use a system of mutually interrelated models with the rat as an experimental animal.
2. The big veins and big arteries should be used as sites of thrombus induction.
3. The use of a well-balanced system of relatively independent challenges, two in veins and three in arteries, is suggested. The challenges in both veins and arteries should be as much mutually related as possible.
4. The models should represent acute experiments of as much global character as possible.
5. The indication parameters have to be as quantitative, simple, and elementary as possible (e.g., temperature as an indicator of blood flow, thrombus weight).
6. The model should be as sensitive to drug effects as possible.

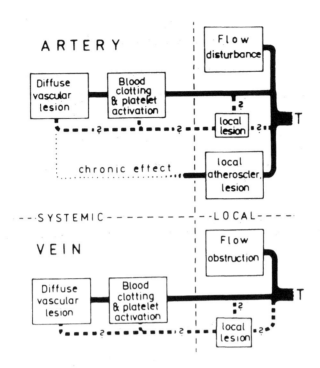

FIGURE 10. The interaction of systemic and local factor groups in the development of arterial and venous thrombosis.

A special problem is the selection of challenges: as a vascular lesion is considered to play the key role in clinical thrombosis the main emphasis should be laid on the selection of a suitable vascular lesion. As the basis for this selection the experience with the test of counting endothelial cell carcasses circulating in blood as a sensitive indicator of a vascular lesion was used in our studies and the method was also included in the battery of routine tests. The so called "hypercoagulability" or "thrombophilia" is considered here almost exclusively to be the result of a vascular lesion, i.e., not excessive local damage but a relatively mild systemic derangement of endothelial function reflected by increased desquamation of a small portion of already defective endothelial cells. It may be expected that this "perturbation" results in a disequilibrium of the endothelial prothrombotic and antithrombotic potential and we do not know whether an increase in the former or a decrease in the latter prevails. Most changes in the blood-clotting system and platelets are of secondary character to this primary defect. It is considered useful to separate the generalized endothelial "perturbation" as a relatively independent change from the additional local vascular lesion caused in arteries most often by defects in atherosclerotic plaques, which are of course, not present in veins (Figure 10). This primary thrombophilic defect which may also be called "endothelial stress" is caused in man, for instance, by smoking, wrong dietary habits, or mental stress. In the present system of models, a well-reproducible nonspecific challenge is used instead, e.g., intravenous administration of hypotonic saline. As localizing factors, partial stasis was used in veins and an artificial stenosis in arteries. Stasis, mostly incomplete, is not uncommon in veins of patients and the high-flow rate is characteristic for the clinical arterial thrombosis. In our model, an intravenous injection of serotonin was used as an additional humoral factor to compensate for the fact that the arterial wall is healthy. In clinical arterial thrombosis the presence of an atherosclerotic vascular defect may increase the sensitivity several times to serotonin released from platelets (Table 7).

These conclusions were not intended to give an impression that the presented solution to the problem is indeed the best alternative. It was an attempt to follow a series of rational

TABLE 7
New System of Models

	Endothelemia	Arterial model	Venous model
Systemic activation	Hypotonic saline i.v.	Hypotonic saline i.v. + serotonin	Hypotonic saline i.v.
Localizing factor	—	Partial occlusion	Partial stasis
Indication	Counting elements	Temperature measurement	Weighing

principles, but other and perhaps more rational approaches may be suggested. A detailed description of the system of models used in the author's laboratory is given in the next chapter.

REFERENCES

1. **Virchow, R.,** Phlogose und Thrombose im Gefässsystem, in *Gesammelte Abhandlungen zur Wissenschaftlichen Medizin,* Meidinger Verlag, Frankfurt, 1856, 219.
2. **Rokitansky, C.,** *Handbuch der (speziellen) Pathologischen Anatomie,* Wien, 1844.
3. **Dupuy, E., Tobelem, G., Soria, C., Pellerin, A., Drouet, L., Bellucci, S., and Caen, J.,** Molecular abnormalities in recurrent thromboembolic disease, *Presse. Med.,* 12, 95, 1983.
4. **Kitchens, C. S.,** Concept of hypercoagulability: a review of its development, clinical application, and recent progress, *Semin. Thromb. Hemost.,* 11, 293, 1985.
5. **Rodgers, G. M. and Shuman M. A.,** Congenital thrombotic disorders, *Am. J. Hematol.,* 21, 419, 1986.
6. **Mannucci, P. M. and Tripodi, A.,** Diagnostic screening of congenital thrombotic syndromes, presented at 11th Int. Congr. on Thrombosis and Haemostasis, Abstr. 918, Brussels, 1987.
7. **Harker, L. A., Ross, R., Slichter, S. J., and Scott, C. R.,** Homocystine-induced arteriosclerosis: the role of endothelial cell injury and platelet response in its genesis, *J. Clin. Invest.,* 58, 731, 1976.
8. **McCully, K. S.,** Homocysteine theory of arteriosclerosis: development and current status, in *Atherosclerosis Review,* Vol. 2, Gotto, A. M. and Paoletti, R., Eds., Raven Press, New York, 1983, 157.
9. **Riedel, M., Ivašková, E., and Seidlová, H.,** HLA and venous thromboembolism, *Tissue Antigens,* 18, 280, 1981.
10. **Coon, W. W.,** Epidemiology of venous thromboembolism, *Ann. Surg.,* 186, 149, 1977.
11. **Allan, T. M.,** ABO blood groups, age and work in ischemic heart disease, *Atherosclerosis,* 21, 459, 1975.
12. **Garrison, R. J., Havlik, R. J., Harris, R. B., Feinleib, M., Kannel, W. B., and Padgett, S. J.,** ABO blood group and cardiovascular disease—Framingham study, *Atherosclerosis,* 25, 311, 1976.
13. **Gallus, A. S.,** Familial venous thromboembolism and inherited abnormalities of the blood clotting system, *Aust. N.Z. J. Med.,* 14, 807, 1984.
14. **Talbot, S., Wakley, E. J., Ryrie, D., and Langman, M. J. S.,** ABO blood groups and venous thromboembolic disease, *Lancet,* 1, 1257, 1970.
15. **Sixma, J. J.,** The prethrombotic state, *Br. J. Haematol.,* 46, 515, 1980.
16. **Penner, J. A.,** Hypercoagulation and thrombosis, *Med. Clin. North Am.,* 64, 743, 1980.
17. **Schafer, A. I.,** The hypercoagulable state. Review, *Ann. Intern. Med.,* 102, 814, 1985.
18. **Collins, G. J., Ahr, D. J., Rich, N. M., and Andersen, Ch.A.,** Detection and management of hypercoagulability, *Am. J. Surg.,* 132, 767, 1976.
19. **Davies, J. A. and McNicol, G. P.,** Detection of a prethrombotic state, in *Haemostasis and Thrombosis,* Bloom, A. L. and Thomas, D. P., Eds., Churchill Livingstone, Edinburgh, 1981, 593.
20. **Breddin, K.,** Detection of prethrombotic states in patients with atherosclerotic lesions, *Semin. Thromb. Hemost.,* 12, 110, 1986.
21. **Astrup, T.,** The haemostatic balance, *Thromb. Diath. Haemorrh.,* 2, 2, 1958.
22. **Spaet, T. H.,** Hemostatic homeostasis, *Blood,* 28, 112, 1966.
23. **Bergentz, S. E., Gelin, L. E., and Rudenstam, C. M.,** Fats and thrombus formation, *Thromb. Diath. Haemorrh.,* 5, 474, 1961.

24. **Nordoy, A., Hamlin, J. T., Chandler, A. B., and Newland, H.,** The influence of dietary fats on plasma and platelet lipids and ADP-induced platelet thrombosis in the rat, *Scand. J. Haematol.,* 5, 458, 1968.

25. **Renaud, S. and Lecompte, F.,** Hypercoagulability induced by hyperlipemia in rats, rabbit and man, *Circ. Res.,* 27, 1003, 1970.

26. **Weaver, M. M. and Ashburn, A. D.,** Effect of circulating red cell mass on diet-induced atrial thrombosis in mice, *Yale J. Biol. Med.,* 3, 148, 1974.

27. **Markwardt, F. and Landmann H.,** Blutgerinnungshemmende Proteine, in *Handbuch der experimentellen Pharmakologie,* Vol. 27, Markwardt, F., Ed., Springer-Verlag, Berlin, 1971, 76.

28. **Gaffney P. J.,** The fibrinolytic system, in *Haemostasis and Thrombosis,* Bloom, A. L. and Thomas, D. P., Eds., Churchill-Livingstone, Edinburgh, 1981, 198.

29. **Bachmann, F.,** Fibrinolysis, in *Thrombosis and Haemostasis 1987,* Verstraete, M., Vermylen, J., Lijnen, R., and Arnout, J., Eds., Leuven University Press, Leuven, 1987, 227.

30. **Ratnoff, O. D.,** Epsilon aminocaproic acid—a dangerous weapon, *N. Engl. J. Med.,* 280, 1124, 1969.

31. **Griffin, J. D. and Ellman L.,** Epsilon-aminocaproic acid (EACA), *Semin. Thromb. Hemost.,* 5, 27, 1978.

32. **Müller-Berghaus, G. and Lasch, H.-G.,** Microcirculatory disturbances induced by generalized intravascular coagulation, in *Handbook of Experimental Pharmacology,* Vol. 16 (Part 3), Springer-Verlag, Berlin, 1975, 465.

33. **McKay, D. G.,** *Disseminated Intravascular Coagulation,* Harper & Row, New York, 1965, 493.

34. **Schafer, A. I.,** Bleeding and thrombosis in myeloproliferative disorders, *Blood,* 64, 1, 1984.

35. **Pearson, T. C., RossRussell, R. W., Symon, L., Wetherley-Mein, G., and Zilkha, E.,** Cerebral blood-flow in polycythaemia, *Lancet,* 2, 161, 1977.

36. **Knizley, H., Jr. and Noyes, W. D.,** Iron deficiency anemia, papilledema, thrombocytosis, and transient hemiparesis, *Arch. Intern. Med.,* 129, 483, 1972.

37. **Mohr, P. and Straib, P. W.,** Thrombozytose bei Colitis ulcerosa und Morbus Crohn, *Schweiz. Med. Wochenschr.,* 100, 1142, 1970.

38. **Ansell, J. and Deykin, D.,** Heparin-induced thrombocytopenia and recurrent thromboembolism, *Am. J. Hematol.,* 8, 325, 1980.

39. **Remuzzi, G., Rossi, E., Misiani, R., Marchesi, D., Mecca, G., de Gaetano, G., and Donati, M. B.,** Prostacyclin and thrombotic microangiopathy, *Semin. Thromb. Hemost.,* 6, 391, 1980.

40. **Moake, J. L., Reedy, C. K., Weinstein, M. J., Colannino, N. M., Azocar, J., Seder, R. H., Hong, S. L., and Deykin, D.,** Unusually large plasma factor VIII: von Willebrand factor multimers in chronic relapsing thrombotic thrombocytopenic purpura, *N. Engl. J. Med.,* 307, 1432, 1982.

41. **Chesterman, C. N., McGready, J. R., Doyle, D. J., and Morgan, F. J.,** Plasma levels of platelet factor 4 measured by radioimmunoassay, *Br. J. Haematol.,* 40, 489, 1978.

42. **Handin, R. I., McDonough, M., and Lesch, M.,** Elevation of platelet factor four in acute myocardial infarction: measurement by radioimmunoassay, *J. Lab. Clin. Med.,* 92, 340, 1978.

43. **Campbell, I. W., Dawes, J., Fraser, D. M., Pepper, D. S., Clarke, B. F., Duncan, L. J. P., and Cash, J. D.,** Plasma beta-thromboglobulin in diabetes mellitus, *Diabetes,* 26, 1175, 1977.

44. **Burrows, A. W., Chavin, S. I., and Hockaday, T. D. R.,** Plasma beta-thromboglobulin concentrations in diabetes mellitus, *Lancet,* 1, 235, 1978.

45. **Preston, F. E., Ward, J. D., Marcola, B. H., Porton, N. R., and Timperley, W. R.,** Elevated beta-thromboglobulin levels and circulating platelet aggregates in diabetic microangiopathy, *Lancet,* 1, 238, 1978.

46. **Bierenbaum, M. L., Fleischman, A. I., Stier, A., Somol, H., and Watson, P. B.,** Effect of cigarette smoke upon *in vivo* platelet function in man, *Thromb. Res.,* 12, 1051, 1978.

47. **Rival, J., Riddle, J. M., and Stein, P. D.,** Effects of chronic smoking on platelet function, *Thromb. Res.,* 45, 75, 1987.

48. **Ludlam, C. A.,** Evidence for platelet specificity of beta-thromboglobulin and studies on its plasma concentrations in healthy individuals, *Br. J. Haematol.,* 32, 233, 1976.

49. **Ludlam, C. A. and Cash, J. D.,** Beta-thromboglobulin: A new tool for the diagnosis of hypercoagulability, in *Haemostasis and Thrombosis, Proceedings of the Serono Symposia,* Vol. 15, Serneri, N., and Prentice, C. R. M., Eds., Academic Press, New York, 1979.

50. **Kjeldsen, S., Gjesdal, K. G., Eide, I., Aakeson, I., Amundsen, R., Foss, O. P., and Leren, P.,** Increased beta-thromboglobulin in essential hypertension: interactions between arterial plasma adrenaline, platelet function and blood lipids, *Acta Med. Scand.,* 213, 369, 1983.

51. **Levine, S. P., Towell, B. L., Suarez, A. M., Knieriem, L. K., Harris, M. M., and George, J. N.,** Platelet activation and secretion associated with emotional stress, *Circulation,* 71, 1129, 1985.

52. **Pumphrey, C. W. and Dawes, J.,** Plasma beta-thromboglobulin as a measure of platelet activity. Effect of risk factors and findings in ischemic heart disease and after myocardial infarction, *Am. J. Cardiol.,* 50, 1258, 1982.

53. **De Boer, A. C., Ping Han, Turpie, A. G. G., Butt, R., Gent, M., and Genton, E.,** Platelet tests and antiplatelet drugs in coronary artery disease, *Circulation,* 67, 500, 1983.

54. **Weksler, B. B. and Goldstein, I. M.**, Prostaglandins: Interaction with platelets and polymorphonuclear leucocytes in hemostasis and inflammation, *Am. J. Med.*, 68, 419, 1980.

55. **Dejana, E., Breviario, F., Bussolino, F., Mussoni, L., and Mantovani, A.**, Pleiotropic effect of interleukin-1 on endothelial cells, presented at 11th Int. Congr. on Thrombosis and Haemostasis, Abstr. 1185 Brussels, 1987.

56. **Montesano, R., Mossaz, A., Ryver, J.-E., Orci, L., and Vassalli, P.**, Leucocyte interleukins induce cultured endothelial cells to produce a highly organized, glycosaminoglycan-rich pericellular matrix, *J. Cell. Biol.*, 99, 1706, 1984.

57. **Warren, J. S. and Ward, P. A.**, Review: Oxidative injury to the vascular endothelium, *Am. J. Med. Sci.*, 29, 97, 1986.

58. **Helin, H.**, Macrophage procoagulant factors—mediators of inflammatory and neoplastic tissue lesions, *Med. Biol.*, 64, 167, 1986.

59. **Niemetz, J. and Fani, K.**, Thrombogenic activity of leukocytes, *Blood*, 42, 47, 1973.

60. **Bengmark, S., Hafström Lo, and Korsan-Bengtsen, K.**, A trial to produce disseminated intravascular coagulation with intravenous infusion of homologous haemolysate and serum in cats, *Acta Chir. Scand.*, 138, 453, 1972.

61. **Born, G. V. R.**, Adenosine diphosphate as a mediator of platelet aggregation *in vivo*: an editorial view, *Circulation*, 72, 741, 1985.

62. **Rickles, F. R. and O'Leary, D. S.**, Role of coagulation system in pathophysiology of sickle cell disease, *Arch. Intern. Med.*, 133, 635, 1974.

63. **Hamer, J. D., Malone, P. C., and Silver, I. A.**, The PO_2 in venous valve pockets: its possible bearing on thrombogenesis, *Br. J. Surg.*, 68, 166, 1981.

64. **T'Sao, C. and Spaet, T. H.**, Ultramicroscopic changes in the rabbit inferior vena cava following partial constriction, *Am. J. Pathol.*, 51, 789, 1967.

65. **Gertz, S. D., Rennels, M. L., and Nelson, E.**, Endothelial cell ischemic injury: protective effect of heparin or aspirin assessed by scanning electron microscopy, *Stroke*, 6, 357, 1975.

66. **Roberge, S., Bazin, M., and Boutet, M.**, Endothelial cell coat modifications in rat thoracic aorta. Effect of ovariectomy and cigarette smoke, *Experientia*, 39, 72, 1983.

67. **Gertz, S. D., Forbes, M. S., Sunaga, T., Kawamura, J., Rennels, M. L., Shimamoto, T., and Nelson, E.**, Ischemic carotid endothelium. Transmission electron microscopic studies, *Arch. Pathol. Lab. Med.*, 100, 522, 1976.

68. **Gutstein, W. H., Farrell, G. A., and Armellini, C.**, Blood flow disturbance and endothelial cell injury in preatherosclerotic swine. *Lab. Invest.*, 29, 134, 1973.

69. **De Bruijn, W. C. and van Mourik, W.**, Scanning electron microscopic observations of endothelial changes in experimentally induced atheromatosis of rabbit aorta, *Virchows Arch. A*, 365, 23, 1975.

70. **Sunaga, T., Yamashita, Y., and Shimamoto, T.**, The intercellular bridge of vascular endothelium, *Proc. Jpn. Acad.*, 45, 627, 1969.

71. **Christensen, B. C. and Garbarsch, C.**, A scanning electron microscopic (SEM) study of the endothelium of the normal rabbit aorta, *Angiologica*, 9, 15, 1972.

72. **Majno, G., Shea, St.M., and Leventhal, M.**, Endothelial contraction induced by histamin-type mediators, *J. Cell. Biol.*, 42, 647, 1969.

73. **Hammersen, F.**, Endothelial filaments and intercellular gaps—A sufficient evidence for contractility?, *Bibl. Anat.*, No 12, 159, 1973.

74. **Chambers, R. and Zweifach, B. W.**, Intercellular cement and capillary permeability, *Physiol. Rev.*, 27, 436, 1947.

75. **Luft, J. H.**, Fine structure of capillary and endocapillary layer as revealed by ruthenium red, *Fed. Proc.*, 25, 1773, 1966.

76. **Behnke, O. and Zelander, T.**, Preservation of intercellular substances by the cationic dye alcian blue in preparation procedures for electron microscopy, *J. Ultrastruct. Res.*, 31, 424, 1970.

77. **Reidy, M. A.**, Biology of disease. A reassessment of endothelial injury and arterial lesion formation, *Lab. Invest.*, 53, 513, 1985.

78. **Hammersen, F. and Hammersen, E.**, Some structural and functional aspects of endothelial cells, *Basic Res. Cardiol.*, 80, 491, 1985.

79. **Gerlach, E., Nees, S., and Becker, B. F.**, The vascular endothelium: a survey of some newly evolving biochemical and physiological features, *Basic Res. Cardio.*, 80, 459, 1985.

80. **Delvos, U. and Müller-Berghaus, G.**, Die Bedeutung des Endothels der Gefässwand für die Aufrechterhaltung der Hämostase, *Klin. Wochenschr.*, 63, 1237, 1985.

81. **Thorgeirsson, G. and Lazzarini Robertson, A. Jr.**, The vascular endothelium—Pathobiologic significance. A review., *Am. J. Pathol.*, 93, 803, 1978.

82. **Ross, R., Faggiotto, A., Bowen-Pope, D., and Raines, E.**, The role of endothelial injury and platelet and macrophage interactions in atherosclerosis, *Circulation*, Suppl. 3, 77, 1984.

83. **Chesterman, C. N. and Berndt, M. C.,** Platelet and vessel wall interaction and the genesis of atherosclerosis, *Clin. Haematol.,* 15, 323, 1986.

84. **Harker, L. A., Ross, R., and Slichter, S. J.,** Chronic endothelial cell injury and platelet factor induced arteriosclerosis, presented at 5th Cong. Thrombosis Haemostasis, Abstr. 38, Paris, 1975.

85. **Ryan, U. S. and Ryan, J. W.,** Cell biology of pulmonary endothelium, *Circulation,* 70 (Suppl. 3) 46, 1984.

86. **Gerritsen, M. E.,** Functional heterogeneity of vascular endothelial cells, *Biochem. Pharmacol.,* 36, 2701, 1987.

87. **Wright, H. P.,** Endothelial turnover, *Thromb. Diath. Haemorrh.,* Suppl. 40, 79, 1970.

88. **Schwartz, S. M. and Benditt, E. P.,** Aortic endothelial cell replication. I. Effects of age and hypertension in the rat, *Circ. Res.,* 41, 248, 1977.

89. **Mason, R. G., Sharp, D., Chuang, H. Y. K., and Mohammad, S. F.,** The endothelium. Roles in thrombosis and hemostasis, *Arch. Pathol. Lab. Med.,* 101, 61, 1977.

90. **Libby, P., Warner, S. J. C., and Birinyi, L. K.,** presented at 11th Int. Congr. Thrombosis and Haemostasis, Abst. 1183, Brussels, 1987.

91. **Kay, A. B., Pepper, D. S., and McKenzie, R.,** The identification of fibrinopeptide B as a chemotactic agent derived from human fibrinogen, *Br. J. Haematol.* 27, 669, 1974.

92. **Rowland, F. N., Donovan, M. J., Picciano, P. T., Wilner, G. D., and Kreutzer, D. L.,** Fibrin-mediated vascular injury. Identification of fibrin peptides that mediate endothelial cell retraction, *Am. J. Pathol.,* 117, 418, 1984.

93. **Ishida, T. and Tanaka, K.,** Effects of fibrin and fibrinogen-degradation products on the growth of rabbit aortic smooth muscle cells in cultures, *Atherosclerosis,* 44, 161, 1982.

94. **Antecka-Genadiew, E., Buczko, W., Stasiak, A., Maciejewski, A., and Wisniewski, K.,** Some pharmacological and biochemical effects of fibrinopeptides A and B in the circulatory system of rats, *Pol. J. Pharmacol. Pharm.,* 35, 359, 1983.

95. **Nawroth, P. P., Handley, D., and Stern, D. M.,** The multiple levels of endothelial cell-coagulation factor interaction, *Clin. Haematol.,* 15, 293, 1986.

96. **Nawroth, P. P., Stern, D. M., Kisiel, W., and Dietrich, M.,** A pathway of coagulation on bovine capillary endothelial cells, *Br. J. Haematol.,* 63, 309, 1986.

97. **Araki, H. and Nishi, K.,** Effects of vascular constriction on occlusive thrombus formation of rat mesenteric artery, *Thromb. Res.,* 44, 39, 1986.

98. **Furchgott, R. F.,** Role of endothelium in responses of vascular smooth muscle, *Circ. Res.,* 53, 557, 1983.

99. **Vanhoutte, P. M.,** Could the absence or malfunction of vascular endothelium precipitate the occurrence of vasospasm?, *J. Mol. Cell. Cardiol.,* 18, 679, 1986.

100. **Brown, Z., Neild, G. H., Willoughby, J. J., Somia, N. V., and Cameron, S. J.,** Increased factor VIII as an index of vascular injury in cyclosporine nephrotoxicity, *Transplantation,* 42, 150, 1986.

101. **Henry, R. L.,** Methods for inducing experimental thrombosis, *Angiology,* 13, 554, 1962.

102. **Deutsch, E.,** Klinische Anwendung der Antikoagulantien. IV. Wirkung der Antikoagulantien auf die experimentelle Thrombose, in *Antikoagulantien, Handbuch der experimentellen Pharmakologie XXVII,* Markwardt, F., Ed., Springer-Verlag, New York, 1971, 332.

103. **Didisheim, P.,** Animal models useful in the study of thrombosis and antithrombotic agents, in *Progress in Haemostasis and Thrombosis,* Vol. 1, Spaet, T. H., Ed., Grune & Stratton, New York, 1972, 165.

104. **Dodds, W. J., Ed.,** *Animal Models of Thrombosis and Hemorrhagic Disease,* DHEW Publ. No. 76-982, National Institutes of Health, U.S. Public Health Service, Washington, D.C., 1976.

105. **Day, H. J.,** Molony, B. A., Nishizawa, E. F., and Rynbrandt, R. H., *Thrombosis, Animal and Clinical Models,* Plenum Press, New York, 1978.

106. **Philp, R. B.,** Experimental animal models of arterial thrombosis and the screening of platelet-inhibiting, anti-thrombotic drugs. A review, *Methods Find. Exp. Clin. Pharmacol.,* 1, 197, 1979.

107. **Colman, R. W., Robboy, S. J., and Minna, J. D.,** Disseminated intravascular coagulation (DIC): an approach. *Am. J. Med.,* 52, 679, 1972.

108. **Saldeen, T.,** Trends in microvascular research, the microembolism syndrome, *Microvasc. Res.,* 11, 227, 1976.

109. **Borgström, S., Gelin, L.-E., and Zederfeldt, B.,** The formation of vein thrombi following tissue injury. An experimental study in rabbits, *Acta Chir. Scand.,* Suppl. 247, 1, 1959.

110. **Aiken, J. W.,** Pharmacological analysis of factors influencing platelet aggregation in stenosed coronary arteries of dogs, *Ann. N.Y. Acad. Sci.,* 454, 131, 1985.

111. **Berman, J. K., Fields, D. C., Judy, H., Mori, V., and Parker, R. J.,** Gradual vascular occlusion, *Surgery,* 39, 399, 1956.

112. **Litvak, J. and Vineberg, A.,** Experimental gradual arterial occlusions with *in vitro* and *in vivo* observations, *Surgery,* 46, 953, 1959.

113. **Friedman M., Byers, S. O., and Pearl, F.,** Experimental production of intra-arterial and intravenous thrombi in the rabbit and rat, *Am. J. Physiol.,* 199, 770, 1960.

114. **Murray, D. W. G., Jaques, M. A., Perrett, T. S., and Best, C. H.**, Heparin and the thrombosis of veins following injury, *Surgery*, 2, 163, 1937.

115. **Best, C. H.**, Heparin and thrombosis, *Br. Med. J.*, 2, 977, 1938.

116. **Aronson, D. L. and Thomas, D. P.**, Experimental studies on venous thrombosis: effect of coagulants, procoagulants and vessel contusion, *Thromb. Haemost.*, 54, 866, 1985.

117. **Wilkinson, A. R., Hawker, R. J., and Hawker, L. M.**, The influence of antiplatelet drugs on platelet survival after aortic damage or implantation of a dacron arterial prosthesis, *Thromb. Res.*, 15, 181, 1979.

118. **Shand, R. A., Butler, K. D., Davies, J. A., Menys, V. C., and Wallis, R. B.**, The kinetics of platelet and fibrin deposition to damaged rabbit carotid arteries *in vivo*: involvement of platelets in the initial deposition of fibrin, *Thromb. Res.*, 45, 505, 1987.

119. **Chung-hsin Ts'ao**, Ultrastructural study of the effect of aspirin on *in vivo* platelet-collagen interaction and platelet adhesion to injured intima in the rabbit, *Am. J. Pathol.*, 59, 327, 1970.

120. **Hirsch, E. and Loewe, L.**, A method for producing experimental venous thrombosis, *Proc. Soc. Exp. Biol. Med.*, 63, 569, 1946.

121. **Bousser, M. G. and Lecrubier, C.**, Platelet aggregation and experimental thrombus formation. Effect of aspirin. *Presse. Med.*, 2, 1687, 1973.

122. **Honour, A. J. and Ross Russell, W. R.**, Experimental platelet embolism, *Br. J. Exp. Pathol.*, 43, 350, 1962.

123. **Rabinovitch, J. and Pines, B.**, The effect of heparin on experimentally produced venous thrombosis, *Surgery*, 14, 669, 1943.

124. **Danese, C. A. and Haimov, M.**, Inhibition of experimental arterial thrombosis in dogs with platelet-deaggregating agents, *Surgery*, 70, 927, 1971.

125. **Piepgras, D. G., Sundt, T. M., and Didisheim, P.**, Effect of anticoagulants and inhibitors of platelet aggregation on thrombotic occlusion of endarterectomized cat carotid arteries, *Stroke*, 7, 248, 1976.

126. **Johnson, A. J. and McCarty, W. R.**, The lysis of artificially induced intravascular clots in man by intravenous infusions of streptokinase, *J. Clin. Invest.*, 38, 1627, 1959.

127. **Welch, W. H.**, The structure of white thrombi, *Trans. Pathol. Soc. Philos.*, 13, 281, 1887.

128. **Williams, A. R.**, Intravascular acoustic microstreaming as an initiator of mural thrombi *in vivo*, presented at 5th Congr. Thrombosis and Haemostasis, *Abstr.* 392, Paris, 1975.

129. **Williams, A. R., Sykes, S. M., and O'Brien, W. D., Jr.**, Ultrasonic exposure modifies platelet morphology and function *in vitro*, *Ultrasound Med. Biol.*, 2, 317, 1977.

130. **Williams, A. R.**, Intravascular mural thrombi produced by acoustic microstreaming, *Ultrasound Med. Biol.*, 3, 191, 1977.

131. **Elcock, H. W. and Fredrickson, J. M.**, The effect of acetylsalicylic acid on thrombosis at microvenous anastomotic sites, *J. Laryngol. Otol.*, 86, 839, 1972.

132. **Moses, C.**, Effect of heparin and dicoumarol on thrombosis induced in the presence of venous stasis, *Proc. Soc. Exp. Biol. Med.*, 59, 25, 1945.

133. **Kiesewetter, W. B. and Shumaker, H. B., Jr.**, An experimental study of the comparative efficacy of heparin and dicumarol in the prevention of arterial and venous thrombosis, *Surg. Gynecol. Obstet.*, 86, 687, 1948.

134. **Hornstra, G. and Vendelmans-Starrenburg, A.**, Induction of experimental arterial occlusive thrombi in rats, *Atherosclerosis*, 17, 369, 1973.

135. **Baumgartner, H. R., Grimm, L., and Zbinden, G.**, Effect of generation of mural platelet thrombi on circulating blood in rabbit aorta, *Experientia*, 29, 442, 1973.

136. **Grover, H. M., Kinlough-Rathbone, R. L., Cazenave, J.-P., Dejana, E., Richardson, M., and Mustard, J. F.**, Effect of dipyridamole and prostacyclin on rabbit platelet adherence *in vitro* and *in vivo*, *J. Lab. Clin. Med.*, 99, 548, 1982.

137. **Clopath, P.**, The effect of acetylsalicylic acid (ASA) on the development of atherosclerotic lesions in miniature swine, *Br. J. Exp. Pathol.*, 61, 440, 1980.

138. **Jarrett, C. L. and Jaques, L. B.**, The antithrombosis activity of heparinoid G 31150, *Thromb. Haemost.*, 10, 431, 1963.

139. **Lavelle, S. M. and McIomhair, M.**, The quantitative reduction by heparin of intravenous thrombosis in normal and hypercoagulated animals, *Ir. J. Med. Sci.*, 149, 266, 1980.

140. **Constantine, J. W., Coleman, G. L., and Purcell, I. M.**, Inversion of an arterial branch. A technique for inducing thrombosis, *Atherosclerosis*, 16, 31, 1972.

141. **Millet, J., Theveniaux, J., and Pascal, M.**, A new experimental model of venous thrombosis in rats involving partial stasis and slight endothelium alterations, *Thromb. Res.*, 45, 123, 1987.

142. **Reyers, I., Mussoni, L., Donati, M. B., and de Gaetano, G.**, Failure of aspirin at different doses to modify experimental thrombosis in rats, *Thromb. Res.*, 18, 669, 1980.

143. **Tanimura, A., Tanaka, S., and Kitazono, M.**, Superficial intimal injury of the rabbit carotid artery induced by distilled water, *Virchows Arch. B*, 51, 197, 1986.

144. **Thomas, D. P., Merton, R., Wood, R. D., and Hockley, D. J.,** The relationship between vessel wall injury and venous thrombosis. An experimental study, *Br. J. Haematol.,* 59, 449, 1985.

145. **Piton, J., Billerley, J., Constant, P., Renou, A. M., and Caillé, J. M.,** Thromboses vasculaires selectives par courant electrique continu: experimentation chez l'animal, *Neuroradiology,* 16, 385, 1978.

146. **Williams, R. D. and Carey, L. C.,** Studies in the production of "standard" venous thrombosis, *Ann. Surg.,* 149, 381, 1959.

147. **Reber, K.,** A device for the production of well-defined lesions of mesenteric blood vessels with resulting platelet thrombi, *Thromb. Diath. Haemorrh.,* 15, 471, 1966.

148. **Bourgain, R.,** An experimental model for the study of arterial thrombosis and atherogenesis, *Acta Clin. Belg.,* 32, 403, 1977.

149. **Hladovec, J.,** Experimental arterial thrombosis in rats with continuous registration, *Thromb. Diath. Haemorrh.,* 26, 407, 1971.

150. **Massad, L., Plotkine, M., Capdeville, C., and Boulu, R. G.,** Electrically induced arterial thrombosis model in the conscious rat, *Thromb. Res.,* 48, 1, 1987.

151. **Romson, J. L., Haack, D. W., Abrams, G. D., and Lucchesi, B. R.,** Prevention of occlusive coronary artery thrombosis by prostacyclin infusion in the dog, *Circulation,* 64, 906, 1981.

152. **Arfors, K. – E., Hint, H. C., and Dhall, D. P.,** Counteraction of platelet at sites of laser-induced endothelial trauma, *Br. Med. J.,* 4, 430, 1968.

153. **Fleming, J. S., Bierwagen, M. E., Losada, M., Campbell, J. A. L., King, S. P., and Pindell, M. H.,** The effect of three antiinflammatory agents on platelet aggregation *in vitro* and *in vivo, Arch. Int. Pharmacodyn. Ther.,* 186, 120, 1970.

154. **Seiffge, D. and Kremer, E.,** Influence of ADP, blood flow velocity, and vessel diameter on the laser-induced thrombus formation, *Thromb. Res.,* 42, 331, 1986.

155. **Weichert, W., Pauliks, V., and Breddin, H. K.,** Laser induced thrombi in rat mesenteric vessels and antithrombotic drugs, *Haemostasis,* 13, 61, 1983.

156. **Meng, K. and O'Dea, K.,** The protective effect of acetylsalicylic acid on laser-induced venous thrombosis in the rat, *Naunyn-Schmiedebergs Arch. Pharmacol.,* 283, 379, 1974.

157. **Josa, M., Lie, J. T., Bianco, R. L., and Kaye, M. P.,** Reduction of thrombosis in canine coronary bypass vein grafts with dipyridamole and aspirin, *Am. J. Cardiol.,* 47, 1248, 1981.

158. **Allison, F., Jr. and Lancaster, M. G.,** Studies on the pathogenesis of acute inflammation. III. The failure of anticoagulants to prevent the leucocyte sticking reaction and the formation of small thrombi in rabbit ear chambers damaged by heat, *J. Exp. Med.,* 114, 535, 1961.

159. **Rosenblum, W. J. and El-Sabban, F.,** Platelet aggregation in the cerebral microcirculation. Effect of aspirin and other agents, *Circ. Res.,* 40, 320, 1977.

160. **Klemm, J.,** Ionisierende Strahlen und terminale Strombahn. Eine mikrocolor-phasenkonstrast-kinematografische Untersuchung an der Kaninchenohrkammer, *Fortscher. Med.,* 86, 154, 1968.

161. **Meng, K.,** Tierexperimentelle Thrombose und Behandlung mit Acetylsalicylsäure, *Med. Welt,* 27, 1359, 1976.

162. **Heiss, M., Haas, S., and Blumel, G.,** The antithrombotic effect of a new thromboxane-synthetase inhibitor (UK-37,248) in comparison with acetylsalicylic acid (ASA) in experimental thrombosis, *Haemostasis,* 12, 102, 1982.

163. **Just, M., Martorana, P. A., and Zoller, G.,** Inhibition of experimental arterial and venous thrombosis by the novel pyridazinone-derivative C 85-3143, *Thromb. Res.,* Suppl. 6, 147, 1986.

164. **Marshall, M. and Hess, H.,** New findings concerning pathogenesis and nonsurgical treatment of peripheral arterial diseases, *Vasa,* 7, 49, 1978.

165. **Sawyer, P. N. and Pate, J. W.,** Bioelectric phenomena as an etiologic factor in intravascular thrombosis, *Am. J. Physiol.,* 175, 103, 1953.

166. **Pflug, J., Calnan, J., and Olsen, E. G. J.,** An experimental model for the study of thrombosis, *Br. J. Surg.,* 55, 706, 1968.

167. **Chiu, H. M., Hirsh, J., Yung, W. L., Regoeczi, E., and Gent, M.,** Relationship between the anticoagulant and antithrombotic effects of heparin in experimental venous thrombosis, *Blood,* 49, 171, 1977.

168. **Carter, C. J., Kelton, J. G., Hirsh, J., and Gent, M.,** Relationship between the antithrombotic and anticoagulant effects of low molecular weight heparin, *Thromb. Res.,* 21, 169, 1981.

169. **Deaton, H. L. and Anlyan, W. G.,** A study of experimental methods for producing thrombosis in small arteries, *Surg. Gynecol. Obstet.,* 111, 131, 1960.

170. **Fahlström, G., Ohman, U., and Magnusson, P. H.,** Intramuscular heparin prophylaxis in experimental thrombosis in rats, *Acta Chir. Scand.,* 136, 489, 1970.

171. **Owen, Ch.A., Jr. and Bowie, E. J. W.,** Effect of heparin on chronically induced intravascular coagulation in dogs, *Am. J. Physiol.,* 229, 449, 1975.

172. **Holden, W. D., Cameron, D. B., Shea, P. C., Jr., and Shaw, B. W.,** Trypsin and thrombin induced venous thrombosis and its prevention with 3,3'-methylenebis (4-hydroxycoumarin), *Surg. Gynecol. Obstet.,* 88, 635, 1949.

173. **Wessler, S.,** Experimentally produced phlebothrombosis in the study of thromboembolism, *J. Clin. Invest.,* 32, 610, 1953.

174. **Mayer, J. E. and Hammond, G. L.,** Dipyridamole and aspirin tested against an experimental model of thrombosis, *Ann. Surg.,* 178, 108, 1973.

175. **Lyman, B. T., Johnson, B. L., and White, J. G.,** Dose-dependent inhibition of experimental arterial thrombosis by carbencillin and ticarcillin, *Am. J. Pathol.,* 92, 473, 1978.

176. **McLetchie, N. G. B.,** The pathogenesis of atheroma, *Am. J. Pathol.,* 28, 413, 1952.

177. **Thomas, D. P. and Wessler, S.,** Stasis thrombi induced by bacterial endotoxin, *Circ Res,* 14, 486, 1964.

178. **De Clerck, F., Goosens, J., Vermylen, J., Hornstra, G., and Reneman, R. S.,** Modification of venous stasis thrombosis in the rat by plateletactive drugs and by heparin, *Arch. Int. Pharmacodyn. Ther.,* 222, 233, 1976.

179. **Wessler, S., Ward, K., and Ho, C.,** Studies on intravascular coagulation. III. The pathogenesis of serum induced venous thrombosis, *J. Clin. Invest.,* 34, 647, 1955.

180. **Fritsch, H., Onderka, M., Zimmermann, R., and Barth, P.,** Kontaktfaktorinduzierte experimentelle Thrombose. Histologische und gerinnungsanalytische Untersuchungen, *Res. Exp. Med.,* 161, 141, 1973.

181. **Hladovec, J.,** A quantitative model of venous stasis thrombosis in rats, *Physiol. Bohemoslov.,* 24, 551, 1975.

182. **Niada, R., Pescador, R., Porta, R., Mantovani, M., and Prino, G.,** Defibrotide is antithrombotic and thrombolytic against rabbit venous thrombosis, *Haemostasis,* 16, (Suppl. 1), 3, 1986.

183. **Wessler, S. and Morris, L. E.,** Studies in intravascular coagulation. IV. The effect of heparin and dicumarol on serum-induced venous thrombosis, *Circulation,* 12, 553, 1955.

184. **Barth, P., Zimmermann, R., Zieboll, J., and Lange, D.,** The antithrombotic effect of acetylsalicylic acid, heparin and phenprocoumon in experimental thrombosis, *Thromb. Diath. Haemorrh.,* 34, 554, 1975.

185. **Peterson, J. and Zucker, M. B.,** The effect of adenosine-monophosphate, arcaine and anti-inflammatory agents on thrombosis and platelet function in rabbits, *Thromb. Diath. Haemorrh.,* 23, 148, 1970.

186. **Zambouras, D. A., Anezyris, P., and Kalakonas, P.,** La cortisone et l'héparine dans les thrombophlébites expérimentales. Etude comparative de leur action, *Presse Med.,* 69, 1134, 1961.

187. **Arfors, K.-E., Bergqvist, D., and Tangen, O.,** The effect of platelet function inhibitors on experimental venous thrombosis formation in rabbits, *Acta Chir. Scand.,* 141, 40, 1975.

188. **Bergqvist, D. and Nilsson, B.,** The influence of low molecular weight heparin in combination with dihydroergotamine on experimental thrombosis and haemostasis, *Thromb. Haemost.,* 58, 893, 1987.

189. **Friedrich, H. W.,** Experimenteller Beitrag zur Thrombocidbehandlung der Thrombose, *Arztl. Wochenschr.,* 5, 178, 1950.

190. **Ostergaard, P. B., Nilsson, B., Bergqvist, D., Hedner, U., and Pedersen, P. C.,** The effect of low molecular weight heparin on experimental thrombosis and haemostasis. The influence of production method, *Thromb. Res.,* 45, 739, 1987.

191. **Ashwin, J. G.,** Elevated incidence of experimental thrombosis after heparin, *Can. J. Biochem. Physiol.,* 40, 1153, 1962.

192. **Seuter, F., Fiedler, V. B., and Philipp, E.,** Nafazatrom, in *New Cardiovascular Drugs,* Scriabine, A., Ed., Raven Press, New York, 1986, 163.

193. **Zimmermann, R., Peter, J., Jung, G., Horsch, A., Mörl, H., and Harenberg, J.,** Antithrombotic and opposite effects of drugs influencing the prostaglandin system, *Thromb. Haemost.,* 46, 179, 1981.

194. **Polterauer, P., Zekert, F., and Gottlob, R.,** Azetylsalizylsäure und Dipyridamol: aggregationshemmung im Experiment am Kaninchen, *Vasa,* 4, 397, 1975.

195. **Zekert, F. and Gottlob, R.,** Eine einfache experimentelle Methode zur quantitativen Bestimmung der antithrombotischen Wirkung von Thrombozytenaggregationshemmern, *Dtsch. Med. Wochenschr.,* 98, 1004, 1973.

196. **Danese, C. A., Voleti, C. D., and Weiss, H. J.,** Protection by aspirin against experimentally induced arterial thrombosis in dogs, *Thromb. Diath. Haemorrh.,* 25, 288, 1971.

197. **Hatanaka, K., Minamiyama, M., Takaichi, S., Tanaka, K., Ishibashi-Ueda, H., Imakita, M., and Yamamoto, A.,** Thrombus formation by the application of thrombin to the outer surface of mouse mesenteric vein: comparison with the application of ADP, *Thromb. Res.,* 40, 731, 1985.

198. **Kojima, S.,** Experimentelle Untersuchungen über Veränderungen des Blutes durch aseptische Thromben-bildung, *Arch. Klin. Chir.,* 174, 216, 1933.

199. **Hladovec, J.,** The effect of ultra-low-dose heparin in experimental venous thrombosis, *Thromb. Res.,* 36, 83, 1984.

200. **Connor, W. E., Hoak, J. C., and Warner, E. D.,** Massive thrombosis produced by fatty acid infusion, *J. Clin. Invest.,* 42, 860, 1963.

201. **Hoak, J. C., Connor, W. E., Eckstein, J. W., and Warner, E. D.,** Fatty acid-induced thrombosis and death: mechanism and prevention, *J. Lab. Clin. Med.,* 63, 791, 1964.

202. **Levison, M. E., Carrizosa, J., Tanphaichitra, D., Schick, P. K., and Rubin, W.,** Effect of aspirin on thrombogenesis and on production of experimental aortic valvular streptococcus-viridans endocarditis in rabbits, *Blood,* 49, 645, 1977.

203. **Butler, K. D. and White, A. M.,** Inhibition of the platelet involvement in the sublethal Forssman reaction by sulphinpyrazone and not by aspirin, presented at Anturan. An international symposium, Hamilton, Bermuda, 1979.

204. **Renaud, S. and Godu, J.,** Thrombosis prevention by acetylsalicylic acid in hyperlipemic rats, *Can. Med. Assoc. J.,* 103, 1037, 1970.

205. **Davidson, E., Howard, A. N., and Gresham, G. A.,** The effect of phenindione on rats fed diets which produce thrombosis and experimental arteriosclerosis, *Br. J. Exp. Pathol.,* 43, 418, 1962.

206. **Faxon, D. P., Sanborn, T. A., Haudenschild, Ch. C., and Ryan, T. J.,** Effect of antiplatelet therapy on restenosis after experimental angioplasty, *Am. J. Cardiol.,* 53, 72 C, 1984.

207. **Freak, M. J.,** Symposium on thrombosis. I. Arterial thrombosis (embolism) in the cat, *J. Small Anim. Pract.,* 7, 711, 1966.

208. **Moe, N.,** Spontaneous and experimental thrombosis in the mouse placenta, *Acta Pathol. Microbiol. Immunol. Scand. (A),* 77, 653, 1969.

209. **Scarpelli, D. G.,** Survey of some spontaneous and experimental disease processes of lower vertebrates and invertebrates, *Fed. Proc.,* 28, 1825, 1969.

210. **Nagaoka, A., Sudo, K., Orita, S., Kikuchi, K., and Aramaki, Y.,** Hematological studies on the spontaneously hypertensive rats with special reference to the development of thrombosis, *Jpn. Circ. J.,* 35, 1379, 1971.

211. **Stephens, L. R., Little, P. B., Wilkie, B. N., and Barnum, D. A.,** Infectious meningoencephalitis in cattle - a review, *J. Am. Vet. Med. Assoc.,* 178, 378, 1981.

212. **Bicher, H. I.,** Anti-thrombotic effect of an heparin-like substance (SP 54) preventing red cell and platelet aggregation, *Arzneim. Forsch.,* 20, 379, 1970.

213. **Schaub, R. G., Ochoa, R., Simmons, C. A., and Lincoln, K. L.,** Renal microthrombosis following endotoxin infusion may be mediated by lipoxygenase products, *Circ. Shock,* 21, 261, 1987.

214. **Perlman, M. B., Johnson, A., and Malik, A. B.,** Ibuprofen prevents thrombin-induced lung vascular injury: mechanism of effect, *Am. J. Physiol.,* 252, H 605, 1987.

215. **Birek, A., Duffin, J., Glynn, M. F. X., and Cooper, J. D.,** The effect of sulfinpyrazone on platelet and pulmonary responses to onset of membrane oxygenator perfusion, *Trans. Am. Soc. Artif. Intern. Organs,* 22, 94, 1976.

216. **Townsend, E. R., Duffin, J., Ali, M., McDonald, J. W. D., Thiesson, J. J., Masterson, J., Klement, P., and Cooper, J. D.,** Preservation of platelets during extracorporeal circulation in sheep: a comparison between aspirin and sulfinpyrazone, *Circ. Res.,* 49, 452, 1981.

217. **Rodvien, R., Robinson, J., Litwak, P., Mitchell, R. R., and Price, D. C.,** Biomaterials: interfacial phenomena and applications, in *Advances in Chemistry Series,* Vol. 199, Cooper, S. and Peppas, N., Eds., American Chemical Society, Washington D. C., 1981.

218. **Mason, R. G., Zucker, W. H., Shinoda, B. H., and Mohammad, S. F.,** Effects of antithrombotic agents evaluated in a non-human primate vascular shunt model, *Am. J. Pathol.,* 83, 557, 1976.

219. **Hanson, S. R. and Harker, L. A.,** Baboon models of acute arterial thrombosis, *Thromb. Haemost.,* 58, 801, 1987.

220. **Wiedeman, M. P., Tuma, R. F., and Mayrovitz, H. N.,** Effects of vasoactive drugs on platelet aggregation *in vivo* and *in vitro, Thromb. Res.,* 15, 365, 1979.

221. **Tuma, R. F., Wiedeman, M. P., and Mayrovitz, H. N.,** Microvascular responses to suloctidil, *Physiologist,* 19, 394, 1976.

222. **Pangrazzi, J., Abbadini, M., Zametta, M., Naggi, A., Torri, G., Casu, B., and Donati, M. B.,** Antithrombotic and bleeding effects of a low molecular weight heparin fraction, *Biochem. Pharmacol.,* 34, 3305, 1985.

Chapter 3

BASIC METHODS

I. MODEL OF VASCULAR LESION

While induction of a vascular lesion is relatively easy, it is much more difficult to demonstrate its presence. The necessity of a quantitative method for the estimation of circulating endothelial cells was obvious at first sight. Such a method would represent a direct indicator of a vascular lesion avoiding morphological examination of the vessel wall. Meanwhile, it has been shown using morphological methods, that a certain degree of vascular lesions is invariably associated with the desquamation of endothelial cells leaving behind typical endothelial defects. Theoretically, it might be possible to show in blood the presence of various constituents of endothelial lining, e.g., components of the surface coat and other materials released from damaged endothelial cells. On the other hand, very similar materials are present mostly in all formed blood elements and tissue cells and many constituents of endothelial cells may be present in blood even under physiological conditions. To demonstrate cells or their formed remnants would represent a much more direct and specific proof of a vascular lesion.

It was mentioned in Chapter 1 that after degeneration or death of the cell its body is displaced by a neighboring replicating cell and desquamates. With a 0.1% daily replication rate, about 50 such elements should enter every milliliter of blood each minute. Desquamated elements are removed by the reticuloendothelial system and their half time in circulation may be estimated at about 5 min. Under such conditions approximately 6 elements should be present in 9 μl plasma (the volume in which the elements are counted). The number actually found under resting conditions in man is less, about 2 elements in 9 μl plasma. Naturally, losses during the isolation have to be expected, but the starting values of the calculation are merely crude approximations. Indeed, the calculated number is still within the same order of magnitude as the actual one. This actual number reflects the normal turn over of cells *in situ*. Under pathological conditions the desquamation would substantially increase involving cells at sites subjected to particular mechanical and metabolic stresses. Such cells which have, more or less, lost their normal properties due to degenerative processes and direct lesions would be most susceptible to desquamation, with the changes again being of physiological (age) or pathological origin.

It is only logical to wonder how such elements have escaped the observation for more than 150 years of hematological studies, perhaps from Virchow's time when K. Vierordt in 1852 published the first quantitative microscopic analysis of blood elements. In fact, they have probably been observed but not recognized as endothelial cells or their remnants. The so-called nonhematological elements rarely occurring in blood smears have been interpreted in various ways. Some were described as more or less elongated elements with an oval or finely granulated nucleus. Occasionally nucleoli were observed. Cytoplasma was described as an irregular ill-demarcated fringe around the nucleus showing fine granulation in Giemsa's staining. Such elements were sometimes thought to be of reticuloendothelial origin. Hesse suggested that they could represent endothelial cells. They were supposed to occur particularly in ulcerative endocarditis, serious blood infections, Hodgkin's disease, and endotheliomas. Similar elements were seen much more frequently in smears obtained from sternal punctures and were again often described as bare nuclei, i.e., remnants of damaged endothelial cells. They were elongated or spindle-shaped, sometimes round and then supposed to come from venous sinuses. In finely structured nuclei, some nucleoli were observed again. Some authors speculated that circulating endothelial cells are closely related to monocytes, while others classified similar elements as tumor cells of various origin-ascribed diagnostic significance. Elements closely resembling anuclear endothelial cell carcasses counted by the present method were sometimes classified as cutaneous scales (keratinized epithelium) (e.g., in the *Sandoz Atlas of Hematology*). It is worth mentioning that the elements described in this section were never obtained by transcutaneous blood collection. It is also important to distinguish between rarely occurring elements, those which are accidental, e.g., admixed with blood during the vessel puncture or another collection procedure, and those which are rare but regularly occurring elements counted after the concentration procedure and whose count in a larger given volume is fairly constant.

Needless to say, the problem of the existence of circulating endothelial cells has always been full of unanswered questions and in general, their identification was highly controversial.

The first author who attempted to estimate circulating endothelial cells intentionally and purposefully was Bouvier[1-4] in the years 1968 to 1970. He supposed that at least some of the previously described cells originated from the vessel wall and based his method on the assumption that the cells might be isolated together with leukocytes. For this purpose he used the so-called Herbeuval's leukoconcentration method[5,6] originally developed for the detection of tumor cells in blood. In principle it was based on the preliminary lysis of red blood cells by saponin followed by the use of a special solution for isolation and fixation of leukocytes. The solution contained polyvinylpyrrolidone and salts in addition to glucose, ascorbic acid, formol, and citrate. Formol served as a fixative and citrate as an anticoagulant. A smear on a glass slide was prepared from this leukocyte suspension obtained by centrifugation and stained by Giemsa's method. Endothelial cells were counted in relation to leukocytes. Under normal conditions no such elements appeared in the blood and were seen only under some pathological conditions. Bouvier together with Gaynor and Spaet,[2,7] showed that the elements were present in clinical thrombosis and experimentally after endotoxin administration. The appearance of elements was described as a "spindle shape, elongated nuclear configuration with a large nucleolus and peculiar wrinkling, and the pale blue cytoplasma with borders difficult to outline". It appeared that almost naked nuclei with only an irregular fringe of cytoplasma had been isolated.

In the following years Bouvier's method was used by Harker et al.,[8] Schwartz et al.,[9] Weber et al.,[10] and Fabiani and Catavitello.[11] In 1973 a new method was developed in the author's laboratory based on the assumed existence in blood of low density anuclear carcasses of endothelial cells which could be isolated not with leukocytes but with platelets and can be concentrated and counted in a hematological chamber under a phase contrast microscope, but only after the preliminary removal of platelets by the addition of adenosine-diphosphate and centrifugation of aggregates. Under such conditions the elements can be easily counted even in normal blood. It is possible that the elements counted by Bouvier were principally the lost nuclei with some remnants of the cytoplasma in contrast to the cell membranes with some cytoplasma seen together with platelets after isolation. Very flat and thin endothelial cells *in situ* have a nucleus markedly projecting into the lumen. There is a large difference in the density between cytoplasma and nuclei and the shear stresses and other mechanical forces effective during their squeezing through the capillaries supposed to maybe cause the rapid loss of nuclei in the circulation. Endothelial contraction, expression by the neighboring cells, and/or the responses of the endothelium to irritation may contribute to the loss. The loss during preparation is not substantial. Scanning electron microscopy clearly showed the site of nuclear loss also connected with the loss of a portion of the cytoplasma (courtesy of Dr. Pelcbauer, CSAV) (Plate 1).* Under physiological conditions only anuclear elements circulate in blood and the slow degenerative changes caused by aging, chronic as well as acute pathological processes, may often cause the loss of nuclei already *in situ*.[12,13] Under pathological conditions, an increase in numbers of anuclear elements as well as nuclei, and

---

* Plate 1 appears after page 50.

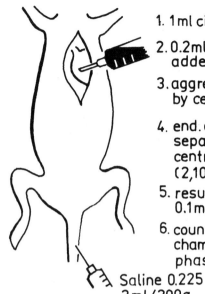

1. 1 ml citrated PRP

2. 0.2 ml ADP (2 mg/ml) added

3. aggregates removed by centrifugation

4. end. cell carcasses separated and concentrated by centrif. (2,100 g 20 min)

5. resuspended in 0.1 ml phys. saline

6. counted in Bürker's chamber under phase contrast

Saline 0.225 %
2 ml/200 g

FIGURE 1.   Schematic diagram of an experiment of counting circulating endothelial elements in rats.

possibly, some nuclear cells may be seen in the circulation. Such nuclei together with nuclear elements which may be, in part, of another origin and are easily differentiated, are isolated by the leukoconcentration method. Gradwohl[14] stated that naked nuclei of different cells could not be differentiated, e.g., nuclei from endothelial cells and smooth muscle cells. Bouvier[1] noted that in electron microscopic (TEM) preparations, the elements are poorly defined probably due to damage and do not allow a good differentiation. Sharnoff[15] described in thromboembolic accidents and generally in thrombophilic states an increased number of megakaryocytes in the pulmonary capillary bed. These elements may easily be related to the circulating naked nuclei and Fagan[16] brought to attention that most such megakaryocytes are, in fact, aggregates of such more or less naked endothelial nuclei.

The method developed in the author's laboratory can be described as follows: the method of counting carcasses of endothelial cells circulating in blood (Figure 1) was described by Hladovec and Rossmann in 1973.[17] Citrated blood (9 parts of blood plus 1 part of 3.8% disodium citrate) was collected from the right hearts of anesthetized rats or from the cubital vein in man with a rigorously siliconized collecting material and preserved at 4°C until the counting carried out after 60 min at the latest. Platelet-rich plasma (PRP) was prepared by centrifugation (395 g for 20 min) at 4°C. Following the addition of 0.2 ml of adenosine-5'-diphosphate (Calbiochem) at a concentration of 2 mg/ml to 1 ml of PRP the mixture was shaken mechanically for 10 min (Figure 2). Another centrifugation (395 g for 20 min) served to remove platelet aggregates. The supernatant was centrifuged at 2100 × g for 20 min and the scanty sediment was carefully suspended in 0.1 ml of 0.9% NaCl by a slow mechanical stirring with a soft polyethylene rod for 1 min. Two platforms of Bürkers's chamber were filled with the suspension and the elements were counted under phase-contrast microscope menader-like in both platforms separately (Figures 3 and 4). The filling and counting was repeated once more. As each platform corresponds to 0.9 μl (3 × 3 × 0.1 mm) and the elements were ten times concentrated, the results were expressed in terms of average element counts in 9 μl PRP from four counts. In the final suspension only anuclear endothelial cell carcasses remained with some of their fragments (not counted) and occasional platelet aggregates of a corresponding size, but of globular form and granular with fuzzy margins.

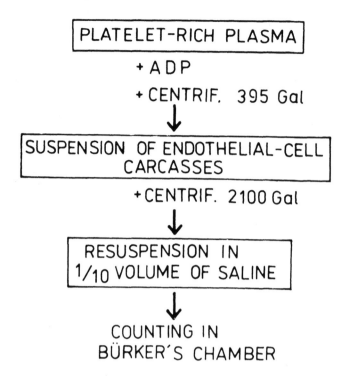

FIGURE 2. Block diagram of the procedure of counting circulating endothelial elements.

BÜRKER'S CHAMBER

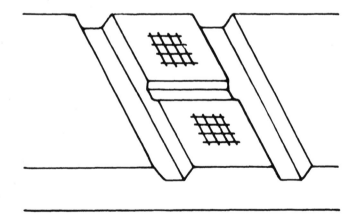

FIGURE 3. The two platforms of a Bürker's chamber.

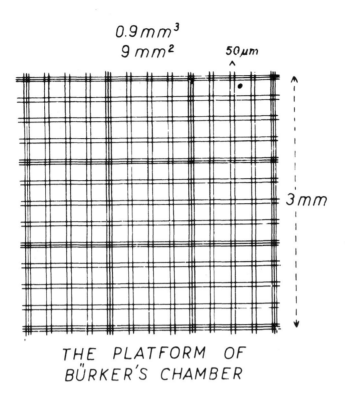

$0.9\,mm^3$
$9\,mm^2$ $50\mu m$

$3\,mm$

THE PLATFORM OF
BÜRKER'S CHAMBER

FIGURE 4.   The Bürker's chamber grid and the relative size of an element
(right upper corner).

Endothelial carcasses are polygonal, flat (15 × 30 μm), very thin (0.5 to 1/μm), often folded, and with rolled in margins (Figure 5) (Plates 2A, 2B, 3).* With very high increased counts, as in late phases of pregnancy and toxemia of pregnancy, the elements are seen in small aggregates (Glawankowa and Popowa).

It is important to note that the elements are easily adsorbed on foreign surfaces and a large portion is lost during blood collection with catheters. ADP has no effect on element counts as the counting can be carried out, although with some difficulty, even in the presence of platelets with identical results.

The method has been adopted in several other laboratories, e.g., by Davis et al.,[18,19] Iwata et al.,[20] Gall et al.,[21] Glawanakowa and Popowa,[22] and in several laboratories in Czechoslovakia. In 1983 Takahashi and Harker[8] published a study addressing a similar subject, which however, in no way could be counted as an attempt at reproduction. Their method was principally different and related to leukoconcentration using density gradients for the isolation of elements which were, moreover, cultured endothelial cells. The authors confirmed the impossibility of demonstrating the presence of nuclear elements in blood under normal conditions using their method and also noticed substantial losses of cells with the platelet fraction. They attempted to base the identification of elements on the immunoreaction of factor VIIIR:AG. This relates to another difficult problem. The identification of elements isolated together with platelets was originally based on the isolation of cells directly from the inner surface of vessels by gently wiping the endothelial lining with swabs wetted in acidified citrate solution and using the same method of isolation and counting as for circulating elements. The shape and size of such elements, both isolated directly and from blood, were compared using hematological staining and phase contrast microscopy (Figures

* Plates 2A, 2B, and 3 appear after page 50.

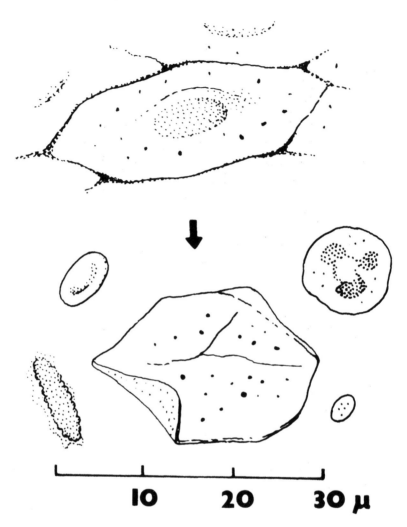

FIGURE 5.   The appearance of endothelial cells *in situ* and in blood together with other formed elements to illustrate their relative size.

17 and 18). They were practically identical. Of course, all elements obtained from the vascular wall and blood were damaged. On the other hand, damaged elements are those which are of interest and undamaged elements are not expected to exist in blood. It is well known from the studies of Chambers and Zweifach carried out before 1947[23] that the surface coat (called by them ''endothelial cement'') is more or less lost after an endothelial lesion and changes in its consistency are probably one of the most important mechanisms in the loss of endothelial lining stability[24] (Figure 6). This is illustrated experimentally by *in vivo* binding of a portion of calcium ions by citrate, EDTA, or lactate (Figure 7). A similar mechanism may be effective in ischemic organs after the accumulation of endogenous lactate. Another mechanism of desquamation may be based on the contraction of cells leading to a widening of interendothelial gaps and the loss of cell coherence. Strong vascular contractions and even dilatations may have a mechanical damaging effect on the endothelial lining.

As changes in the consistency of the cell coat are universally present in an endothelial lesion, it can be expected that its constituents would be released into the blood. Thus, it is known that increases in blood levels of factor VIIIR:AG could serve more or less as an indicator of a vascular lesion suffering, nevertheless, from low specificity.[25] The presence of this factor on the circulating elements isolated with platelets was demonstrated by Iwata

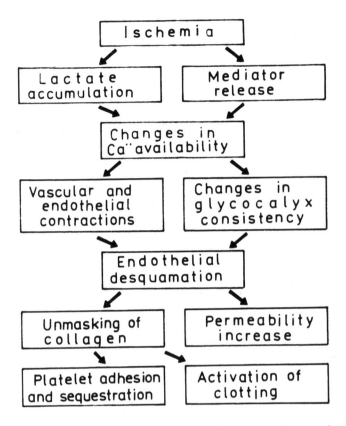

FIGURE 6.   Block diagram of the changes in glycocalyx consistency and subsequent endothelial desquamation in ischemia.

et al.[20] and Davis et al.[19] In this laboratory the method was used beside other immune reactions, in cooperation with the immunological department (Dr. V. Hašková). None of them were sufficiently specific, showing no identification but degree of damage. Similarly, it was impossible to reliably demonstrate the presence of dipeptidyl peptidase and amino-peptidase M said to be specific for endothelium (cooperation with Lojda).[26,27] Morphological markers such as Weibel-Pallade bodies could not be regularly expected in damaged elements that have lost a portion of the cytoplasm. The activity of alkaline phosphatase in blood after a standard endothelial lesion by citrate was shown, in cooperation with Mrhová, to increase whereas in aortic tissue its activity decreased (Figure 8). No significant changes were observed in acid phosphatase, adenosine-monophosphate, and adenosine-triphosphate. An increase of a plasminogen activator was observed in blood after citrate with the use of the euglobulin lysis test in rats (Figure 9). Many other tests are theoretically possible such as those for the presence in blood of angiotensin-converting enzymes, thrombospondin, prostacyclin derivatives, special collagen and glycosaminoglycan fractions, etc. None of them can be expected to be sufficiently specific and positive findings would represent an indirect piece of evidence only. Such indirect evidence was also increased permeability in the pulmonary vascular bed after a standard vascular lesion by intravenous administration of 100 mg/kg homocysteine to rats. The increased permeability was demonstrated by intra-venous administration of Evans blue, extraction of stained homogenized lung tissue, and photometry (Figure 10). The same stimulus caused simultaneous activation of stasis throm-bosis (ligature of an intestinal loop combined with intravenous injection of a kaolin sus-pension, transection of mesenteric vessels in a Petri dish containing distilled water followed by hemoglobin photometry) and increased platelet sequestration. This corresponded in other

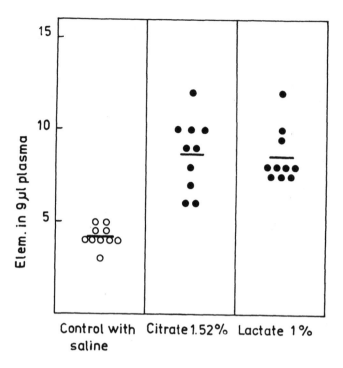

FIGURE 7.   The increase of element counts after a challenge with intravenous citrate and lactate in rats.

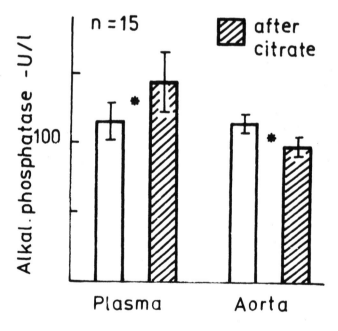

FIGURE 8.   The increase of alkaline phosphatase in plasma concomitant with its decrease in the vessel wall after an intravenous citrate injection in rats.

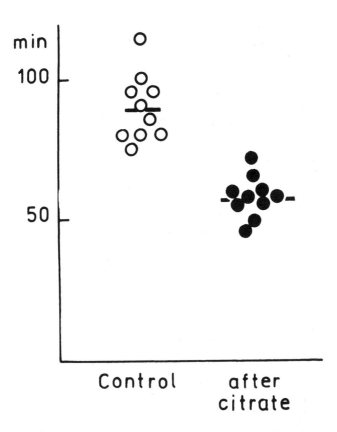

FIGURE 9. The decrease of euglobulin lysis time in rats after an intra-venous citrate challenge.

experiments with an increase in circulating endothelial elements. In general, the same agents, such as citrate, lactate, epinephrine, hypotonic saline, homocysteine, vasoactive drugs, etc., that produced an increase in circulating endothelial elements with a maximum attained 5 min after intravenous injection (Figure 11) induced at the same dose also platelet seques-tration, i.e., an acute transitory decrease of platelets (counted by Piette's method[28]). As shown with Cr^{51}-tagged platelets, the decrease was caused by transitory platelet sequestration predominantly in the pulmonary microcirculation and probably corresponded to the platelet adhesion at sites in the lining unmasked by desquamated endothelial cells (Figure 12). In this platelet sequestration model not only the challenging agents but also protective drugs and their dosages were often the same as in the endothelemia model. The sequestered platelets formed local aggregates and after a short delay were released again into the circulation. This is also the most probable origin of circulating platelet aggregates as demonstrated by the Wu-Hoak method. A parallel increase in circulating elements isolated with platelets and circulating platelet aggregates after smoking was demonstrated by Davis et al.[19] An acute decrease in the fibrinogen level (gravimetric method) was also observed after a standard lesion by intravenous administration of citrate, probably based on the infiltration into the vessel wall (Figure 13). A marked compensatory increase in the fibrinogen level was noted several days later. The endothelial lesion induced by hypotonic saline led to a parallel increase in circulating elements and activation of both arterial and venous thrombosis (Figure 14). This type of challenge was used in both thrombosis models in the present studies.

All these and many other kinds of indirect evidence from pharmacological studies have supported the identification of circulating elements with endothelial cell carcasses. On the other hand, the final proof of their identity by morphologic, immunologic, and histochemical

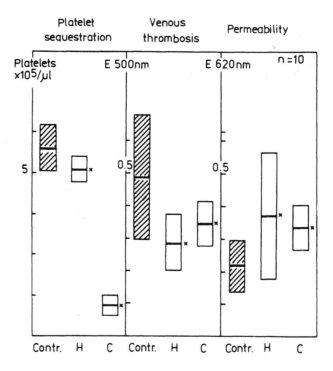

FIGURE 10.   The parallel changes in platelet sequestration, activation of venous thrombosis, and permeability increase in lungs after an i.v. injection of homocysteine or citrate in rats (H: homocysteine 100 mg/kg, C: citrate 1.52%, 2 ml/200g).

or biochemical methods, supposing the integrity of cells, is extremely difficult. In fact, looking for a similar proof may be misplaced in damaged elements. Irrespective of the designation of elements, the method already serves as a very sensitive indicator of a vascular lesion which has been an urgent necessity for a long time.[17] The method is very simple and well reproducible. It could be easily used in pharmacological and clinical studies.

Under pathological conditions the elements come predominantly from the microcirculation (largest surface) of the most affected region, e.g., the values are high behind an ischemic organ (Figure 15). This was shown experimentally after ligating one or both femoral arteries in rats. On the contrary, venous occlusion invariably produced decreased counts. The explanation is not known. Meanwhile, the lesion that would effectively increase endothelial counts has to be rather extensive and not too intensive. In animal experiments the site of the administration of challenging agents and the volume of administered fluid may have a marked influence on the source of cells. Thus, after intravenous injection of challenging agents, the cells come preferentially from the pulmonary microcirculation, as shown indirectly in Figure 25.

The elements in various animal species (mammals) are of practically the same size and shape. Moreover, they also show similar basal counts (Table 1). The values in man range between 1.7 and 3.5 elements in 9 µl plasma evidently depending on age (increases with age), sex (lower in young women than in men, high in pregnant women),[22,29] and they increase during the daytime. Treatment by various drugs may have a modifying influence (e.g., estrogens increase the sensitivity to some challenges while corticoids and immunosuppressive agents decrease the values).[30] The table of values in various species illustrates that the relation of the endothelial surface to blood volume is universal and almost constant like *in situ* survival of cells. In fact, the mesothelial cells covering the body cavities and even epithelial linings may share similar properties with the endothelium such as stability

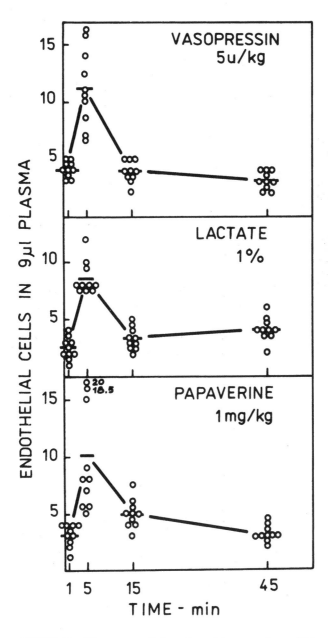

FIGURE 11.   Time course of element count increase after various challenges in rats.

and its regulation. Without special methods morphologically indistinguishable elements can be obtained, e.g., from the peritoneal cavity of rats with swabs wetted by acidified citrate solution, or quantitatively, by an intraperitoneal injection of 10 ml saline with the addition of challenging and/or protective agents, mixing by a short gentle kneading of the abdomen, and collection of 1 ml fluid by another puncture 1 min later. Following 0.1% 2Na-EDTA the counts were approximately doubled as compared with those of controls, just like after acidified citrate 1.52%, methionine or homocysteine 50 mg/kg in 10 ml saline, and epinephrine 1 μg/kg in 10 ml saline (Figure 16). Pyridoxine (10 mg/kg) blocked the effect of methionine just as in the endothelial model (Figure 17). This also shows that the desquamating activity of homocysteine and methionine does not need systemic administration and is effective directly on epithelial linings.

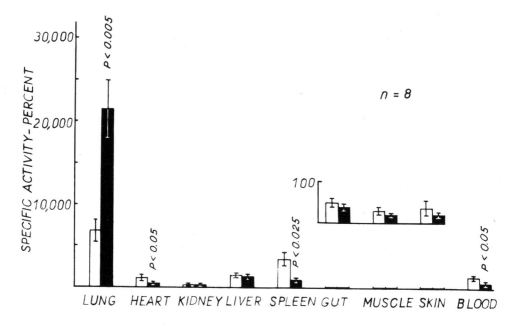

FIGURE 12.   Distribution of radiolabeled platelets after intravenous 1.52% citrate administration (full columns) in different organs of rats as an indicator of platelet sequestration.

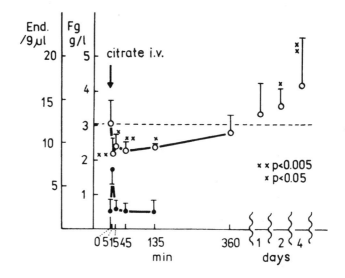

FIGURE 13.   Decrease in fibrinogen level after an intravenous injection of 1.52% citrate (open circles) and a corresponding increase in endothelial element counts (full circles). Fg: fibrinogen.

The agents capable of inducing increased endothelemia in animal studies were of various kinds, e.g., citrate, lactate, adrenaline and other catecholamines,[31] nicotine,[32] hyper- and hypotonic saline,[31] calcium chloride solutions,[33] homocysteine and homocystine,[34] methionine as a source of homocysteine,[35] hydrogen peroxide,[36] various endotoxins,[31] collagenase, and many other agents (Table 2). They were administered to anesthetized rats into the tail vein in a relatively large volume of 2 ml/200 g, 5 min before the blood collection from the heart after the thoracic cavity has been opened. With this volume well reproducible results could be obtained. Administration of saline served as a control. After intravenous admin-

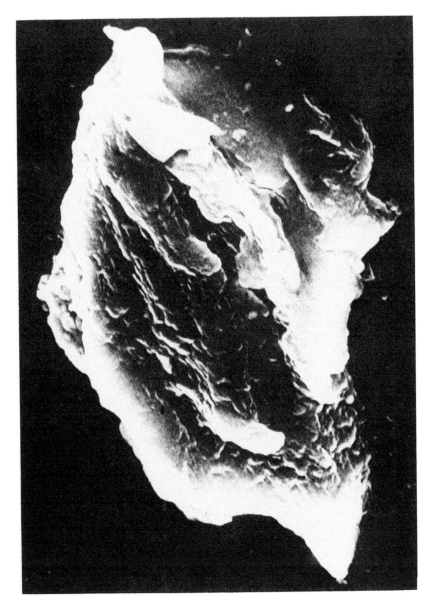

Plate 1. Scanning electron microscopic appearance of a desquamated endothelial cell with a membrane defect after the loss of nucleus.

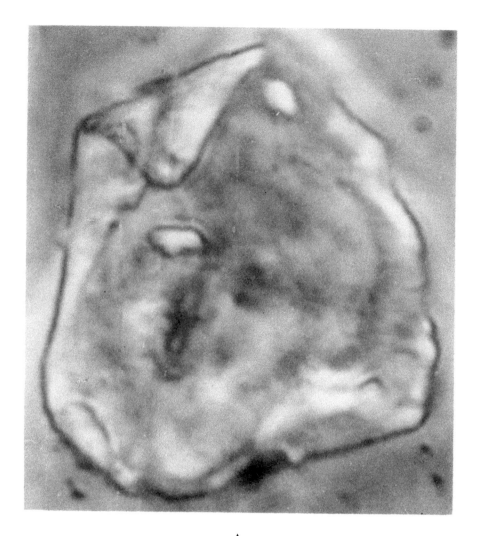

A

Plate 2. Phase contrast appearance of elements. A: Positive. B: Negative.

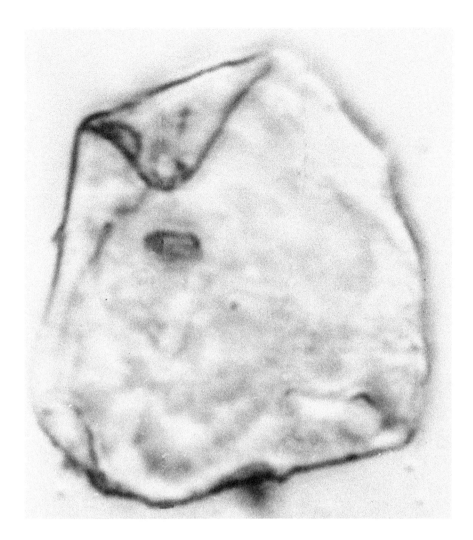

Plate 2B.

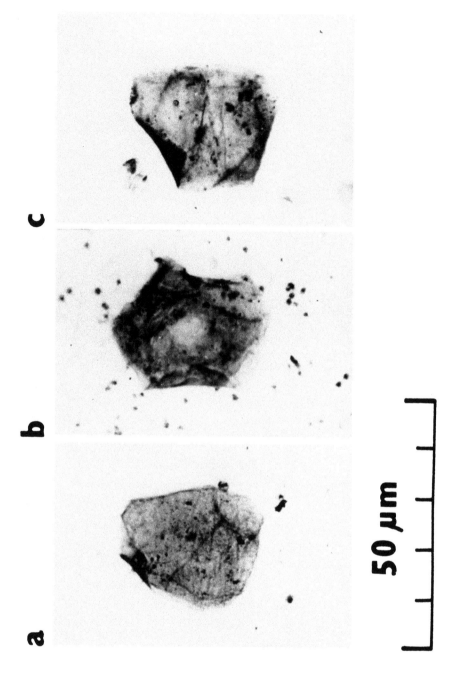

50 μm

Plate 3. Elements after staining with hematoxyline-eosine. The middle one was isolated directly from the aortic surface.

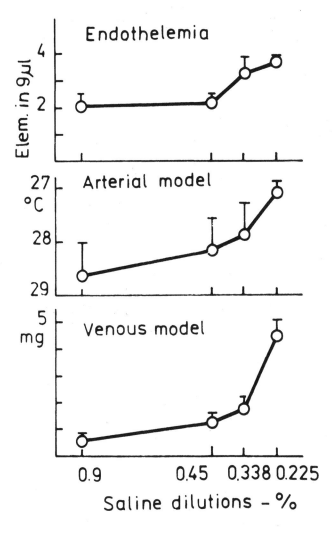

FIGURE 14. Parallel changes in endothelial, arterial, and venous models after increasingly hypotonic intravenous NaCl solutions in rats.

istration of the challenge increased element counts were observed for 15 to 20 min with a maximum after 5 min (Figure 24). Methionine was used as an oral challenge if administered 60 min before blood collection and this challenge was also applied in clinical studies as a more sensitive "endothelial vulnerability test" instead of estimating mere basal values (Figure 18). The increase in element counts was prolonged for several hours. The drugs that were investigated for a modifying effect on the response to a standard challenge were administered intravenously every 5 min, or orally by a gastric tube 60 min before the intravenous challenge. Many challenging and protective agents had a two-phase effect with increasing doses (Figure 19). Thus, citrate, 2Na-EDTA, and lactate may decrease the basal values at very low dosages and induce desquamation at high doses. The effect of such agents is probably due to the binding of a fraction of calcium ions indispensable for the stability of endothelial lining. The adverse drug effect can be antagonized by the administration of calcium, which also has a two-phase effect. There obviously exists a concentration of calcium ions optimal for the endothelial stability. Like challenging agents, many stabilizing agents (with the exception of, e.g., calcium-channel blockers) such as acetylsalicylic acid have a marked and often rather narrow optimum dose range of the protective effect and with increasing doses their effect may be completely reversed so that they themselves may cause

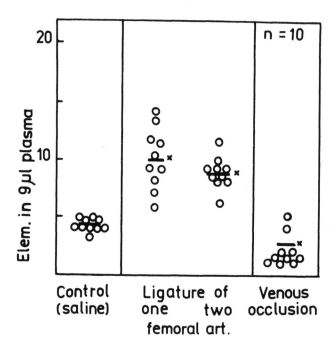

FIGURE 15.   Effect of ischemia and stasis on endothelial element counts.

TABLE 1
Circulating Endothelial Elements
in Some Mammals

	n	$\bar{x}$	SD
Dog	6	2.25	0.60
Rat	18	1.94	0.42
Mouse	6	4.38	1.80
Guinea pig	10	2.10	0.74
Man	8	2.57	0.97

desquamation (Figure 20). Another notable example is warfarin which has in doses lower than those possessing an anticoagulant effect, a marked stabilizing activity due to the relation to bioflavonoids. Thus in the anticoagulant dose range it might exert adverse effects on the endothelium and increase the occurrence of capillary bleeding (Figure 21). The drugs used for general anesthesia in rats have no modifying influence on the results of the test (Table 3). The most potent stabilizing and destabilizing agents are probably some prostanoids the effect of which was noted already at picograms per kilogram doses. Of special interest is the destabilizing effect of hydrogen peroxide and the possibility to antagonize its effect by oxygen-free radical scavengers (Figure 22). In general, a stabilizing effect can be observed after most cardiovascular drugs including all antiplatelet agents if administered at doses in the clinical range. The effect could be used to study their acute immediate activity not affected by drug metabolism or passage into tissues (Table 4). Thus, the endothelium may function as a first-line target model. The stabilizing effect probably has much in common with the activity of membrane-stabilizing agents and the so-called cytoprotective agents.

Some effect of stabilizing agents on endothelial counts can be observed even after *in vitro* addition, probably due to a change in the affinity of elements to each other and to foreign materials. However, this effect is noted with concentrations higher than those that can be obtained after *in vivo* administration.[37]

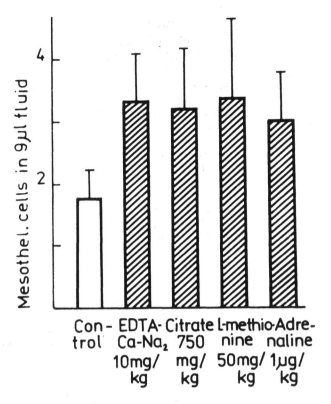

FIGURE 16. Effect of i.p. EDTA, citrate, methionine, and adrenaline on the desquamation of mesothelial cells in the peritoneal cavity.

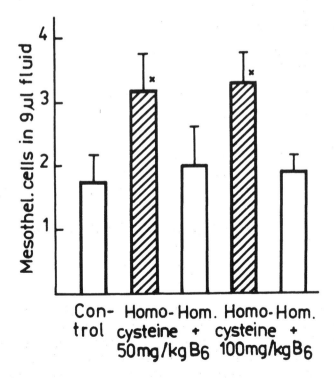

FIGURE 17. Effect of i.p. homocysteine on desquamation of mesothelial cells in the peritoneal cavity and its inhibition by pyridoxine.

TABLE 2
Drugs Inducing
Endothelial Lesions

Vasoactive drugs
  Vasodilating drugs
  Vasoconstricting drugs
Peptides
  Vasopressin
  Angiotensin II
  Bradykinin
  Protamine
Enzymes
  Hyaluronidase
  Proteases
Ca^{2+}-Chelating agents
  Na-EDTA
  Citrate
  Lactate
Hypo- and hypertonic solution

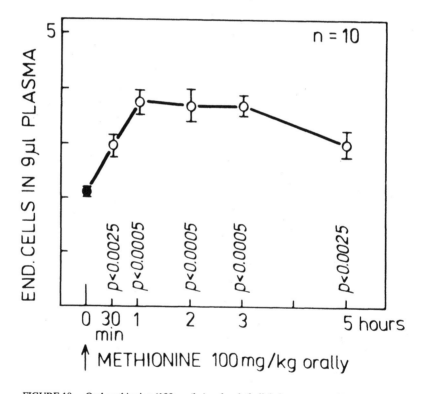

FIGURE 18.   Oral methionine (100 mg/kg) and endothelial element count in rats.

In man, the counting of circulating elements isolated together with platelets can serve diagnostic purposes. Increases were observed after myocardial infarctions and severe angina pectoris attacks,[38] after smoking[39] (Figure 23), strenuous ergometer exercise[40] (Figure 24), mental stress (calculations within a limited time period) (Figure 25), vasodilating infusions, toxemia of pregnancy,[22] etc. More sensitive than merely basal values may be, as already mentioned, the functional test using oral administration of methionine as a challenge, e.g., after oral contraceptives (Figure 26), in hypertonics, etc.

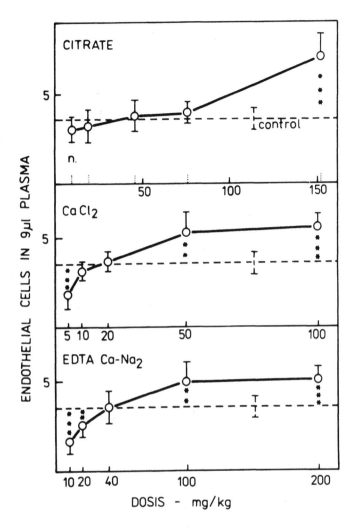

FIGURE 19. Protective and desquamating effect of i.v. calcium chelating agents with low and high doses in rats, respectively.

II. ARTERIAL THROMBOSIS MODEL

The multifactorial character of thrombosis, and particularly localization in large arteries, have already been accepted in the introduction as the main premises for the design of adequate models. Only then can a sufficient sensitivity and reactivity to important factors contributing to the simulated situation, i.e., clinical arterial thrombosis, be ensured. Previous models developed in the author's laboratory had serious drawbacks: arterial thrombosis in a short plastic prosthesis with built-in electrodes for conductivity measurements in the rabbit carotid artery[41,42] had the advantage of continuous and objective registration of the process but suffered from using foreign material at the site of thrombus formation thus almost excluding important vascular factors. The model of electrically induced and thermometrically indicated thrombosis in the rat's carotid artery[43] avoided the previous disadvantage but excessive damage to the vessel produced a situation dissimilar to clinical thrombosis (Figure 27). Such serious lesions have a tendency to emphasize special mechanisms of thrombus development which probably have more in common with hemostatic processes and result in a relatively low sensitivity to antithrombotic agents, that to be effective have to be given at doses about one order of magnitude higher as compared with the usual clinical dose range. This sensitivity loss was sometimes mistakenly regarded as being related to species differences.

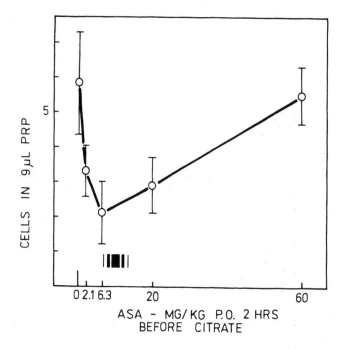

FIGURE 20.   A conspicuously narrow dose optimum of ASA effect on endothelial stability after i.v. citrate in rats (black block: the usual clinical single dose).

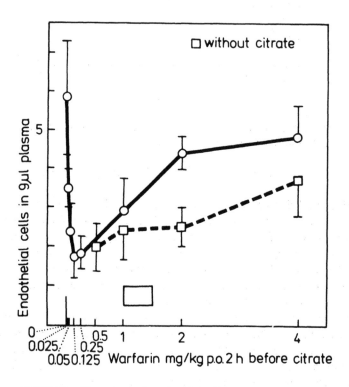

FIGURE 21.   The optimum dose of warfarin effect on endothelial stability in rats. Oblong: clinical dose.

TABLE 3
Influence of General Anesthesia on
Circulating Endothelial Elements

	Control (saline) n = 6 x̄ ± SD		Endothelemia increase after citrate i.v. n = 6 x̄ ± SD	
Urethane	2.02	0.61	4.32	0.97
Ether (inhalation)	2.10	0.22	4.80	0.67
Thiopental	1.98	0.11	4.58	0.19
Pentobarbital	1.80	0.57	4.75	0.76

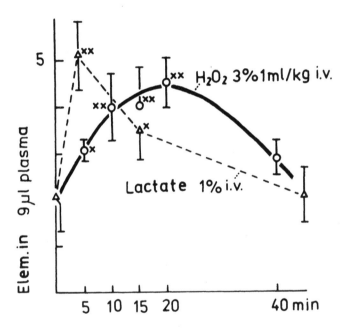

FIGURE 22. Effect of i.v. hydrogen peroxide on endothelial stability in rats in comparison with that of i.v. citrate.

Similar criticism may be applied to many other models described in the literature. Some recently published models are based not on complete occlusion of the vessel by thrombus but on continuous detachment of loose platelet emboli. This might be a good model for the study of the pathogenesis of transient ischemic accidents in neurology but not for an acute occlusive process. Special mechanisms and factors are obviously needed to stabilize such small embolizing thrombi against rapid lysis and to stimulate their further unlimited growth *in situ*. Similar models can be classified as platelet aggregation *in vivo* or as "prethrombosis models".

Three independent factors were used for thrombus induction in the present arterial model:[44]

1. The first factor was the partial mechanical occlusion of the vessel to simulate stenosis caused by an atherosclerotic plaque. It led to hemodynamic changes in the stenosed

TABLE 4
Drugs with a Stabilizing
Effect on Endothelial Lining

Antithrombotics
   Antiplatelet agents
   Heparin
   Oral anticoagulants
Cardiovascular drugs
   Adrenolytics
   Calcium channel blockers
   Antiserotonins
   Cardiotonics
   Antiarrhythmics
   Antihistamins
   Vasodilating agents (e.g., nitrites)
Membrane active agents
   Local anesthetics
Radioprotectives
Antiphlogistics
   Venoprotective agents
Antioxidants
Immunosuppressives
Autacoids (prostacyclin)

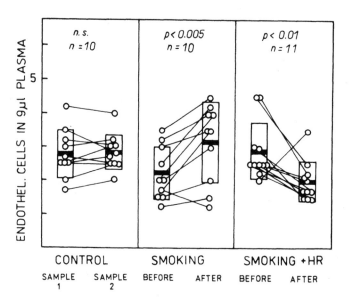

FIGURE 23.   Effect of smoking two cigarettes on endothelial stability in volunteers (HR: hydroxyethylrutoside preparation used to prevent the effect of smoking).

portion of the artery: the increased rate of blood flow resulted in a greater impact of platelets at the critical sites of the vessel wall, in the development of eddy currents behind the stenosis, and often even in a boundary layer formation with local pockets of relative stasis.

2.   The second factor was the generalized low-intensity vascular lesion. This is the supposed mechanism in the development of the humoral thrombophilic state. Some aspects of this mechanism may be more or less known, such as platelet and blood-clotting

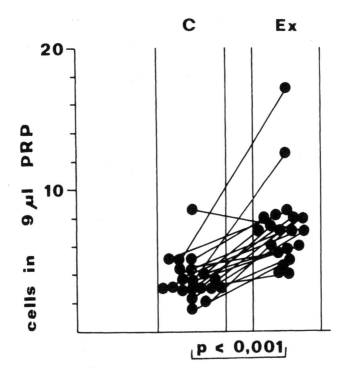

FIGURE 24.   Effect of physical exertion on a bicycle ergometer on endothelial stability in volunteers.

activation. However, it is possible that unknown factor(s) may pass into the circulation which could, for example, depress some defensive endothelial functions, or in turn, stimulate procoagulant ones. In clinical practice such a generalized state may be caused by the presence of life style errors (diet, smoking, and stress), intercurrent infections, immune reaction, etc. The most easily reproducible challenge was chosen in the rat model: Hypotonic saline (0.225% NaCl) causing an endothelial lesion as evidenced by an increase in circulating endothelial cell carcasses.

3.   The third factor was the injection of 20 μg/kg serotonin. This agent was supposed to represent the universal arterial thrombosis-stimulating factor. Using the electrical thrombosis model, a series of supposed or possible thrombosis-enhancing agents was investigated.[45] Whereas thrombin, adenosine diphosphate, epinephrine, and ellagic acid possessed no prothrombotic effects, or on the contrary, exerted inhibitory activity, serotonin alone at relatively high doses of 160 μg/kg and more potentiated thrombosis, i.e., significantly shortened thrombosis times (Figures 28 and 29). Antiserotonin lisuride shortened thrombosis times probably by inhibiting endogenous serotonin. The reason why only serotonin had prothrombotic effects can be tentatively explained by pointing out that all other tested agents are effective alone producing a generalized platelet aggregation in the circulation with the resultant consumption of a portion of platelets and a refractory state of the remaining ones. Similar consequences may be seen in the blood-clotting system. Serotonin is not very active as an aggregant alone and may have, under special circumstances, no aggregant effect at all. On the other hand, it is known to strongly potentiate the effects of other aggregants and in this way could step into play at the site of developing thrombus potentiating the activity of other locally released mediators. In atherosclerotic arteries the ability of the endothelium to cope with relatively large quantities of serotonin released locally from platelets could be seriously compromised. As no atherosclerotic vessels are present in the model

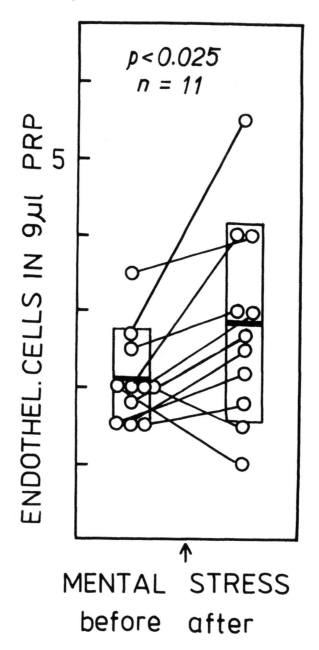

FIGURE 25. Effect of mental stress (calculation) on endothelial stability in volunteers.

using young healthy animals, normal disposal of serotonin is overcome by externally administered drug.

For a long time it was suspected that the passage from the defensive phase of the hemostatic mechanism to pathological thrombosis may be caused by some factor or factors that may be called "triggering" factors. Serotonin accumulated in platelets in relatively large quantities and released under pathological conditions may correspond to the definition. The question may be asked why states connected with high serotonin levels in the blood such as chromaffinomas, are not particularly prone to thrombotic accidents. Chronically

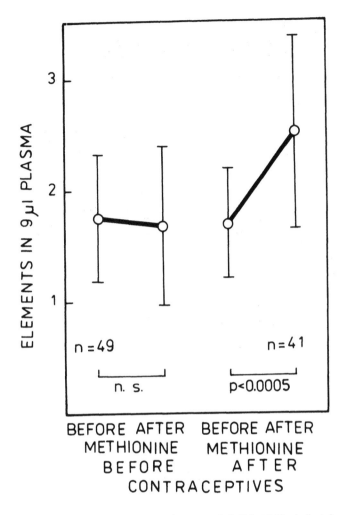

FIGURE 26. Effect of contraceptives on endothelial stability indicated by oral methionine tolerance test.

increased levels of serotonin in the blood would lead to a compensatory increase in the activity of the mechanism for its removal from blood. However, the effect of serotonin in arterial thrombosis is supposed to be of an acute and local character.

The detailed procedure used to induce arterial thrombosis can be described as follows: female rats, weighing 180 to 220 g, were used under urethane anesthesia (1.875 g/kg s.c.), with ten animals in a group. Rectal temperature was measured at the onset of the experiment using the sublingual probe of the thermistor thermometer (Ellab). The probe was provided with a plastic arrest leaving only 8 mm free to prevent deeper insertion, with deeper ''core'' temperature being more stable and less easily influenced by blood flow changes. The animals were not covered by any insulating material. Room temperature was maintained at 22 to 22.5°C. With a different room temperature, new controls would be required. After having obtained the starting rectal temperature the abdominal cavity was opened and a portion of the aorta was isolated from the surrounding tissue with as little trauma as possible. A mini-bulldog clip was placed on the aorta just under the origin of the left renal artery. One branch of the clip was provided with a short piece of catheter to limit the minimal distance of the branches to 0.7 mm. This distance was chosen after a series of preliminary experiments. In this way, the aorta was constricted so that a very narrow slit remained open. Hypotonic saline (0.225% NaCl, i.e., two times 1:1 diluted physiological saline) 2 ml/200 g body

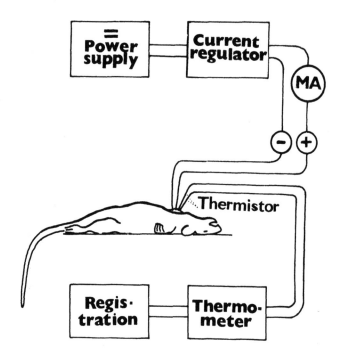

FIGURE 27.   Schematic diagram of arterial thrombosis model using electric current induction in rat carotid artery.

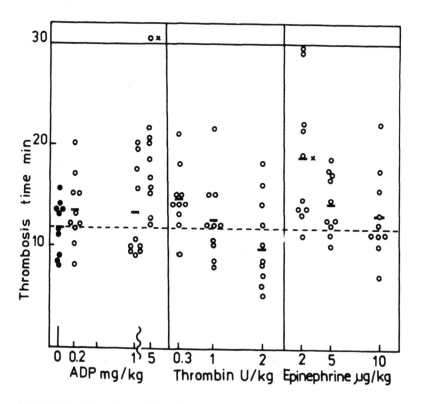

FIGURE 28.   Effect of potential prothrombotic agents in the electrically induced arterial thrombosis model in rats.

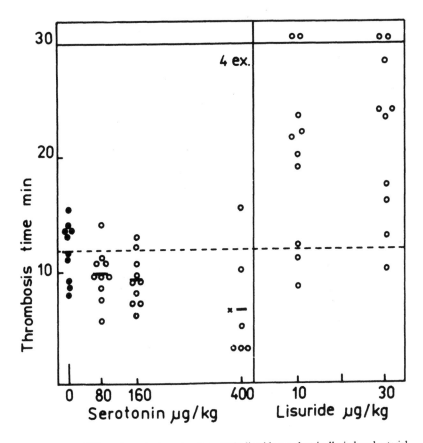

FIGURE 29. Effect of serotonin and antiserotonin lisuride on electrically induced arterial thrombosis model in rats.

weight together with 20 µg/kg serotonin creatinine sulfate (5-HT) was injected 5 min later via the femoral vein within approximately 20 s. The abdominal cavity was closed provisionally, and 60 min after the injection, the rectal temperature was measured for the second time. This was the general procedure but some modifications were used during some studies, as specified further on (Figure 30).

After the ligation of the aorta the rectal temperature decreased in anesthetized animals rapidly attaining about a 4°C difference after 60 min (Figurre 31). Partial occlusion by the clip resulted in a slower decrease almost leveling off at the 60 min interval and leaving a final difference between partial and total occlusion of about 2°C. This also represented the range within which all further drug effects took place. If partial occlusion was combined with intravenous administration of hypotonic saline only, a significant decrease in the 60-min temperature was observed (Figure 32). This decrease was somewhat more pronounced if 5-HT was injected instead of hypotonic saline. On the other hand, if both agents were administered in combination, complete occlusion was attained with a temperature decrease identical to that after complete ligation. Histological preparations stained with hematoxylin-eosin demonstrated a multilayer platelet deposit producing partial or complete obstruction of the lumen in 5-HT as well as in the 5-HT plus hypotonic saline groups. Some adhering platelets were observed in histological preparations even in the group with a mere clip. The question arose whether other agents producing a generalized mild endothelial lesion could be substituted for hypotonic saline (Figure 33). The selection of hypotonic saline as a standard challenging agent was based on its easy reproducibility and high sensitivity to low doses of heparin.[46] In the present model, an endothelial lesion similar to that obtained with hypotonic

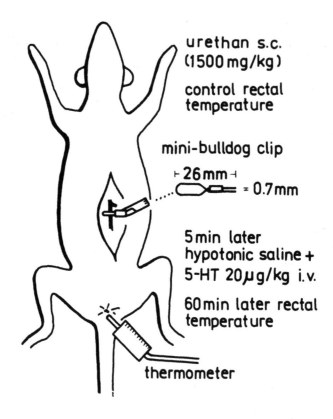

FIGURE 30.   Schematic diagram of the new model of arterial thrombosis
in rats (stenosis plus systemic administration of hypotonic solution together
with serotonin).

saline was produced with nicotine (0.0125 mg/kg administered intravenously in combination with 5-HT, 5 min after clip insertion), oral methionine (100 mg/kg 1 h before 5-HT injection), and with calcium chloride (50 mg/kg in distilled water in combination with 5-HT, 5 min after the clip insertion). However, epinephrine at pharmacological doses (1 μg/kg intravenously together with 5-HT) was ineffective and citrate (1.52%, 2 ml/200 g intravenously together with 5-HT) inhibited the effect of the combination clip plus 5-HT.

Another question was the possibility of replacing 5-HT by other agents ((Figure 34). Platelets contain relatively large amounts of 5-HT, somewhat less histamine, some epinephrine, produce ADP, and under the influence of thrombin traces in their immediate environment, thromboxane A_2. Most of these agents, with the possible exception of histamine, have proaggregatory activity. Nevertheless, besides 5-HT only histamine had notable activity in the model.

To investigate the possible role of 5-HT vasoactivity in the model a nitrate preparation, pentaerythritol tetranitrate (PETN) was at a dose of 0.3 mg/kg administered orally 1 h before sham operation or clip insertion (Figure 35). Whereas 5-HT alone did not influence the sham-operated controls, PETN produced a significant temperature increase not affected by the addition of 5-HT. In animals with aortic clips, PETN showed an insignificant tendency to increases in temperature, probably by decreasing peripheral resistance. On the whole, the effect of 5-HT was preserved at a somewhat higher level after the addition of PETN.

Furthermore, the effect of intravenously administered 5-HT on blood pressure in corresponding doses was measured directly in anesthetized rats. A decrease was observed with a maximum of 1.3 to 6.7 kPa (10 to 50 torr) lasting several seconds and returning to normal levels within 30 to 120 s. This decrease was followed by a much more prolonged moderate

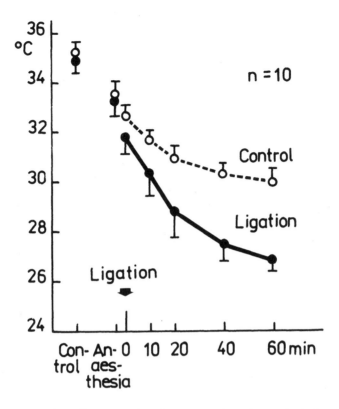

FIGURE 31.   Time course of rectal temperature change in control animals and those with complete aortic occlusion.

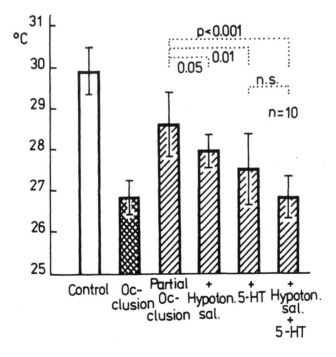

FIGURE 32.   Effect of partial aortic occlusion combined with i.v. hypotonic saline and/or serotonin on 60 min-rectal temperature in rats.

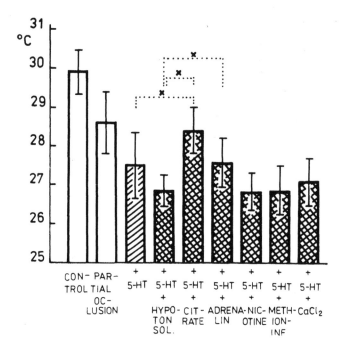

FIGURE 33.   Effect of substitution by other agents of hypotonic saline in the arterial thrombosis model.

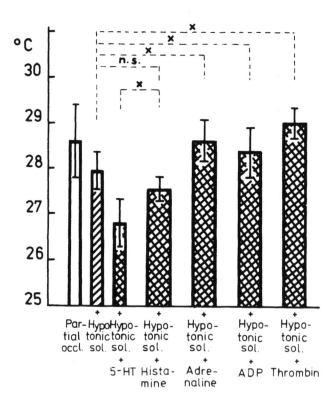

FIGURE 34.   Effect of substitution by other agents of serotonin in the arterial thrombosis model.

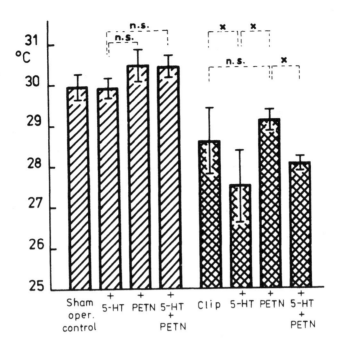

FIGURE 35.   Effect of oral PETN on sham-operated rats and those with clip-induced stenosis.

increase (0.7 to 1.3 kPa, i.e., 5 to 10 torr) lasting for 20 to 40 min. Such pressure changes could not influence temperature measurement 60 min after 5-HT injection. This does not rule out the possibility that some local vasoconstriction could participate in this model, and all the more, in clinical arterial thrombosis. It is generally accepted that arterial spasms and arterial thrombosis are closely interrelated.

Hypotonic saline induced a significant increase in plasma hemoglobin from 4.89 ± 2.34 to 10.26 ± 3.90 mg/ml (n = 8) 5 min after the intravenous administration. If, however, freshly hemolyzed blood (0.1 ml/200 g of erythrocyte suspension hemolyzed with 0.1 ml of distilled water within 30 min, adjusted to isotonicity with 0.1 ml of 1.8% saline and made up with physiological saline to the volume of 2 ml) was injected intravenously in rats, hemoglobin concentration rose in the 5 min sample to 8.93 ± 2.03 mg/ml. This dose of hemolyzed blood did not replace hypotonic saline as a thrombogenic factor if combined with the aortic clip and 5-HT injection resulting in a final temperature of $27.41 \pm 0.31°C$ (n = 6). At the same time, it was effectively replaced, e.g., by intravenous nicotine or oral methionine which are both devoid of hemolytic activity. Consequently, hemolysis did not contribute significantly to the prothrombotic effect of hypotonic saline.

III. VENOUS THROMBOSIS MODEL

Most of the contemporary models of venous thrombosis are based on the Wessler's principle, i.e., a combination of stasis with blood-clotting activation. This activation is mostly achieved directly, i.e., by the introduction of serum, serum products, or active surfaces into the circulating blood. An attractive alternative is the use of a vascular lesion thus producing an effective activating surface and decreasing simultaneously the natural defensive potential of the endothelium. This also resembles more closely the natural situation in clinical practice.

On the other hand, two types of vascular lesions should be distinguished under such conditions. One is local, predisposing a limited area of the endothelium to the process

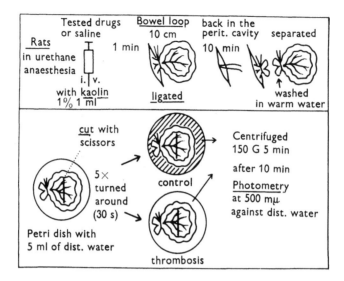

FIGURE 36.   Schematic diagram of venous thrombosis model carried out on mesenteric vessels in rats.

of thrombus formation. The other one is systemic or very extensive leading to a generalized humoral change. Another important aspect is the intensity or severity of the lesion. No parallelism exists between the supposed severity, i.e., more or less profound destruction of the vessel wall, and thrombotic tendency. If a humoral thrombophilic state is looked for, a mild but extensive endothelial lesion possibly of systemic character is the best choice. A local lesion predisposing to thrombosis appears, for example, less important in deep vein thrombosis than in superficial thrombophlebitis. Even then a relatively mild extensive lesion corresponds better to the clinical situation resulting in an endothelial functional defect or unmasking of subendothelial collagen. As deep vein thrombosis is clinically a much more important condition than superficial thrombophlebitis, it was preferable to use this kind of mild systemic lesion. In order to retain at least partial uniformity of the challenge, hypotonic saline was used in the venous model for this purpose just as it was used in the arterial model. This challenge was combined with the incomplete stasis induced by a one-sided venous ligation.

Another problem was the site of thrombus induction. In earlier models developed in this laboratory either accumulation of radiofibrinogen in rabbit central ear veins[47] or thrombus formation in the vessels of rat intestinal loops were used.[48] The indication in the latter method was based on blood extravasation from mesenteric vessels severed in a standard way and followed by hemoglobin photometry. Capacitance vessels of various sizes had the decisive role in this method. The systemic mild vascular lesion combined with local stasis was already used for thrombus induction (Figure 36). Systemic administration of hypotonic saline was used in a modification of the method developed especially for testing low doses of heparin (Figure 37). Nevertheless, the method was abandoned as a component of a standard battery of models. The main cause was the localization of thrombosis: only relatively large veins should be used as corresponding best to the clinical situation. The resulting new model was carried out as follows.[49]

Female Wistar rats weighing 180 to 220 g were operated on under urethane anesthesia (1.875 g/kg of urethane subcutaneously). The animals were given intravenously hypotonic saline (0.225% NaCl, 2 ml/200 g body weight) into the femoral vein. One minute later, the abdominal cavity was opened, the inferior vena cava isolated from surrounding tissue, and a tight ligature was applied with a cotton thread just below the left renal vein (Figure

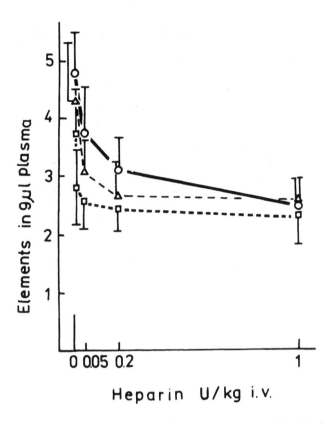

FIGURE 37. The effect of heparin in the mesenteric vessel model of venous thrombosis using three types of challenges. Solid line: citrate, thin broken line: epinephrine, thick broken line: hypotonic saline.

38). The abdominal cavity was closed provisionally and reopened 10 min later. The vena cava was then ligated 2 cm below the first ligature. After ligating the remaining 2 to 3 bigger branches leading to the vascular segment, the latter was removed and opened by a longitudinal incision in a Petri dish provided with a white background. The thrombus was removed and placed into a wet chamber (another Petri dish containing a saline-soaked filter paper, covered with a lid, and maintained at room temperature). Thrombus weighing was carried out 2 h later. Clot retraction which was very fast during the first 10 min was practically finished at that time and the wet weight was relatively constant thereafter. The weight variability of control thrombi was investigated in six independent experiments with six animals in each. The mean weight with a standard deviation was 4.04 ± 0.33 mg. The sham-operated controls were given physiological saline instead of hypotonic saline. In such controls small thrombi were often present and the mean thrombus weight with SD was 0.52 ± 0.24 mg.

The tested agents were administered either intravenously into the femoral vein 5 min before the hypotonic saline injection or orally by a gastric tube 60 min before thrombus induction.

In contrast to other models of this kind, acetylsalicylic acid and sulfinpyrazone were effective. Heparin was effective already at doses below 0.1 U/kg i.v.

The multifactorial character of thrombosis was represented in this model by incomplete stasis (central ligation of the vena cava was present during the critical period of thrombus formation) and by the vascular lesion as an indirect source of humoral activation. As compared with the method of Reyers, this vascular lesion was of a systemic character and was relatively mild but well defined. In Reyers' method the time period of thrombus formation

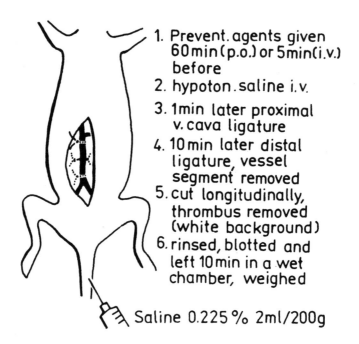

1. Prevent.agents given 60 min (p.o.) or 5 min (i.v.) before
2. hypoton. saline i.v.
3. 1 min later proximal v. cava ligature
4. 10 min later distal ligature, vessel segment removed
5. cut longitudinally, thrombus removed (white background)
6. rinsed, blotted and left 10 min in a wet chamber, weighed

Saline 0.225% 2ml/200g

FIGURE 38.   Schematic diagram of the new venous thrombosis model in rats (stasis in vena cava plus hypotonic saline).

was much more prolonged (60 min as compared with 10 min) but the role of the vascular lesion was ill defined: some of the lesion was unquestionably caused by the vessel preparation, manipulation, and ligation. Even stasis may contribute to the lesion by a derangement in the nutrition of the vessel wall, by the delay in the removal of metabolic products, etc. There is probably little endothelial desquamation and platelet contribution as evidenced by the lack of sensitivity to acetylsalicylic acid, also observed in a similar model combining stasis with saline flushing of the vessel. Whatever the model, insufficient definition of the vascular lesion could cause a decreased reproducibility. Moreover, the whole process is of a local character while clinical deep vein thrombosis is, in general, connected with a systemic humoral thrombophilic state.

Another problem to discuss is the presence of some fibrin clots even in the sham-operated animals receiving physiological saline instead of hypotonic saline. This residual clot is relatively resistant to the action of antithrombotic agents including heparin. A hypothesis is suggested that the residual thrombus represents the hemostatic, i.e., defensive component of thrombus formation related to the damage by vessel manipulation. Its complete suppression probably may not be desirable as the aim of prophylaxis is, according to this hypothesis, to prevent unlimited thrombus growth. Of course, very high doses of heparin, i.e., over 50 U/kg, would prevent the formation of even this residual thrombus but would also cause a severe hemostatic defect. In addition, this may provide an explanation for the insensitivity of Reyers' model to ASA.[50,51]

As has been mentioned, antiplatelet agents are, in general, effective in the suggested new model. They were much less effective if, instead of a mild vascular lesion, the process of activation was cut short by the administration of kaolin as a contact factor activator. This shows that the activity of antiplatelet agents is based predominantly on the protection of the vessel wall, and possibly on the prevention of some consequences of platelet interaction with the damaged vessel wall. This interaction might result in the release of some platelet constituents enhancing thrombogenesis, possibly identical with already known factors (PF 3, PF 4, serotonin, TXA_2, PAF) or may be unidentified as yet. There appears to be some activity of antiplatelet agents even in the short cut modification: this may be related to the local contribution of the vascular lesion and interacting platelets. Its detection is attributable only to the quantitative character and high sensitivity of the model.

IV. POSSIBLE ADDITIONAL MODELS

The models described so far were designed to form a battery which would be interrelated by some common factor. Thus they share the systemic challenging agent (i.v. hypotonic saline), and experimental animals (species, sex, weight). Arterial and venous models have additional localizing factors (partial stasis, partial occlusion). There is only one additional factor in arterial thrombosis: 5-HT. The indication methods are always quantitative and as simple as possible. Both arterial and venous models should mimic the thrombotic accidents in relatively large arteries and veins which are of main clinical interest. Basically, the endothelemia test is not a model of thrombosis, but rather one of a predisposing situation or prethrombosis. It was included in the battery for two reasons:

1. The aspect of the vascular lesion in thrombogenesis has been neglected so far despite its evident contribution particularly to the activity of antithrombotics.
2. The method made the basis for the design of both thrombosis models and hence is conceptually and genetically related to them.

Needless to say, many more prethrombosis models could be suggested for use in testing antithrombotics, most of them based on secondary consequences of the systemic endothelial lesion (radiofibrinogen uptake,[47] acute platelet sequestration,[52] increased platelet turnover,[53] circulating platelet aggregates, release of some platelet constituents, etc.). All of them would require suitable systemic challenge, preferably identical to those used in the endothelemia model (intravenous administration of citrate, lactate, epinephrine, hypotonic saline, nicotine, etc.).

On the other hand, special questions would require special models. Not always is the main interest directed to thrombotic occlusion of large vessels. Thus, the study of thrombotic ischemic accidents (TIA) in neurology requires models making it possible to study microembolism of platelet thrombi from the damaged inner surface of a large artery. To do so, a stenosis of the coronary artery[54] or its lesion by electric current may be used.[43,55] To study methods of preventing occlusions of artificial prostheses and catheters, corresponding artificial surfaces as sites of thrombus induction should be used. Many modifications of such methods have been described in the literature. To solve some particular problems of the mechanism of thrombus formation, models located in the microcirculation could be useful because of easy observation of effects of topically administered agents. Interpretation of such analytical tests should be correspondingly careful. The necessity of using special models in the study of DIC and its prevention is evident and it would be advisable to study some special surveys.

In general, the search into thrombotic processes has suffered, until now, from insufficient discrimination between various kinds of clinical situations and corresponding models. There does not exist a general simple pattern of thrombus developments, and if some common concept is accepted as a working hypothesis, it should be sufficiently diversified and adaptable to various situations. Otherwise, the conclusions should be restricted only for clinical situations as closely related to the model conditions as possible.

V. THE USE OF NEW MODELS IN THE DRUG SCREENING

The described models were used in a screening of antithrombotics and potential antithrombotics whose results are presented in the following section. Throughout the screening

TABLE 5
Control Values in Three Standard Models

	Endothelemia	Arterial model	Venous model
Control with saline x̄ ± SD	2.08 ± 0.38	28.65 ± 0.60 (partial occlusion)	0.52 ± 0.24 (sham operated)
Control with challenge (thrombosis control) x̄ ± SD	3.69 ± 0.18 (hypotonic saline) 5.03 ± 0.38 (citrate)	27.10 ± 0.20	4.45 ± 0.57

female rats, Wistars, weighing 180 to 220 g were used as experimental animals. While in methodological studies ten animals were included in a group, in the drug screening the corresponding number was six. In most experiments oral route of administration by gavage was used 1 h in advance of thrombus induction, if not otherwise specified. Significance of differences was tested by variance analysis with Duncan's test while the t-test was used in combination studies. Significant differences were considered those with $p < 0.05$ and marked with a small cross in diagrams. The curves show means with standard deviations. The controls, i.e., both those with physiological saline instead of hypotonic saline (controls without thrombosis, denoted with broken line and T−) and those with thrombosis (broken line and T+) were repeated six times within approximately 2 years necessary to complete the screening. Means of all six estimations were used in diagrams (Table 5). In combination studies a broken line shows the dose-to-effect curve of one drug while the other administered is at a constant dose. In more interesting interactions the order of drugs was rearranged. The effect of combinations is indicated by a thick line.

REFERENCES

1. **Bouvier, C. A., Gaynor, E., Cintron, J. R., Bernhardt, B., and Spaet, T. H.,** Circulating endothelium as an indication of vascular injury, in *Vascular Factors and Thrombosis*, Koller, F., Brinkhous, K. M., Biggs, R., Rodman, N. F., and Hinnom, S., Eds., Schattauer Verlag, Stuttgart, 1970, 163.
2. **Bouvier, C. A.,** Role des lésions endothéliales dans la thrombogenèse, *Médic. Hyg.*, 30, 653, 1972.
3. **Gaynor, E., Bouvier, C. A., and Spaet, T. H.,** Vascular lesions: possible pathogenetic basis of the generalized Shwartzman reaction, *Science*, 170, 986, 1970.
4. **Gaynor, E., Bouvier, C. A., and Spaet, T. H.,** A technique for locating rare cells in the circulation for ultramicroscopy, *Proc. Soc. Exp. Biol. Med.*, 113, 520, 1970.
5. **Herbeuval, R. and Herbeuval, H.,** Technique de concentration leucocytaire pour la mise en évidence de cellules anomales dans le sang, *C. R. Acad. Sci.*, 250, 3070, 1960.
6. **Herbeuval, H. and Fourot, M.,** Etude comparative de l'endothélium vasculaire et sa lasale, sur coupe et en leucoconcentration, *C. R. Soc. Biol.*, 158, 137, 1964.
7. **Gaynor, E., Bouvier, C. A., and Spaet, T. H.,** Circulating endothelial cells in endotoxin-treated rabbits, *Clin. Res.*, 16, 535, 1968.
8. **Takahashi, H. and Harker, L. A.,** Measurement of human endothelial cells in whole blood, *Thromb. Res.*, 31, 1, 1983.
9. **Gerrity, R. G., Richardson, M., Caplan, B. A., Cade, J. F., Hirsh, J., and Schwartz, C. J.,** Endotoxin-induced vascular endothelial injury and repair II. Focal injury, en face morphology, (3 H)-thymidine uptake and circulating endothelial cells in the dog, *Exp. Mol. Pathol.*, 24, 59, 1976.
10. **Weber, G., Losi, M., Toti, P., and Vatti, R.,** Circulating endothelial-like cells in arterial peripheral blood of hypercholesterolemic rabbits, *Artery*, 5, 29, 1979.
11. **Fabiani, F. and Catavitello, R.,** Présence de cellules endothéliales circulantes après lésions vasculaires aiguës, *Médic. Hyg.*, 37, 886, 1979.
12. **Gutstein, W. H., Farrell, G. A., and Armellini, C.,** Blood flow disturbance and endothelial cell injury in preatherosclerotic swine, *Lab. Invest.*, 29, 134, 1973.

13. **Davenport, W. D. and Ball, C. R.,** Diet-induced atrial endothelial damage, *Atherosclerosis,* 40, 145, 1981.
14. **Gradwohl, R. B. H.,** *Clinical Laboratory, Methods and Diagnosis,* C. V. Mosby, St. Louis, 1943.
15. **Sharnoff, J. G. and Kim, E. S.,** Evaluation of pulmonary megakaryocytes, *Arch. Pathol. Lab. Med.,* 66, 176, 1958.
16. **Fagan, D. G., Goodall, H. B., and Al Hasso, A. R. A.,** The occurrence of nuclear masses in the pulmonary capillary bed in infants, presented at 7th Europ. Conf. Microcirc. Part II., Aberdeen, *Bibl. Anat.,* 12, 41, 1973.
17. **Hladovec, J. and Rossmann, P.** Circulating endothelial cells isolated together with platelets and the experimental modification of their counts in rats, *Thromb. Res.,* 3, 665, 1973.
18. **Davis, J. W., Shelton, L., Eigenberg, D. A., and Hignite, Ch.E.,** Lack of effect of aspirin on cigarette smoke-induced increase in circulating endothelial cells, *Haemostasis,* 7, 66, 1987.
19. **Davis, J. W., Shelton, L., Eigenberg, D. A., Hignite, Ch.E., and Watanabe, I. S.,** Effects of tobacco and no-tobacco cigarette smoking on endothelium and platelets, *Clin. Pharmacol. Ther.,* 37, 529, 1985.
20. **Iwata, Y., Kuzuya, F., Hayakawa, M., Naito, M., Shibata, K., and Endo, H.,** Circulating endothelial cells fail to induce cerebral infarction in rabbits, *Stroke,* 17, 506, 1986.
21. **Gall, A., Sinzinger, H., Widhalm, K., and Silberbauer, K.,** Circulating endothelial cells and platelet half-life in hyperlipoproteinemia and atherosclerosis, presented at the 6th Int. Symp. on Atherosclerosis, Abstr. 387, West Berlin, 1982.
22. **Glawanakowa, W. and Popova, W. G.,** Untersuchungen über die Desquamation des Gefässendotheliums bei EPH-Gestosen, *Cor Vasa,* 30, 140, 1988.
23. **Chambers, R. and Zweifach, B. W.,** Intercellular cement and capillary permeability, *Physiol. Rev.,* 27, 436, 1947.
24. **Gordon, P. B., Levitt, M. A., Jenkins, C. S. P., and Hatcher, V. B.,** The effect of the extracellular matrix on the detachment of human endothelial cells, *J. Cell. Physiol.,* 121, 467, 1984.
25. **Brown, Z., Neild, G. H., Willoughby, J. J., Somia, N. V., and Cameron, S. J.,** Increased factor VIII as an index of vascular injury in cyclosporine nephrotoxicity, *Transplantation,* 42, 150, 1986.
26. **Lojda, Z.,** Proteinases in pathology. Usefulness of histochemical methods, *J. Histochem. Cytochem.,* 29, 481, 1981.
27. **Lojda, Z.,** Die Histochemie der Proteasen, *Acta Histochem.,* 30, 9, 1984.
28. **Piette, M. and Piette, C.,** Numération des plaquettes sanguines utilisant un liquid hypotonique à base de chlorhydrate de procaine, *Sang,* 30, 144, 1959.
29. **Hladovec, J., Koutský, J., Přerovský, I., Dvořák, V., Novotný, A.,** Oral contraceptives, methionine and endothelial lesion, *Vasa,* 12, 117, 1983.
30. **Hladovec, J., Jirka, J., Přerovský, I. and Málek, P.,** Decrease of endothelaemia during immunosuppression, *Biomed. Pharmacother.,* 25, 204, 1976.
31. **Hladovec, J.,** Circulating endothelial cells as a sign of vessel wall lesion, *Physiol. Bohemoslov.,* 27, 140, 1978.
32. **Hladovec, J.,** Endothelial injury by nicotine and its prevention, *Experientia,* 34, 1585, 1978.
33. **Hladovec, J.,** Vasotropic drugs — a survey based on a unifying concept of their mechanism of action, *Arzneim. Forsch.,* 27, 1073, 1977.
34. **Hladovec, J.,** Experimental homocystinemia, endothelial lesions and thrombosis, *Blood Vessels,* 16, 202, 1979.
35. **Hladovec, J.,** Methionine, pyridoxine and endothelial lesions in rats, *Blood Vessels,* 17, 104, 1980.
36. **Hladovec, J.,** Protective effect of oxygen-derived free radical scavengers on the endothelium *in vivo,* *Physiol. Bohemoslov.,* 35, 97, 1986.
37. **Hladovec, J.,** Differentiation of *in vitro* and *in vivo* effects of a flavonoid on endothelial cell counts, *Arzneim. Forsch.,* 27, 1142, 1977.
38. **Hladovec, J., Přerovský, I., Staněk, V., and Fabián, J.,** Circulating endothelial cells in acute myocardial infarction and angina pectoris, *Klin Wochenschr,* 56, 1033, 1978.
39. **Přerovský, I. and Hladovec, J.,** Suppression of the desquamating effect of smoking on the human endothelium by hydroxyethylrutoside, *Blood Vessels,* 16, 239, 1979.
40. **Hladovec, J. and Přerovský, I.,** Effects of hydroxyethylrutosides on circulating endothelial cells in experimental animals and man, in *Hydroxyethylrutosides in Vascular Disease.* Condensed Proceedings of an international symposium, Moretonhampstead, The Royal Society of Medicine, International Congress and Symposium Series, No. 42, 1981, 19.
41. **Hladovec, J. and Mansfeld, V.,** Konduktometrische Registrierung der Blutgerinnung *in vivo,* *Blut,* 5, 282, 1959.
42. **Hladovec, J., Lehký, T., and Rybák, M.,** Studium der antithrombotischen Wirksamkeit von Plasmin mit Hilfe einer neuen Methode, *Z Gesamte Inn. Med.,* 15, 1125, 1960.
43. **Hladovec, J.,** Experimental arterial thrombosis in rats with continuous registration, *Thromb. Diath. Haemorrh,* 26, 407, 1971.

44. **Hladovec, J.,** A new model of arterial thrombosis, *Thromb. Res.,* 41, 659, 1986.

45. **Hladovec, J.,** The effect of some platelet aggregating and potential thrombosis-promoting substances on the development of experimental arterial thrombosis, *Thromb. Diath. Haemorrh.,* 29, 196, 1973.

46. **Hladovec, J.,** The effect of ultra-low-dose heparin in experimental venous thrombosis, *Thromb. Res.,* 36, 83, 1984.

47. **Hladovec, J., Přerovský, I., and Roztočil, K.,** The influence of inflammation on the ^{125}I-fibrinogen uptake test in experimental thrombosis, *Angiologica,* 10, 93, 1973.

48. **Hladovec, J.,** A quantitative model of venous stasis thrombosis in rats, *Physiol. Bohemoslov.,* 24, 551, 1975.

49. **Hladovec, J.,** A sensitive model of venous thrombosis in rats, *Thromb. Res.,* 43, 539, 1986.

50. **Reyers, I., Hennissen, A., Donati, M. B., Hornstra, G., and de Gaetano, G.,** Aspirin and the prevention of experimental arterial thrombosis: difficulty in establishing unequivocal effectiveness, *Thromb. Haemost.,* 54, 619, 1985.

51. **Reyers, I., Mussoni, L., Donati, M. B., and de Gaetano, G.,** Failure of aspirin at different doses to modify experimental thrombosis in rats. *Thromb. Res.,* 18, 669, 1980.

52. **Hladovec, J., Svobodová, J., and Rossmann, P.,** Influence of citrate on platelet adhesion to the endothelial surface, *Physiol. Bohemoslov.,* 19, 421, 1970.

53. **Hanson, S. R., Harker, L. A., and Bjornsson, T. D.,** Effect of platelet-modifying drugs on arterial thromboembolism in baboons. Aspirin potentiates the antithrombotic actions of dipyridamole and sulfin-pyrazone by mechanism(s) independent of platelet cyclooxygenase inhibition, *J. Clin. Invest.,* 75, 1591, 1985.

54. **Folts, J. D., Crowell, E. B., and Rowe, G. G.,** Platelet aggregation in partially obstructed vessels and its elimination with aspirin, *Circulation,* 54, 365, 1976.

55. **Shea, M. J., Driscoll, E. M., Romson, J. L., Pitt, B., Lucchesi, B. R.,** The beneficial effects of nafazatrom (Bay G 6575) on experimental coronary thrombosis, *Am. Heart J.,* 107, 629, 1983.

Chapter 4

EFFECTS OF ANTITHROMBOTICS AND RESULTS OF DRUG SCREENING

I. ACETYLSALICYLIC ACID (ASA)

The story of acetylsalicylic acid (ASA) began to unfold a long time ago. Since its introduction to the market under the name Aspirin in 1899 by Bayer, it has been one of the most effective nonsteroid anti-inflammatory drugs (NSAID), also classified by pharmacologists as analgesics-antipyretics. Its range of indications is fairly wide and the drug was for many years and still is one prescribed and taken in the largest quantities. Its recently introduced additional use as an antithrombotic started after World War II. The idea originated from some clinicians, e.g., Gibson,[1] who came to believe, without a particularly rational background, that the drug might be effective as an antithrombotic. Its weak effects as antivitamin K and on the prolongation of bleeding are by no means impressive. Gibson treated a large number of patients with alleged success, unfortunately not satisfying the requirements of a controlled clinical trial. In fact, these criteria were, at that time, not yet well defined. At the same time, platelets and their functions came into the focus of increased attention, at first as various adhesivity tests. Bounameaux[2] showed the effectiveness of salicylate in an *ex vivo* study already in 1954. After the introduction of the photometric aggregation method by Born in 1962,[3] the effectiveness of ASA in this test was simultaneously demonstrated in several laboratories in 1968.[4-7] The first relatively well-controlled clinical trials were published in 1974.[8] In 1968, the effectiveness of ASA was also demonstrated in an animal model.[7] In 1971 Vane[8] demonstrated that the drug inhibits tissue cyclo-oxygenase while Smith and Willis[9] described the same effect in platelets. It was Moncada et al. who in 1979[10] presented an attempt at a unified concept of aspirin action based on the inhibition of eicosanoid production. Nevertheless, despite a wide acceptance,[11,12] this concept is probably not the only explanation of aspirin activity, and possibly not even the most plausible one. The mechanism of antithrombotic activity of ASA remains, in general, insufficiently clarified. Despite this shortcoming, ASA is now the most widely acknowledged platelet-inhibiting drug used on a large scale in many countries and in a number of both acute and chronic clinical situations. Thus, its always broad indications have become still significantly broader making ASA one of the most successful drugs ever invented. Of course, there exist various side effects, but in view of the massive use and abuse, this is not surprising and does not belittle its value as a relatively nontoxic drug.

The case of ASA illustrates the numerous pitfalls confronting the investigators of antithrombotics. The most important one is probably the divergence of *in vitro* and *in vivo* activity.

ASA is effective *in vitro* under various conditions and on various platelet functions. These effects are not necessarily related to the clinical effect, or perhaps may be related to a portion of clinical effects only in special indications. This lack of a close correlation comes as no surprise. *In vitro* effects are generally used in the screening of new antithrombotic drugs. It is well known that a tiny fraction of drugs effective under such conditions is clinically useful. Many drugs are effective *in vitro* under suitable conditions, often at relatively high concentrations which cannot be attained after clinical administration. *In vivo* thrombogenesis is always due to several mechanisms which may be mutually interchangable. Consequently, the most effective agents are those that are effective simultaneously in many ways or that affect some relatively unspecific and very general operating mechanisms. ASA is an excellent example of such a drug: all hopes to restrict its mechanism of action to one single activity fail, particularly if the knowledge of all its possible activities is still far from being complete. This is no agnosticism: any new piece of knowledge is extremely useful and the only danger comes from a premature oversimplified interpretation and possible abandonment of further efforts.

The *in vitro* antiplatelet activity of ASA can be tentatively classified into four groups according to the effects on "activation", adhesion, aggregation, or release.

A. ACTIVATION

The term "activation" is not very clearly defined. Does activation exist in advance of adhesion, or is it only its consequence? Logically, low degree activation might result in an increased reactivity to stimuli, but on the contrary a high degree might bring about a refractory state. ASA was generally considered as a drug effective on processes taking place later on in the process of thrombogenesis, i.e., on aggregation and release. This is based on its lack of effect on platelet survival and on the systemic release of some platelet constituents (beta-thromboglobulin, PF 4). On the other hand, some studies suggest that ASA might also influence some parameters usually serving as indicators of activation such as shape change. In the study of Simrock et al.[13] single doses of 7 to 15 mg/kg were necessary in man to attain this effect lasting about 8 to 12 h.

It is necessary to remember that platelet survival methods are extremely sensitive to technical details of the procedure and are not easy to interpret. The endothelial lesion that could possibly affect the results should be very extensive (not necessarily intensive) and other possible mechanisms of platelet-level regulation should be kept in mind, e.g., sequestration by the reticuloendothelial system, the rate of new platelet formation. Meanwhile, there is not much agreement about the value of the method.[14] It is probably poorly related to thrombotic processes and at most reflects some activities that may be called "prethrombotic" and are more closely related to defensive hemostatic mechanisms.

In conclusion: while some effect of ASA on platelet activation is possible, it has not been unequivocally demonstrated due to the poor definition of activation and lack of suitable methods.

B. ADHESION

The effect of ASA on platelet adhesivity illustrates the evolution of methods from the most simple to increasingly sophisticated ones in an effort to come nearer to the *in vivo* situation. The effect on adhesion to glass surfaces was alternately shown in some studies to be denied by others. It was probably the lack of uniformity in experimental conditions that made all comparisons very difficult. In fact, similar methods were more useful in the diagnosis of hemostatic defects than in thrombophilia. Later on, collagen-covered glass was used yielding more reliable results. Of course, collagen does not have the same activity as subendothelial tissue. Further refinement came with the use of everted vessel segments *in vitro* introduced by Baumgartner.[15] The equivocal results obtained with this technique called for a better definition of the flow conditions, hematocrit, type of anticoagulant used, etc. Under such specified conditions, ASA was in general ineffective when administered alone at concentrations corresponding to those attainable after a usual *in vivo* dosage. However, ASA may potentiate the effect of dipyridamole. In some studies ASA produced increased adhesion and had a positive effect only on secondary aggregation and "thrombus" growth. Both *ex vivo* platelets and aortic samples of rabbits were used by Davies and Menys[16] to test adhesion after prolonged adminstration of ASA. No influence on adhesion was observed in contradiction to studies demonstrating increased adhesion.

Most studies failed to consider the possibility that the relationship between ASA concentrations and activity may be rather complicated. Such a two-phase effect with increasing doses was best seen in studies of endothelial stability where a clear-cut narrow optimum dosage was observed (Figure 20 in Chapter 3). A similar two-phase effect was documented

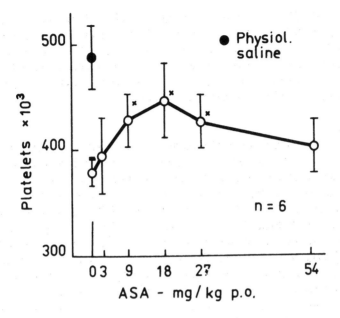

FIGURE 1. Effect of oral ASA on citrate-induced platelet sequestration in rats.

in the platelet sequestration method *in vivo* after a citrate challenge (Figure 1). This was an acute transitory decrease in platelet counts after a systemic mild endothelial lesion induced by the intravenous injection of challenging agents such as citrate, lactate, and epinephrine. While an optimal effect was seen after oral administration of approximately 12 mg/kg, the effect decreased as the dose was increased. This may be interpreted as a combined effect on endothelial stability and platelet activation/adhesion. In fact, both aspects of drug effects are not separable in this *in vivo* adhesion model. The presence of a two-phase effect with increasing doses in the endothelial model can be used as an argument against the suggested role of a thromboxane-prostacycline balance because thromboxane could hardly be involved in this model.

In conclusion, ASA may be positively effective in adhesion tests as soon as they are designed to more closely resemble the *in vivo* situation including the dosage. ASA, when given at relatively high dosages or added at high concentrations might increase adhesion under special experimental conditions which, however, does not imply that a corresponding prothrombotic activity could be expected under clinical conditions.

C. AGGREGATION

The effect of ASA in aggregation tests is also complex and not easy to interpret.[17,18] The inhibition of *in vitro* aggregation by ASA was described by many authors using various aggregating challenges, ASA concentration, species for blood collection, anticoagulants, indication devices (photometric, impedance measuring), etc. ASA inhibited, in general, the second, i.e., release-dependent wave, not the first one of ADP-induced aggregation. It was effective against epinephrine and collagen-induced aggregation in a dose-related manner. It inhibited the effect of thrombin on aggregation but only at its relatively low concentrations. In *in vitro* experiments with collagen the inhibition was dose-related and obviously dependent on the release of ADP. In *ex vivo* studies the activity of ASA was often similar to that *in vitro*, and a good correlation seemed to exist between the concentrations effective *in vitro* and those which could be attained *in vivo*. This, of course, might have some significance for the control of effective concentrations after *in vivo* administration, but not for the estimation of the probable antithrombotic effect. Seuter[19] published a comparison of a series of 22 drugs both *in vivo* and *ex vivo* in rabbits using collagen for aggregation induction. He observed some species (rabbit/rat) differences after oral administration and the *in vitro* vs. *ex vivo* effect was different with many drugs. On the whole, ASA was superior in relation to the prolongation of effect and therapeutic width.

D. RELEASE

When the inhibitory activity of ASA on the release of platelet constituents is considered, it would be appropriate to distinguish the release after adhesion from that after aggregation.[18] Whereas in adhesion of isolated platelets, ASA is probably ineffective as a release inhibitor, it is fairly efficacious in a situation characterized by aggregation, and thus, by the precedent release of mediators in sufficient local concentrations (ADP ?). Thus, ASA appears to act predominantly on pathologic thrombus formation and less on the primary and defensive hemostatic processes dependent on platelet activity. This may be an advantage even though some authors judged ASA a weak antithrombotic agent. In other words, an ideal antithrombotic agent should only suppress selectively the second part of the whole process and should exert no antihemostatic activity. Unfortunately, ASA administration could lead sometimes to a hemorrhagic tendency, a fact showing that under special conditions it could even affect the first phase. It may be argued that the first phase could play an unfavorable role in the process of atherogenesis which compared with thrombosis would present somewhat different predisposing conditions in this respect. Unfortunately, no drug with a predominant inhibitory effect on the first phase is probably available, hence, the suggestion cannot be verified. Meanwhile, ASA has been reported by some to possess in experimental models an antiatherosclerotic effect and by others no effect.

It would seem that all controversies emerging from *in vitro* studies could be resolved by the use of *in vivo* models. While this may be true theoretically, in practicality it is not. A large number of models have been used for the estimation of ASA antithrombotic activity, based on very different mechanisms and also offering the most diverse interpretations.

As has been said, the credit for the first use of ASA in an *in vivo* model goes to Evans et al.[7] in 1968. In their study concerning mainly *in vitro* and *ex vivo* aggregation experiments they also used an extracorporeal shunt model in rabbits. After a very high single dose of 200 mg/kg ASA inhibited platelet deposition. Of course, similar models have a limited value as equivalents of clinical thrombosis.

Approximately at that time Didisheim[20] published the result of his study using electric current to induce the formation of white bodies in the mesenteric arteries of rats. Oral administration of ASA at doses from 20 to 400 mg/kg was not significantly effective as far as the overall effect is concerned. However, 20 mg/kg resulted in some tendency to shorten the outstaying of thrombi *in situ*. Unfortunately, the method was not sufficiently quantitative and the formation of unstable transitory platelet thrombi at the site of the lesion in the microcirculation again constitutes a poor model of clinical thrombosis.

Many studies using microcirculatory models followed. ASA was almost ineffective in the study of Honour et al.[21] who used a Perspex® capsule on the brain surface of rabbits to observe platelet thrombi after a lesion inflicted by electric current and local administration of ADP. In addition, the rabbits were sensitized by alloxan. Whereas ASA given orally at a dose of 42 mg/d was ineffective alone and did potentiate dipyridamole activity. The estimation of effectiveness was based on the ADP concentration necessary to induce aggregation at the site of injury. The very complex and artificial character of the procedure, an unsuitable dosage of ASA, and the localization in the microcirculation make it a far cry from clinical thrombosis. It is rather an analytical test showing a special aspect of the process and one more adequately classified as a "prethrombosis" model.

Remarkably different results were seen in other microcirculatory thrombosis models with ASA. Thus, Rosenblum and El-Sabban[22-24] did not observe any effects in the cerebral microcirculation of mice employing quite adquate doses of ASA, i.e., 1, 10 and 25 mg/kg. For thrombus induction they used UV-irradiation in sensitized animals. On the other hand, Michal and Geissinger,[25] using venules of the hamster cheek pouch after iontophoretic administration of ADP, demonstrated a marked effect of ASA as well as a synergism with calcium dobesilate. Bourgain et al.[26] used rat mesenteric artery damage by electric current and superfusion by ADP to demonstrate a significant effect of ASA. Spilker and van Balken[27] showed that prolonged administration of ASA (200 mg/kg) significantly increased the threshold for the induction of thrombotic occlusion by the electric current stimulation of mesenteric and brain surface microvessels. Bousser and Lecrubier[28] demonstrated the activity of ASA in rabbit cerebral cortical microcirculation.

Another group of authors concentrated on different types of models using large vessels. Peterson and Zucker[29] studied the antithrombotic activity of ASA in rabbit veins. A severe lesion was produced by sodium morrhuate. Because the method was not sufficiently quantitative, the dose/effect relation could not be established even though some antithrombotic effect was seen. In 1971, Danese et al.[30] used dog arteries injured either by a sclerosing agent (0.1 N sulfuric acid) or endarterectomy. A relatively large dose of 40 mg/kg ASA was administered orally for 3 d. Complete occlusions only were significantly inhibited. The vascular lesion was rather drastic with both modifications. Zekert and Gottlob[31] designed a vein thrombosis model in rabbits using injury by silver nitrate and indication by Cr^{51}-tagged erythrocytes. ASA was effective alone at high doses (100 mg/kg), or in combination with dipyridamole. The lesion was severe and the dosage was high. Similarly, after a severe lesion (endarterectomy) ASA (10 mg/kg 2 h in advance) did not prevent carotid occlusions in the studies of Piepgras et al.[22] After a similarly severe lesion (surgical and chemical), prolonged administration of ASA (32 mg/kg daily for 5 d in advance) exerted a significant preventive effect in the study of Dyken et al.[33] A relatively severe enzymatic lesion of the vessel wall was likewise produced in the peripheral arteries by pronase in the studies of Mayer[34] and with much the same model, by Lyman.[35] Incomplete prevention of thrombosis was observed by very large doses of ASA in the study of the former group and no effect at all in that of the latter.

In a group of models more appropriately called DIC-models, ASA was often, but not invariably effective. In the study of Renaud and Godu[36] based on the use of very high oral doses of ASA (100 to 200 mg/kg) in hyperlipemic rats and after an endotoxin challenge, ASA proved to be effective as shown by a semiquantitative evaluation. Rüegg et al.[37] used sodium arachidonate and Tomikawa[38] used ADP, collagen, and lactic acid as a challenge. In both studies ASA was either ineffective, or without any prominent effect. On the other hand, Lindsay et al.[39] also used arachidonic acid, and in their hands, ASA was effective already at a dose of 20 mg/kg. Partial protection against the endotoxin effect was afforded by ASA in the study of Fleming et al.[40] Srivastava[41] used the induction with collagen and epinephrine in mice and ASA was markedly effective in the prevention of mortality or paralysis at a dose of 15 mg/kg while 25 and 100 mg/kg had decreasing effects in this order.

A similar problematic relation to clinical thrombosis emerged from the study of Haft[42] with epinephrine-induced myocardial necrosis. ASA decreased the number of platelet aggregates in the myocardial microcirculation.

A very specialized kind of test was that of MacDonald[43] who prolonged the survival of renal allografts in presensitized dogs by heparin, and to some extent, also by ASA at relatively high doses (ca. 60 to 100 mg/kg). Of course, in such complex and specialized models many activities other than antithrombotic may come into play.

An interesting morphological study using, unfortunately, very high doses of ASA (300 mg/kg), was carried out by Chung-hsin Ts'ao.[44] After ASA he observed a less compact deposition of partially not degranulated platelets at the site of injury induced by a ligation and concluded that ASA inhibited both the platelet adhesion to collagen and release.

In his morphological study in rabbits, Sheppard[45] demonstrated that ASA (200 to 300 mg/kg) inhibited platelet adhesion to collagen but not to the basal membrane and microfibrils of the internal elastic lamina.

Often no effects of ASA were observed when relatively severe lesions had been inflicted. Thus, Elcock and Fredrickson[46] using very high doses of about 200 mg/kg ASA did not prevent occlusions of divided and reanastomosed small veins in rabbits. Almost negative results were obtained in the study of Marbet and Duckert[47] using jugular veins of rats. They were dabbed by a formalin-methanol solution. In addition, ellagic acid was administered intravenously. ASA, when given at a dose of 100 mg/kg orally 24 h in advance, was almost ineffective. This is not surprising in view of an excessive lesion and inappropriate drug administration. An insignificant preventive trend was described by Barth et al.[48] in Wessler's type of a model (venous stasis and administration of a purified activation product) using jugular veins of rabbits. Such models are obviously more suitable for testing anticoagulants than ASA.

In many laboratories various kinds of AV-shunts made from artificial materials were used. ASA was mostly ineffective or effective only at a very high dose level. Thus, ASA was ineffective at a dose of 140 to 150 mg/kg in the model of Graudins et al.[49] based on platelet deposition in a PVC catheter introduced into the superior vena cava of rabbits. Some effect was observed by Gurewich and Lipinski[50] in the carotid artery thrombosis of rabbits, but suloctidil was more effective. Smith and While[51] observed no significant effect of ASA using an AV-shunt with an inserted cotton thread in rats. However, low dose ASA effectively prevented thrombus formation in hemodialysis patients.[52]

Very similar models were used in the studies of Benis et al.,[53] and later, Mason et al.[54] In his experiments with monkeys, Mason used the introduction into the AV-shunt of a similar special device to produce turbulence employed previously by Benis. When administered at a dose of 30 mg/kg/d ASA decreased the formation of thrombotic deposits only partially in the study of Mason while Benis injected ASA directly into the shunt without any effect.

Dikshit[55] in cats, Paris et al.[56] in rats, and Umetsu[57] in rats inserted threads into AV-shunts. Dikshit observed with ASA ED_{50} of about 20 mg/kg, Umetsu noted 42% inhibition of thrombus formation after 100 mg/kg of ASA, and the most interesting results were obtained by Paris noting an optimum effective relatively low dose of 3.12 mg/kg ASA and decreasing activity with both lower and higher doses. His speculation about the role of PGI_2 in this effect was based on the assumption of prostacyclin as a circulating hormone which is no longer accepted. In fact, a similar optimum of about 10 mg/kg ASA was reported also by Lewis et al.[58] in a very different experimental setting, i.e., hamster cheek preparation and stimulation by electric current to produce and count white bodies in the microcirculation.

Philp[59] cited Herrmann et al. as also using AV-shunt model just as Rosenberg et al. Both induced thrombi in rabbits. The former observed little effect by weighing thrombi after 100 and 200 mg/kg ASA and the latter found a consistent antithrombotic activity after only 25 to 50 mg/kg of ASA.

Cattaneo et al.[60] investigated thrombus weights as well as platelet survival after the introduction of a polyethylene tubing into the carotid or femoral arteries of rabbits. Very high doses of ASA (200 mg/kg for 5 d) were only effective while sodium salicylate showed even more effect. As usual the objections may be directed against the use of artificial surfaces, insufficiently quantitative methods, and high doses of ASA. No effect on platelet survival was noted. The weak effect of ASA was explained by the predominant thrombin dependence of the model. About a 40% inhibition of thrombus formation was observed by Lavelle and MacIomhair[61] in the rat vena cava after an introduction of platinum wire.

In two studies ASA had only a prothrombotic activity. Kelton et al.[62] observed, in a mechanically induced thrombosis of rabbit veins, a thrombosis increasing effect of ASA at a dose of 200 mg/kg i.v. and tried to interpret this by the inhibition of PGI_2 synthesis in the vessel wall. This interpretation is not very convincing as the dose of 10 mg/kg, while having no thrombogenic activity in the study, inhibited PGI_2 synthesis as well. In fact, Dejana et al.[63] described almost full inhibition of prostacyclin synthesis already after 25 mg/kg, while this dose did not adversely influence platelet adhesion to the rabbit aorta both *in vitro* and *in vivo*. It should be also remembered that Kelton used intravenous administration of ASA and later it will be shown that this could cause a local injury of the vessel wall.

Zimmermann et al.[64] observed an insignificant and transitory thrombogenic effect of ASA (100 mg/kg orally) using the perivascular damage with silver nitrate in rabbit jugular veins. This effect was only reported with the first dose, repeated administrations were ineffective.

Silver et al.[65] used forceps to inflict a mechanical lesion of intermediate severity to the central ear artery of rabbits, together with a semiquantitative morphological evaluation of platelet adhesion to the subendothelium. ASA was significantly effective at a dose of 8 mg/kg. Even though this method could draw some criticism on account of its cumbersome evaluation and its not representing proper thrombus formation (only one or two layers of platelets were deposited), the relatively low effective dose indicated an improved design.

Using a somewhat different model, Hanson and Harker[66] observed a similar phenomenon in baboons. While not estimating the degree of vessel obstruction, they did find increased consumption and decreased survival of platelets due to sequestration in an AV-shunt. When alone ASA was ineffective, but it did potentiate the effect of dipyridamole. Meanwhile, many experimental studies as well as clinical experience show that dipyridamole is frequently more effective if artificial surfaces are involved in thrombogenesis.

An attempt to tackle a more specific and complex problem was made in the studies of Moschos et al.[67,68] The authors were unable to prevent thrombotic occlusions of coronary arteries in dogs by prolonged administration of ASA (approximately 30 mg/kg) but demonstrated an improved clinical condition, i.e., decreased mortality and frequency of arrhythmia, as well as an occasionally smaller infarction size probably due to the prevention of microthrombi formation in the myocardium. Levison et al.[69] decreased the thrombogenesis in rabbit bacterial endocarditis with ASA. The effect of ASA on experimental atherosclerosis was studied by Pick et al.,[70] and Clopath[71] with some positive results.

In his model using dogs with an artificial stenosis of coronaries Folts et al.[72] showed an improved clinical condition after 35 mg/kg of ASA coinciding with the prevention of cyclic flow reductions.

In agreement with a more recently emerging general tendency, Millet et al.[73] used a relatively low degree venous wall lesion in a model similar to that of Reyers et al.[74,75] The lesion was produced by flushing a rat venous segment with physiological saline. After 100 mg/kg ASA in the study of Millet and both 2.5 and 200 mg/kg in the study of Reyers, no effect whatsoever was observed. Intermediate doses were not investigated. Both studies were characterized by a not very well-defined local lesion and partial stasis. Reyers had difficulties in establishing ASA activity even in a cooperative study. The model represents venous thrombosis suitable rather for testing anticoagulants.

Laser-induced lesions were increasingly more popular, probably because of the relatively well reproducible dosage of the stimulus. The method was already used for testing ASA by Fleming et al.[40,76] in 1970 in the rabbit ear chamber. ASA was partially effective at relatively low doses (2 and 4 mg/kg/min by intravenous infusion). It was, at the same time, less effective than indole.

Laser-induced lesion of rat mesenteric arteries was furthermore used by Seiffge and Weithmann.[77] ASA was effective at a relatively low dose of 10 mg/kg. The method involved a good quantitative evaluation based on the number of laser shots necessary to produce a definite thrombus. ASA had a synergistic effect with pentoxifylline. From the point of view of interpretation, a disadvantage was the localization in the microcirculatory bed.

Weichert and Breddin[78] also used laser-induced thrombosis in the rat mesenteric micro-circulation and observed a dose-related activity of ASA starting from the dose of 50 mg/kg.

A remarkable improvement in the design of thrombosis models can be registered in the studies of the research group working in Bayer's pharmacological research. They subjected the problem to systematic investigation and developed and tested a number of models demonstrating the effects of ASA with increasing adequacy. At first, they used iontophoretic administration of ADP in the rat microcirculation. ASA was effective only at the 100 mg/kg dose level. Later the group used laser-induced lesions in the microcirculation of rats to concentrate on larger vessels, mostly the jugular veins of rats.[79] Laser application became better standardized and the weighing of thrombi was introduced for evaluation. ASA was effective if administered orally just before the laser stimulus at a dose as low as 10 mg/kg, and the effect having attained about 50% inhibition at most, did not increase further with increasing doses. The negative results with ASA of some previous investigators were tentatively interpreted as an insufficiently quantitative character of methods. A further methodological development by Meng and Seuter[80] was the use of a relatively less severe lesion to the rat carotid artery by local chilling combined with partial occlusion by a silver clip. The weight of thrombi was again determined. The method made it possible to estimate even a partial effect. ASA was significantly effective already after 3 mg/kg with an optimum after 10 to 30 mg/kg was orally administered. The formation of nonocclusive thrombi was inhibited by 70 to 90% but the incidence of occlusive thrombi (about 20%) had not changed. This might be related, according to the authors, to the still relatively high degree of damage to the vessel wall. Of course, the chilling to $-15°C$ affects the wall throughout its total thickness. A very similar effectiveness of ASA was observed if the same method was applied to rat jugular veins (50% inhibition of thrombus formation after 30 mg/kg of ASA orally). In comparison, other NSAID such as indomethacin and phenylbutazone had approximately the same antithrombotic activity while having been more effective as antiphlogistics. Of course, an antiphlogistic activity is a very complex quality depending on the method used. With full justification, Meng discussed the controversial requirement in some studies of complete inhibition of thrombus formation after a very severe damage.

On the whole, the methods of this group, while bringing a significant improvement, may still be criticized for all the attention being paid to the separate local vascular damage (still relatively excessive) with a consequent necessity to exaggerate the intensity of the challenge.

In his earlier studies the author, Hladovec,[81] used a method based on inducing thrombosis in the rat carotid artery by electric current. The process of occlusion was continuously registered by measuring contact temperature distally from the site of damage. Intravenously administered ASA was effective but after relatively high doses only (60 mg/kg) (Figure 2). The same method was used also by Philp[82] with similar results after ASA. The necessity to use high doses was the consequence of the relatively severe damage inflicted to the vessel wall and this later caused a search for a new method.

Orally administered ASA inhibited platelet sequestration *in vivo* (i.e., an acute transitory decrease in platelets after parenteral administration of an agent producing a mild systemic endothelial lesion) with a marked optimum around 8 to 12 mg/kg with hypotonic saline as the challenging agent (Figure 52).[83] By contrast, intravenously administered ASA (as calcium salt) when administered alone and at a relatively high dose exerted an adverse effect enhancing platelet sequestration. It should be remembered that ASA is an acidic compound able to directly damage the endothelial lining similar to all kinds of epithelia. This is in agreement with studies of other authors observing the direct effect of ASA on endothelium.[84] An unfavorable effect of an increased local concentration of calcium cannot be excluded. After oral administration the unfavorable local effect is less apparent because of the binding of dissociated ASA to suitable protein carriers. The same negative effect was observed in the

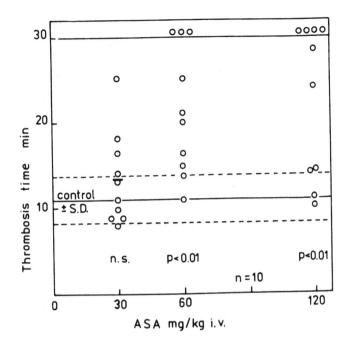

FIGURE 2. Effect of i.v. ASA on electrically induced arterial thrombosis.

endothelem test (Figure 3) when ASA was administered against a challenge or alone.[85] This adverse direct effect of relatively high concentrations of ASA probably represents the main mechanism of the toxic action of ASA on the mucous membranes of the gastrointestinal tract. In the venostatic thrombosis model used previously as a standard method (a systemic mild vascular lesion combined with stasis in the mesenteric circulation of the rat, evaluated as the blood lost from severed vessels by photometric estimation) ASA had no adverse effects but was only weakly effective (inhibition by about 30% at most) in the short cut modification with kaolin suspension used as the challenge.[85]

A new battery of models was introduced in 1986 based on an improved design and more rational consideration. ASA was tested in all models after oral administration 1 h in advance of thrombus induction (Figure 4). It was possible to demonstrate a satisfactory dose-to-effect relationship in all three models and the dosages were, in general, close to the clinical dose range. In the endothelemia model, the effect was independent of the type of challenge used (citrate or hypotonic saline) and the fully effective doses were about 8 mg/kg. A special experiment showed that the effect was relatively short-lived and was no more demonstrable 12 h after the administration (Figure 5). In the arterial thrombosis model (a combination of a partial aortic occlusion with a mild systemic endothelial lesion by i.v. hypotonic saline with 5-HT added) the effective dose was about 5 mg/kg and the drug was also effective in the venous thrombosis model (a mild systemic challenge with a partial venous occlusion) where a significant effect was already observed after 1 mg/kg, about 60% inhibition after 10 mg/kg, and full inhibition after 30 mg/kg. The relatively high activity in all three models and particularly in the venous one was rather surprising. The venous model was based on an indirect challenge and a mild diffuse vascular lesion was used to induce activation of blood clotting and platelets. ASA might have influenced this initial phase without substantially interfering with the phase of fibrin thrombus growth. On the other hand, serious local damage to the vessel wall is not desirable and such model design might be much closer to the clinical situation. The results also show that ASA could find a reasonable application

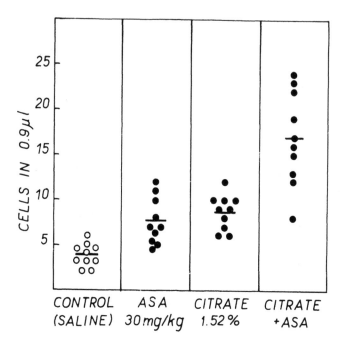

FIGURE 3.   The endothelial element count-increasing effect of i.v. ASA at a relatively high dose alone or in combination with a citrate challenge.

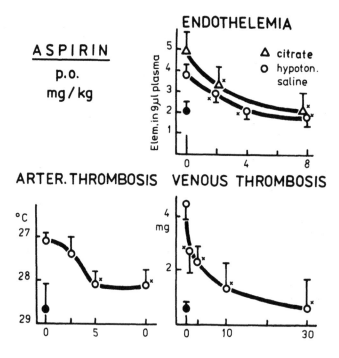

FIGURE 4.   Effect of ASA in the standard battery of tests.

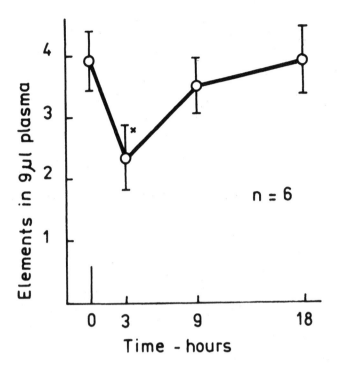

FIGURE 5.   Duration of ASA effect on endothelial stability after 8 mg/ kg p.o. 1 h in advance of the citrate challenge.

even in the prevention of venous thrombosis, at least in cases with increased contribution of vascular lesions and platelets.

In an effort to throw some light on the contribution of the prostaglandin or eicosanoid system to the effect of ASA, sodium salicylate was tested in a way similar to ASA (Figure 6). It became evident that the salicylate was effective in all tests of the battery and the differences with respect to ASA were only quantitative. Even in the endothelial stability test, a significant positive effect was observed amounting to about 80% inhibition. The effective dose was, in general, 4 to 5 times higher than in the case of ASA with a somewhat larger difference in the arterial in comparison with the venous model. Both are, of course, acute models and any speculations regarding the effect on coagulation factor synthesis in the liver would be out of place.

What is then the mechanism of ASA and salicylate effect? The eicosanoid system can hardly contribute to the salicylate effect even though some competitive inhibitory effect was described against cyclo-oxygenase. In fact, there has never been enough evidence showing that the eicosanoid system is related to *in vivo* thrombogenesis in a decisive manner. The results of both experimental and clinical studies were rather equivocal in this respect and *ex vivo* changes in the blood levels of PG-metabolites may be secondary and not causally related to the process of thrombosis. An example of this lack of hard evidence is the study of Bourgain et al.[86] which can be readily interpreted as an argument against the key role of eicosanoids. It is also evident that the results of *in vitro* or *ex vivo* aggregation studies are in doubtful relation to those emerging from clinical trials. It is not only the question of ASA dosage which cannot be answered by any speculation about the tromboxane-prostacyclin balance, but it is also the duration of the antithrombotic effect of ASA which is much shorter in the clinical practice than in *ex vivo* tests. Several authors have already expressed their doubts about the simplistic interpretation of ASA activity by way of the eicosanoid system.[13,66,87-89] Also the importance of acetylation capacity of ASA is questionable as shown

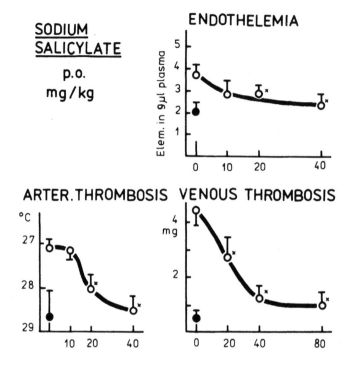

FIGURE 6.   Effect of sodium salicylate in the standard battery of models.

by the high activity in platelet aggregation tests of ASA analogues with acetyl groups in position two of the benzene ring but without the available acetyl radical.[90] Besides, acetylation is not specific and many other proteins can be modified in their biological activity in this way. The relative unimportance of the eicosanoid system is demonstrated, inter alia, by the existence of congenital defects in cyclo-oxygenase activity without any thrombophilic tendency and the mere fact that ASA so effectively inhibits cyclo-oxygenase without having a corresponding radical effect on hemostasis (except rarely in some individuals) or on thrombus formation after severe vascular damage. Even if the effect on arachidonic acid metabolism is accepted as important it must not necessarily be mediated by the inhibition of cyclo-oxygenase activity and lipoxygenase pathway may be involved.[87,91]

The mechanism of the antithrombotic ASA effect remains to be clarified. Cattaneo et al.[60] and de Gaetano[92,88] turned the attention to the influence on fibrinolysis. Collier[93] expressed the opinion that the effect of ASA (as well as of other NSAID) is of a general regulatory character which he defines as an "antidefensive" activity, that is the inhibition of the activation of cellular blood and vessel wall components (platelets, leukocytes, endothelial cells) engaged in various pathological conditions including the process of thrombosis. He suspected that some very basic and common mechanisms may be involved concerning the terminal mediation of various converging pathways. This may represent the effect on the cell membrane properties, possibly related to the acidic character of salicylates capable of forming soluble salts with calcium. It is in this way that they might influence the stability of the glycocalyx component of the membrane which is very dependent on the presence of calcium ions. In fact, practically all NSAID are known to possess membrane-stabilizing effects on red blood cells; they inhibit, e.g., the increase in erythrocyte sedimentation after various agents. At present, it is known that calcium has an optimum concentration both in blood and in tissues, that it may exert a sealing effect on membranes at low, and an opposite effect at high concentrations. This is illustrated e.g., by the endothelemia model (Figure 19 in Chapter 3). The two-phase effects with increasing doses might be more easily related to this phenomenon than to the hypothetic thromboxane-prostacyclin balance. It might be of interest to remember that Irino et al.[94] found that salicylates inhibit *in vitro* platelet aggregation by decreasing the active influx of extracellular Ca^{2+} into platelets stimulated by ADP.

In sufficiently quantitative and sensitive models ASA did not block thrombus development completely, but only by about 60%. Meanwhile, this inhibition may be complete if ASA is combined with other agents as will be shown in another chapter (e.g., in combination with dipyridamole, sulfinpyrazone, prenylamine, and metipranolol). This incomplete effect of ASA alone is probably important for understanding ASA activity, and once more, a hypothesis has been put forth suggesting that complete inhibition of thrombogenesis is probably not the desirable objective of preventive agents. The reason for this is that it would be necessarily accompanied by an increased bleeding tendency, as if one portion of the antithrombotic effect would inhibit the thrombophilic tendency whereas the other, appearing only after higher doses, would correspond to the suppression of the defensive and useful hemostatic function. Similar partial inhibition was observed by Meng and O'Dea[79] speculating that experimental studies without a significant effect of ASA have used methods with an insufficient discriminatory capacity in this respect, so that partial inhibitions went unnoticed. Another example was the activity of low and very low dose heparin producing incomplete suppression of venous thrombus formation, but effective at the same dose as a clinically preventive antithrombotics. Complete suppression may be desirable only under special conditions such as an already present thrombus growth or thrombogenesis on artificial surfaces when ASA is used in combination with dipyridamole.

The treatment of various models used in the study about ASA and described in this survey may be somewhat hypercritically judged. On the other hand, without a critical approach it would be entirely impossible to get oriented in the mess of contradictory findings. ASA presents an excellent opportunity to survey thrombosis models in their effectiveness to discover useful antithrombotic drugs. ASA is, or at least was, at the time of writing the present survey, the best and most widely acknowledged anitplatelet antithrombotic for clinical purposes. The models which would be sufficiently sensitive to ASA should be, in accordance, the most suitable ones for screening antithrombotic agents. The precondition is that the model would be of a sufficiently global character.

In conclusion, it was possible to show that the antithrombotic activity of ASA may be demonstrated at dose levels closely corresponding to the clinical dose range, the dose-effect relationship can be established, and even some hints to its mechanism of action can be made with subsequent suggestions for its optimal use.

II. DIPYRIDAMOLE

Dipyridamole, a pyrimido-pyrimidine derivative, was originally used since 1961 as a vasodilating agent with main indications in coronary diseases. It is this origin as a vasodilating agent that dipyridamole has in common with some other drugs exerting antithrombotic effects, such as pentoxifylline, suloctidil, ketanserin, calcium channel blockers, beta-adrenolytics, etc. Nevertheless, the favorable clinical effect of dipyridamole based on vasodilatation, e.g., in angina pectoris, has never been positively proven and the rationality of such indications remains questionable. Of course, other mechanismsm might contribute to some favorable effects. Already in the phase of testing as a vasodilating agent, it was supposed that the main mechanism of action might be accumulation of adenosine in the plasma due to the inhibition of its cellular uptake and metabolism (deamination) e.g., in erythrocytes and endothelial cells. In this way, the well known vasodilating effect of adenosine could be potentiated. First experimental studies suggesting the use of dipyridamole as an antithrombotic appeared in 1965[95] and the following years saw an explosion of interest in this use of the drug even before that of aspirin. Experimental and clinical studies amounted to several thousands, but in spite of that, and just as in the case of aspirin, it is still uncertain how the drug acts or whether its clinical use is fully justified.

Dipyridamole has a relatively short-lived effect after both oral and parenteral administration. The high variability of its effectiveness, attaining differences of one order of magnitude, is caused mainly by its low solubility with subsequently difficult absorption in the gastrointestinal tract. When in blood, the drug is almost completely bound to plasmatic proteins and is eliminated mainly by glucuronidation in the liver. The enterohepatic circulation contributes to the variability of effects. A small portion is excreted by the kidney.

The mechanism of the supposed antithrombotic effect has given rise to several hypotheses, all of them built on the increase in the level of the natural antiaggregating agent, cyclic adenosine-monophosphate (cAMP). Thus, it was suggested that dipyridamole may cause inhibition of cAMP-phosphodiesterase degrading cAMP. Nevertheless, with the normal clinical dosage, the necessary concentrations could hardly be attained and this mechanism cannot be relevant to the *in vivo* effect of the drug. It was not easy to demonstrate the antiaggregatory effect of dipyridamole *in vitro*, either. Some authors have shown that it is effective with low concentrations of aggregating agents, against spontaneous aggregation often observed after venipuncture, and particularly, with whole blood impedance aggregometry. This is most probably related to the release of ADP from erythrocytes, or on the contrary, the uptake of adenosine by these cells. There is no question that the sensitivity of *in vitro* tests to dipyridamole is very dependent on specific experimental conditions. The release inhibition of platelet constituents is also much more readily demonstrable with whole blood. All results point to the most probable and now the most widely accepted explanation of the dipyridamole effect as the inhibition of adenosine transport and its uptake in cellular elements. This hypothesis was already formulated in connection with the vasodilating activity. The increasing plasma adenosine level may also act by stimulating adenylate cyclase, thus increasing the cAMP production. The third hypothesis of the dipyridamole effect was based on the interaction with the prostanoid system. It was suggested that dipyridamole might act by potentiating the effect or synthesis of prostacyclin, inhibition of its metabolism, stimulation of arachidonic acid metabolism, or even inhibition of thromboxane activity and production. The results of such studies are not questioned here but as all these processes are closely interconnected with platelet activation and vascular lesions, indirect or secondary effects cannot be excluded. Direct effects are not very likely. Dipyridamole is no exception among other cardiovascular drugs; they often have multiple mechanisms of action with some prevailing under particular conditions. It may be noted here that even the possibility of an antioxidant (free oxygen radical scavenging) effect could be taken into consideration under some conditions.

Actual experimental conditions are also responsible for the variable results of some other *in vitro* and *ex vivo* tests such as adhesion to different surfaces including glass, extracellular matrix of cultivated endothelial cells, and the subendothelium of damaged everted vessels. All of them can serve to emphasize the necessity to use proper *in vivo* models.

The first experimental *in vivo* study was based on previous investigations of Born et al.[96,97] who found in 1962 that adenosine and its more stable analogue 2-chloroadenosine inhibited formation of unstable and repeatedly embolizing thrombi (white bodies) in small superficial pial arteries of the rabbit's brain surface after a mechanical injury. At that time, it was already known that the supposed coronaro-dilating activity of dipyridamole (Persantin®) was probably based on the sparing effect on adenosine. Emmons et al.[95,98] in 1965 used virtually the same method in rabbits pinching with forceps at a variable force small cerebro-cortical arteries of rabbits. Dipyridamole had a transient effect completely blocking white body formation if given after the injury at a dose of 1.5 mg/kg and more intravenously. Even after lower doses, the quality of thromboembolic masses was definitely changed. If administered before the injury dipyridamole delayed and shortened the period of white body formation, but a marked loss of activity was observed if the drug was administered more than 1 h in advance. With a minor injury, dipyridamole decreased the potentiating effect of ADP, ATP, and particularly of 5-HT on the white body formation. Even topical external application was effective. The authors observed dissociation between the antihemostatic and antithrombotic activity, the latter not being accompanied by the former. It is necessary to stress that the method, even though very interesting from the theoretical point of view, did not allow far-reaching conclusions for clinical use as the authors rightly pointed out. The method likewise is not very quantitative and may be greatly influenced by subjective factors. It does not represent the relatively more stable thrombosis in large arteries, either. The local lesion is relatively severe.

Another model described by Arfors et al.[99] was based on the use of a ruby laser for producing an endothelial lesion in arterioles of the rabbit ear chamber. Dipyridamole, at a dose of 2.5 mg/kg i.v., was effective in decreasing the number of emboli but the effect was again very transient lasting only 20 to 30 min. On the other hand, the loss of the local reactivity of platelets at the site of an already present injury was much more prolonged. It is not surprising to see that dipyridamole was effective in this model as an injury of cellular elements including red blood cells with their active nucleotide metabolism had to be expected. Otherwise the model has much in common with that of Emmons et al.,[95,98] bringing an improved reproducibility of the dosage of the injurious challenge.

Approximately at the same time, 1968, Philp and Lemieux[100] published their study based partially on the same method as that of Emmons. The results after intravenous administration of 10 mg/kg of dipyridamole in rabbits and rats just before inflicting the lesions were much less remarkable, but some positive trends were noticeable.

Didisheim experimented in 1968[20] with rats and their mesenteric microcirculation. Arterial (100 to 325 μm of inner diameter) lesions were produced by electric current. Duration of mural thrombi in situ, repeated embolizations, and complete occlusions were recorded. Whereas heparin was found ineffective and warfarin possessed even unfavorable effects, aspirin had some insignificant favorable effects on complete occlusions. At a dose of about 17.5 mg/kg i.v., dipyridamole produced a relatively short-lived but profound effect under the same conditions. The author has also mentioned that repeated injections were more effective than a single administration. He had some doubts whether or not this was due to the inhibition of the usually noted marked local vasoconstriction. In some studies he attempted to eliminate hypotension as a contributing factor. The deep hypotension after injection of procaine into the cisterna magna had no antithrombotic effect.[101] On the other hand, the possibility of a local effect against the spasm was not ruled out. In another study[101] he used a rather different model: a teflon femoral AV-microshunt in rats. The tubing was compressed for 10 s. Dipyridamole significantly inhibited "thrombogenesis" in the tubing showing that local vasoconstriction with an effect on blood flow is not decisive for thrombogenesis and the vasodilating activity of dipyridamole is probably not involved. In a series of studies Didisheim et al.[102,103] investigated the antithrombotic activity of two pyrimido-pyrimidine derivatives closely related to dipyridamole (RA 233 and RA 433) and selected on the basis of cAMP phosphodiesterase inhibition. For this purpose, they used the same AV-shunt model. While both compounds were effective, the morpholine derivative RA 433 was more potent. This is in contrast with the results of Hassanein[104] who noted an opposite relation of both drugs in vitro, a finding illustrating, as Didisheim pointed out, the hazards of predicting the clinical effectiveness of any drug only on the basis of in vitro observations. In fact, Elkeles et al.[105] found that RA 433, compared with dipyridamole, is much more effective in vitro and about equally effective in vivo. Hampton et al.[106] came to similar conclusions while studying the effects of a large series of dipyridamole analogues: there was no correlation between their in vitro and in vivo activity with VK 744 having been the most active in vitro but ineffective in vivo. The authors stress that the relevance of platelet function tests to thrombogenesis is questionable. Honour et al.[107,108] used a special modification of a pial artery model in rabbits with a very complicated combination of alloxan priming, electrical stimulation, and topical administration of ADP. In their experiments, oral dipyridamole and in later studies particularly the analogue SH 1117, were effective in suppressing the sensitivity-increasing effect of alloxan. Of course, alloxan has a general injurious effect on endothelium. Their results point to the key role of a vascular lesion in the antithrombotic activity of dipyridamole. While very interesting from the theoretical point of view, similar studies using small arteries of the microcirculation with no stable thrombus formation and a low degree of quantitation should be used for the prediction of clinical effectiveness with utmost caution.

Negative results with dipyridamole were obtained by Danese et al.[30] They used two canine models, both based on a relatively severe vascular injury, i.e., endarterectomy or 0.1 N sulfuric acid instillation into the large arteries (femoral, carotid, or axillary). Dipyridamole was administered at a dose of approximately 8 mg/kg orally for 3 d. The presence of thrombosis and the approximate degree of occlusion was estimated. Aspirin decreased the degree of occlusion. The failure of dipyridamole to exert any effect at all was explained by the authors either by species or model differences or the timing of administration resulting in possible low blood concentrations. However, the main cause may be the extremely severe vascular lesion having nothing in common with the clinical situation as well as an insufficiently quantitative model. It is interesting to note that the same author obtained significantly positive results with dipyridamole in a similar model in dogs (intimectomy). In this study, a marked divergence was observed in the effect of drugs on the appearance of platelet aggregates on the vascular surface and the occurrence of occlusive thrombi showing that both processes do not necessarily go in parallel.

In a group of models based on the introduction of foreign surfaces into the circulation, Cucuianu et al.[109] studied the effect of dipyridamole in various *in vitro* tests as well as on thrombotic deposit formation in rabbit extracorporeal shunts coated with gammaglobulin and with flow reduced by clamping. The tubing with deposits was weighed. Dipyridamole and two of its analogues were effective. The effectiveness of RA 433 which otherwise showed little *in vivo* activity was explained by the inhibition of platelet interaction with foreign surfaces.

Haft et al.[110] observed a significant decrease in the frequency of myocardial necrosis in dogs after epinephrine injections. Dipyridamole and aspirin showed a marked inhibitory effect which the authors ascribed to the prevention of the appearance of platelet aggregates in the myocardial microcirculation. Of course, other mechanisms might also be involved. Under somewhat similar conditions, Moschos et al.[67] using an electrically induced thrombus formation in the proximal coronary artery of dogs injected radio-labeled platelets. Aspirin and dipyridamole (the latter at a dose of ca 5 mg/kg) administered orally for 7 d decreased the occurrence of platelet microthrombi in the myocardial microcirculation without influencing the development of major thrombi. The frequency of arrhythmia and mortality also decreased. It may be remembered that no effect of dipyridamole on infarct size was observed by Watanabe et al.[111]

Mayer and Hammond[34] tested dipyridamole and aspirin in a dog model inflicting severe enzymatic damage to femoral arteries by instillation of pronase. Dipyridamole (250 mg/d) prevented subsequent thrombotic occlusions by 70%.

Dragojevic et al.[112] administering 10 mg/kg dipyridamole p.o. daily for 10 d prevented thrombotic accretions on a Teflon® strip inserted and fixed in the left atrium of dogs.

Negative results were obtained by Turina et al.[113] after introducing a helically bent probe made of platinum-iridium wire into the heart of dogs and after the preventive oral administration of 6 mg/kg dipyridamole daily. The failure might have been due to species and dose differences, or a too strong stimulus. Under similar conditions a combination of dipyridamole with anticoagulants is usually indicated.

O'Sullivan and Vellar[114] prevented electrically induced thrombosis in the rabbit's vena cava by 5 mg/kg dipyridamole. A combination with aspirin was also effective. It is important to stress here that it was venous thrombosis that was effectively prevented in this case. Hasegawa et al.[115] also reported complete suppression of thrombosis on Teflon® grafts introduced into the superior vena cava of dogs by daily administration of 10 mg/kg dipyridamole i.v. More than 50% of control grafts were occluded within 10 d to 18 months and the remaining had thick thrombotic deposits. These positive results stimulated the study of Polterauer et al.[116] who prevented thrombotic occlusions in jugular veins of rabbits after their damage by silver nitrate. Thrombotic deposition was measured by the accumulation of Cr^{51}-labeled erythrocytes. Dipyridamole was effective at a dose of 5 mg/kg orally twice, i.e., 16 and 3 h before the surgery. A combination of aspirin (100 mg/kg) was also effective. Of course, the lesion was very severe. On the other hand, the authors emphasized the quantitative character of the method.

Dipyridamole was tested in an AV-shunt of rhesus monkeys by Mason et al.[54] Special "captured vortex" devices made of polystyrene were inserted into the shunt between the aorta and inferior vena cava. Oral administration of 2 mg/kg dipyridamole on the test day and 1 d before decreased the thrombotic deposition in the shunt as measured gravimetrically. Like other similar studies, one showed dipyridamole quite effective in models using foreign surfaces and flow disturbances as prothrombotic factors.

Rüegg[37] observed about 50% protection in rabbits from arachidonic acid-induced sudden death (100 mg/kg orally). This is principally a disseminated intravascular coagulation method (DIC), just as that employed in the studies of Tomikawa et al.[342] who used dipyridamole with negative results in lactic acid-induced DIC, whereas Yoshikawa et al.[117] observed a protective influence of dipyridamole against endotoxin-induced DIC in rats. Similar endotoxin DIC in rabbits was used by Gurewich and Lipinski.[118] Ortega[119] induced mouse DIC by epinephrine and collagen injections and Slabber et al.[120] prevented endotoxin-induced glomerular fibrin deposits. In all these studies dipyridamole possessed a partial positive effect. Negative dipyridamole effects were noted in a mouse model with DIC caused by injection of collagen with epinephrine by Dikshit et al.[121]

The studies of Rosenblum and El-Sabban[122] designed to assess the effect of dipyridamole on white body formation in the pial microcirculation on the brain surface of mice induced by fluorescein and UV-irradiation were essentially negative. This is just another example of divergent results as compared with Honour et al.[108,123] whose positive results were mentioned above.

Umetsu and Sanai[124] induced thrombosis in an extracorporeal shunt with a silk thread in rats. The absence of dipyridamole effect was explained by a relatively long period (6 h) between administration (100 mg/kg orally) and thrombus induction, with the effect of dipyridamole known as being relatively transitory. A shunt method was used also by Hanson et al.[66] in baboons. A decrease a radiolabeled platelets was noted in the circulation as a consequence of sequestration in the shunt. Dipyridamole alone (2.5 mg/kg orally) or in combination with aspirin (20 mg/kg orally) was effective. A plastic catheter was inserted into the rabbit's carotid for induction of thrombosis by Gurewich and Lipinski[50,118] and Louie and Gurewich.[125] Dipyridamole was moderately effective but its action was markedly potentiated by low doses of ASA. A foreign material was also introduced into the femoral arteries of dogs (polytetrafluoroethylene grafts) and the deposition of radiolabeled autologous platelets was estimated in addition to graft weight. Dipyridamole (50 mg, i.e., ca 2 mg/kg orally) was effective, but less than calcium antagonists.[126] Groves et al.[127] using a balloon catheter induced vascular damage in rabbits. Doses as low as 2.5 to 12.5 mg/kg of dipyridamole were effective in preventing thrombosis. Silver et al.[65] stressed the necessity to use a relatively mild mechanical lesion inflicted to the rabbit ear artery with forceps. Dipyridamole was not effective at a dose of 1.5 mg/kg i.v., but if administered at the same dose five times within 3 d, it did prevent platelet adhesion to the vessel wall as estimated by morphological methods (SEM).

Folts[128] used dipyridamole unsuccessfully in a model based on cyclic blood flow reduction associated with "acute thrombus formation" followed by embolization from mechanically stenosed arteries of monkeys, rabbits, dogs, and pigs. No stable occluding thrombi were observed and this defined the limits of the predicting capacity of the method. Dipyridamole was not effective at a dose of 2 mg/kg i.v. alone and in combination with low dose ASA. Fuster et al.[129] supported clinical studies of this group with the prevention of aorto-coronary bypass occlusions by experiments in dogs. After saphenous vein bypass graft surgery and injection of radiolabeled autologous platelets, the thrombogenesis was estimated by scintigraphy *in vivo*. The administration of dipyridamole (55 mg/d) combined with ASA (325 mg/d) resulted in marked improvement in comparison with the control.

Another possibility to exploit favorable effects of dipyridamole may be its addition to the blood in extracorporeal circulation thus decreasing platelet losses.[130] Similarly, dipyridamole decreased the frequency of retinal embolism associated with a cardiopulmonary bypass in the dog[132] and in the pig.[131]

Coeugniet[133] pointed out the remarkable activity of dipyridamole in immunological reactions, endotoxin effect, and lymphokine production in lymphocytes.

Somewhat peripheral to the focus of attention of this survey were several studies investigating the effect of dipyridamole in the models of atherosclerosis based on the thrombogenic theory. In some studies the effect of dipyridamole pointed in a favorable direction, e.g., prevention of homocysteine-induced endothelial lesions with subsequent intimal proliferation in baboons and rats.[134,135] On the other hand, no effect on proliferative changes was observed by Friedman and Burns[136] or the effect of dipyridamole was distinctly unfavorable.[137] Experimental conditions were very different in all such studies and the results are hardly comparable. The problem is closely related to the much disputed question of possible inhibition of proliferative tissue reaction by dipyridamole.

In the author's laboratory dipyridamole was investigated with the use of several models. The effect on platelet adhesion *in vivo* (platelet sequestration) was studied in rats. The acute decrease in platelet counts after a suitable challenge (in this case 1.9% citrate solution, 2 ml/200 g i.v.) known to also induce endothelial lesions was favorably influenced by dipyridamole attaining the control values obtained after physiological saline injection (Figure 7). The effect was dose-dependent with a marked maximum around 10 mg/kg p.o. administered 1 h in advance.

If ADP was added to 1.52% citrate (0.25 mg/kg ADP) a much deeper decrease in platelet count was observed, a phenomenon minimally influenced by dipyridamole showing that the main effect of the drug is probably localized at the level of endothelium and not on circulating platelets (Figure 8).

In an electrical model of thrombosis, dipyridamole administered intravenously into rats 1 min before the challenge was significantly effective already at a dose of 0.1 mg/kg whereas at a dose of 10 mg/kg full effect was attained according to its definition (Figure 9).[81] This is quite in accord with the results obtained in the more recently used arterial thrombosis model. It is interesting to remember that in the case of ASA the effective dose was 60 mg/kg i.v. in the electrical model and about 7 mg/kg orally in the model used more recently showing that with an excessive challenge the effect of ASA decreases more than that of dipyridamole.

The results attained with the presently used standard battery of tests are shown in Figure 10.[138] Dipyridamole was administered orally, if not indicated otherwise in the diagrams. In the endothelemia model the drug was effective in protecting endothelium against the desquamating effect of both citrate and hypotonic saline equally at very low doses (0.2 mg/kg p.o.). In arterial thrombosis, intravenous and oral administrations were equally effective

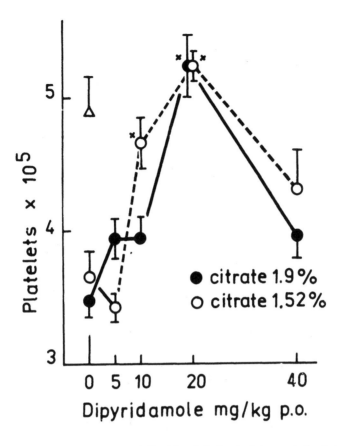

FIGURE 7.   Effect of oral dipyridamole in the platelet sequestration test after the challenge with two citrate concentrations.

showing full suppression of occlusive thrombus formation at doses between 6 and 9 mg/kg. Surprisingly, the drug was also effective in the venous thrombosis model at a still lower dose level (1 mg/kg p.o.), however, without attaining full suppression of the process. Of course such partial effect might be important if the challenging stimulus is not too strong. Meanwhile, the intravenously administered drug was fully effective at the same dose level. This is in accordance with numerous studies described in the survey also showing a preventive effect against venous thrombosis. Explanation of the difference between the oral and parenteral administration in the venous model is not easy, but it may be caused by a different component of the molecule effective in the venous model as compared with the arterial one possibly related to an increased binding to proteins or even metabolic changes after oral administration which may be deleterious to the component effective in the arterial model. No matter which way it is, the dosages in the endothelial model and in the venous one are lower or equal, respectively, to clinical dosages. The arterial model shows that the dose increase (2 to 3 times) would be worthwhile to test clinically if dipyridamole is given alone, and of course, if the increased dose is not contraindicated for adverse side effects. On the other hand, the main future of dipyridamole lies probably in the combination with aspirin making this increased dosage unnecessary.

To summarize, in most *in vivo* experimental models, dipyridamole was quite effective as an antithrombotic. Very probably, most negative studies used inadequate doses or, as an experimental correlate of indications, an unsuitable experimental design. It is not possible to suspect all positve studies of an experimental bias. This survey may give some hints as to the suitable dosage and indications. While the fully effective dosage was very variable, in sufficiently sensitive models it was about 5 to 10 mg/kg orally.

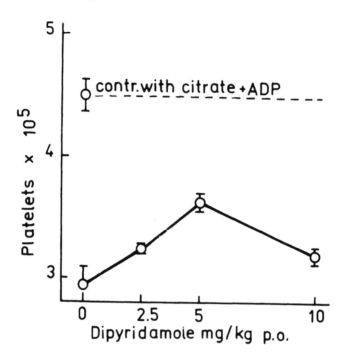

FIGURE 8. Effect of oral dipyridamole on the platelet sequestration after the challenge with the combination of citrate plus ADP.

The effect of dipyridamole has, by all indications, a strong component affecting the vessel wall and exerts a relatively weaker influence on platelets. It is effective in preventing thrombotic depositions on various artificial surfaces. This may be caused by the rough and incompatible nature of surfaces damaging erythrocytes mechanically and indirectly by adverse flow conditions. The effect on release and removal of nucleotides from blood from damaged erythrocytes is probably favorably influenced by dipyridamole in the sense of Born's theory concerning the role of nucleotides (ATP, ADP, cAMP, and adenosine) in thrombogenesis.[140]

It may be concluded that the use of dipyridamole has a good rational base but the drug should be indicated in special situations and not indiscriminately. Combinations are particularly advantageous. It is true that there has been some skepticism regarding the clinical value of dipyridamole as an antithrombotic, voiced e.g., by Loeliger[141] and FitzGerald.[142] True, some clinical studies with dipyridamole were a disappointment, but then they generated unjustified expectations and their design was often defective. It would be desirable to base further clinical trials on a higher level of information including that obtained in experimental studies.

III. SULFINPYRAZONE

Sulfinpyrazone was used since 1957 as an uricosuric agent and for several years was marketed as such to be later replaced by more effective drugs. The drug is a pyrazolidine derivative closely related to phenylbutazone. Even though it is one of the nonsteroid anti-inflammatory drugs (NSAID) or analgesic antipyretic drug, its anti-inflammatory activity is relatively weak in most models. It is well and rapidly absorbed in the gastrointestinal tract attaining maximum plasma concentrations in 1 to 2 h. In the plasma, it is almost completely bound to proteins. Duration of the effect is much more prolonged than corresponds to the actual blood levels. This is often explained by its later appearing and relatively more active metabolites, particularly the oxidative product sulfide. However, only several percent of the

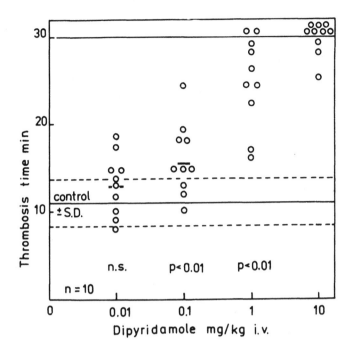

FIGURE 9.   Effect of i.v. dipyridamole on the electrically induced arterial thrombosis.

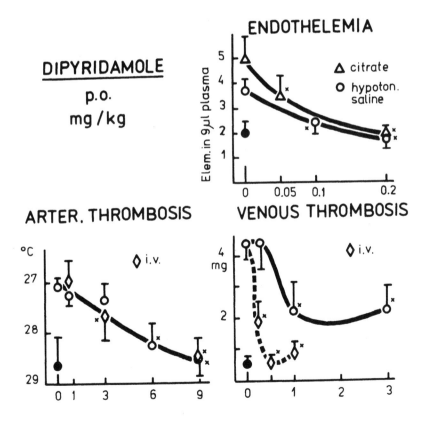

FIGURE 10.   Effect of dipyridamole in the standard battery of models.

drug are subjected to biotransformation, a large proportion being excreted as an unchanged compound in the urine. The activity of metabolites is estimated by *in vitro* methods not allowing authoritative conclusions about their actual value. The drug produces no tendency to bleeding.

First studies of its possible antithrombotic effects originated from clinicians. On the one hand, there was the impression that the drug might have favorable effects in some peripheral arterial diseases; on the other, increased platelet survival was found in patients treated for such diseases.[143] Studies of the latter group were followed by many others attmepting to support their findings. Thus, Steele et al.[144,145] found that in groups of patients suffering from diseases connected with thromboembolic phenomena, platelet survival was shortened[146] and this defect was corrected by sulfinpyrazone.[144,145] However, the method was not well reproducible due to technical differences in the procedure.[14] The survival studies were supported by clinical ones employing AV-shunts[147,148] showing favorable results, and later by a number of *in vitro* as well as *in vivo* studies seeking to define some rational basis for therapeutic use of the drug. These attempts were quite unsuccessful for a long time. The drug was effective as an *in vitro* antiaggregant only at very high concentrations which could never be attained with clinical dosages. Initially, sulfinpyrazone was also completely ineffective in *ex vivo* samples. Only after the lowering of the stimulus intensity (low concentrations of collagen) was it possible to demonstrate some *in vitro* and *ex vivo* activity particularly marked if arachidonic acid was used as an aggregation stimulus. However, this led to somewhat hasty conclusions that the main effect of the drug is directed against prostanoid production. It was found that the drug possessed, just as most NSAID, a competitive inhibitory activity against cyclo-oxygenase. Originally, the drug was found to have no effect on the release of platelet constituents, but later, inhibition of the release of radiolabeled serotonin was observed *ex vivo*. Together with the finding of the inhibitory effect on serotonin uptake in platelets, this led to another theory about the serotoninergic mechanism of its action. An *ex vivo* effect was furthermore observed using the so called ''spontaneous aggregation''. As far as another platelet function, adhesion to the subendothelium, and other surfaces is concerned, the sophisticated but very artificial models using everted vessels first showed a positive antiadhesive effect of sulfinpyrazone at relatively high concentrations, but later, some improvements of the method such as removal of citrate from the system, or on the contrary, addition of erythrocytes, led to negative results.

Such *in vitro* models represent at their best only a glimpse at a much more complex interaction of platelets with the vessel wall. Still more often they show some artifactual situation developing after the tearing out of samples from dynamic *in vivo* balances.This does not mean that a complete mosaic could not be reconstructed from many such glimpses in the future. On the other hand, for the time being, conclusions obtained in such studies should be taken with due caution.

In almost all *in vivo* models sulfinpyrazone was proved to be effective even though high doses were often necessary. Most authors noted an absence of correlation between *in vivo* and *in vitro* findings. The first experimental *in vivo* study was carried out by Mustard et al.[149] using an AV-shunt in rabbits and platelet survival as an indicator of thrombogenesis. The authors reported a significant influence on platelet survival in normal rabbits but only after prolonged treatment (4 weeks) by sulfinpyrazone twice daily at a dose of 10 mg/kg/d subcutanaeously. When administered at a dose of 20 mg/kg/d s.c., there was some trend to decrease thrombus weight without a simultaneous flow change. The effect of sulfinpyrazone was dependent neither on serum uric acid levels nor on the presence of atherosclerotic changes. The authors also found increased uptake of serotonin by platelets later confirmed by other authors. The relative lack of an effect on thrombus formation in the shunt was correctly interpreted not as the absence of an antithrombotic effect as no vessel wall, and particularly, no diseased vessel wall was involved.

Renaud et al.[150] used a relatively complicated method with endotoxin DIC in hyperlipemic rats. Oral administration of sulfinpyrazone was effective at extremely high doses (100 mg/kg). Endotoxin shock and generalized Shwartzman reaction were also inhibited in rabbits in the study of Evans and Mustard.[151] Many attempts to use DIC models for testing sulfinpyrazone appeared later, particularly those with arachidonic acid injection causing a pulmonary distress with subsequent death of animals of various species. This model was supposed to be specific for TXA_2 production,[152] but considerable objections have been raised.[153] The model may reflect bronchoconstricting and vasoconstricting activity as well as a mediation by products of the lipoxygenase pathway. It was used for testing sulfinpyrazone e.g., by Rüegg,[37] Kohler et al.,[154] Philp et al.,[82] and Vigdahl.[155] The drug orally administered was effective at doses between 10 and 30 mg/kg.

A different methodology was chosen by Duling et al.[156] who used an electrical stimulation and microelectrophoretic administration of vasoactive agents in the microcirculation of the hamster cheek pouch. The drugs were administered orally 1 h before thrombus induction and sulfinpyrazone at a dose of 20 mg/kg was effective in preventing white body formation. A similar method was used by Lewis and Westwick in 1975.[157] Instead of mechanical injury and iontophoretic administration, they used electrical lesions inflicted by a KCl-electrode to count thrombi developing during the first 4 min after stimulation. The latter was graded by duration. Already from a dose of 20 mg/kg orally sulfinpyrazone caused a significant decrease in white body formation. ASA was somewhat more effective and a bell-shaped dose-effect curve was obtained with a maximum around 10 mg/kg. A tendency to a similar optimum was observed with sulfinpyrazone. The authors were also able to measure the vessel diameter.

Laser or mechanical stimulation was used in a similar hamster preparation by Wiedman in 1979,[158] also including a bat wing model to his series of methods. Sulfinpyrazone at a dose of 50 mg/kg i.v. or i.p. influenced white body formation both in the hamster and the bat. Thrombus growth only and not the formation of initial aggregates was influenced.

Another microcirculation model was developed by Adams and Mitchell in 1979[159] in rabbit pial arteries injured by forceps and combined with topical ADP administration. Whereas heparin remained almost without effect, sulfinpyrazone was effective at the dose of 40 mg/kg, i.e., a relatively high dose level.

Several groups of investigators used the model of thrombosis induced by electric current in the rat originally described by Hladovec.[160] In the study of Philp et al.,[82] sulfinpyrazone was effective at a dose of 100 mg/kg i.v., ASA only at the level of 200 mg/kg, and VK 744 (a dipyridamole analogue) was effective at approximately the same doses as sulfinpyrazone. The method is quantitative and objective but the degree of inflicted damage to the vessel wall is too high. The same method was used by Vigdahl et al.[155] In their hands sulfinpyrazone was significantly effective at a dose of 25 mg/kg orally 4 h before thrombus induction. ASA was only effective at a much higher dose level.

A mechanical lesion of the aorta (crushing with forceps) was used in the rat by Wilkinson[161] and thrombus formation was estimated by platelet loss and survival of radiolabeled platelets. Sulfinpyrazone and ticlopidine were effective (sulfinpyrazone after 60 mg/kg orally).

Arfors et al.[162] inflicted severe trauma to rabbit femoral veins by morrhuate and combined it with stasis. Sulfinpyrazone, like ASA, dipyridamole, and VK 744 were without effect and the author stressed the agreement of this result with an ineffectiveness of platelet-inhibiting agents in clinical venous thrombosis. On the other hand, these clinical studies were based on the prevention of postoperative venous thrombosis often associated also with a severe vascular lesion just as in the model of rabbits. An increasing degree of venous vascular damage is probably connected with a decreasing relative platelet contribution to the thrombotic process. A similar decreasing activating effect on platelets may be related to decreasing extensity of the lesion.

Several models designed for sulfinpyrazone testing included the use of various AV-shunts, extracorporeal circulations, and generally, thrombus formation on artificial surfaces. These experimental studies were preceded by the positive clinical studies of Kaegi et al.[147,148] and Pineo et al.[163] demonstrating prevention of occlusion of the AV-shunts by sulfinpyrazone. The first experimental study with AV-shunt was the negative or almost negative study of Mustard et al.[149] In another study, Mason et al.[54] used AV-shunts in monkeys including the insertion of a "captured vortex" device. All the tested antiplatelet agents were effective including ASA, dipyridamole, and sulfinpyrazone. The last one was not very effective, but the dose was relatively low (3 mg/kg/d orally). In the study of Wilkinson et al.,[161] a Dacron® prosthesis was inserted into the aorta of dogs and platelet survival was determined with radiolabeled platelets together with the platelet loss. Sulfinpyrazone at a dose of 60 mg/kg orally (twice daily) significantly increased platelet survival and decreased total platelet loss. Birek et al.[164] studied decreases in platelet counts during perfusion of a membrane oxygenator in sheep. Sulfinpyrazone prevented platelet loss and the increase in pulmonary vascular resistance after the addition of 1000 to 1500 mg/h to the perfusate. Heparin was without effect. Townsend et al.[165] also estimated the preservation of platelets during an extracorporeal circulation in sheep. A membrane oxygenator was inserted into the veno-venous shunt. Sulfinpyrazone, 1.5 g, was given intravenously and improved platelet preservation while ASA (50 mg/kg i.v.) was without effect. Both drugs prevented the increase in vascular pulmonary resistance. The author suggested a very different action of both drugs, with sulfinpyrazone affecting aggregation and primary platelet adhesion. Hanson et al.[66] investigated the activity of sulfinpyrazone in an AV-shunt in baboons. The rate of platelet utilization was assessed by the disappearance of radiolabeled platelets from the blood. Sulfinpyrazone was already effective at a dose of 20 mg/kg/d p.o., while ASA and dazoxiben were ineffective and dipyridamole somewhat more effective than sulfinpyrazone. However, ASA potentiated the effect of sulfinpyrazone. The authors concluded that the prostanoid system is of no importance in their model. While the mechanism of sulfinpyrazone action was not explained, it was suggested that it may predominantly influence endothelium. Meanwhile, the same conclusion was reached in another study of this group[166] in which sulfinpyrazone (100 mg/kg/d orally) was effective in preventing endothelial lesions in baboons administered homocysteine by chronic infusion. The degree of lesions was evaluated by morphometry. In addition, sulfinpyrazone normalized platelet survival. *In vitro* effects of homocysteine in endothelial cell cultures were more problematic and the authors suggested the existence of some indirect mechanism.

An interesting group of models, quite different from those generally used for testing antithrombotics, were based on the effect of sulfinpyrazone on inflammatory reactions and particularly those associated with the activation of the immune system. This effect is probably related to the contribution of platelets. Butler et al.[167,168] and Butler and White[169] studied the inhibition of Arthus reaction in guinea pigs. Sulfinpyrazone at a dose of 50 mg/kg i.v. inhibited the resulting thrombocytopenia. Some other antiplatelet agents were also effective (ASA 10 mg/kg, indomethacin), but dipyridamole was ineffective. In some experiments platelet sequestration in the lungs was quantitatively assessed by radiolabeled platelets. Whereas with some drugs, a correlation of *in vivo* and *in vitro* or *ex vivo* studies with platelet aggregation was present to some extent, with sulfinpyrazone it was not. Of course, immune reaction of Arthus type is a very complex process and sulfinpyrazone might have interfered at various stages (production of mediator effects on various targets except platelets, etc.). A similar complexity has to be accepted in response to the Forssman reagent where sulfinpyrazone was also effective, but in general, high doses were necessary. However, its favorable effect in models of allograft rejection (Sharma et al.,[170] in dogs, Vaessen et al.,[171] in rats, and Jamiesson,[172] in rats) might have some implication for clinical therapy.

Rügg[37] pointed out that sulfinpyrazone at a dose of 30 mg/kg orally is capable of restoring the blood fibrinolytic activity after a kaolin-induced rat paw edema. Whether this is connected with the anti-inflammatory activity, effect on leukocytes, or direct induction of fibrinolysis was difficult to decide. By any means, the dosage is very high.

A series of models was developed for testing sulfinpyrazone in connection with the somewhat problematic results of the large clinical study of secondary myocardial infarction prevention (ART) concluded in 1975.[173] The favorable effect was suspected to be based on a mechanism other than antithrombotic, or at least on the prevention of some special consequences of platelet thrombus formation. Thus, Moschos et al.[174,175] found that sulfinpyrazone prevented arrhythmias, ECG changes, and ionic shifts in the myocardium after the occlusion of a coronary by balloon catheters in dogs. The dose was 300 mg for 7 d. A similar antiarrhythmic effect was observed in the canine coronary occlusion-reperfusion model (30 mg/kg/d) by Povalski,[176] in cats by Kelliker,[177] and in pigs by Stäubli et al.[178] Inhibition of cyclical flow changes caused by formation and embolism of platelet thrombi in dogs with a mechanical coronary stenosis was observed by Folts.[179] The effective dose was 30 mg/kg i.v. Adrenochrome-induced arrhythmias in rats were prevented by sulfinpyrazone in the study of Beamish et al.,[180] isoproterenol-induced myocardial necrosis was inhibited by high doses (100 mg/kg orally) in the study of Hashimoto and Ogawa,[181] and the severity of myocardial infarction induced by coronary ligation or isoproterenol administration was reduced in rats by Innes and Weisman.[182] Russell[183] observed a decrease in arrhythmias in dogs with occluded coronaries after 30 mg/kg of sulfinpyrazone i.v. and suggested that a decreased heart rate might be responsible.

Clopath and Horsch[184] noted some antiatherosclerotic activity of sulfinpyrazone at very high doses in rats and rabbits but not in swine.

More recently, there have only been a few experimental studies on sulfinpyrazone published with more attention paid, probably not quite deservedly, to drugs influencing the prostaglandin system.

The studies carried out in the author's laboratory included the effect of *in vivo* platelet sequestration in rats. A marked effect was observed of relatively low doses of the drug (1 mg/kg orally) (Figure 11).[185] Here, it should be remembered that this is not a thrombosis model. It shows the transient adhesion of platelets on a slightly injured systemic endothelium resulting in a very limited desquamation with a subsequent acute decrease in platelet counts. Basically, this adhesion is a defense reaction and may also be followed by some aggregation on adhering platelets. The small aggregates either disintegrate on the spot or after embolization into the periphery.

The effect on the endothelial stability test with an extended series of doses is shown in another diagram (Figure 12).[186] It is evident that a much less marked optimum (bell-shaped curve) is observed as compared with ASA. The drug was effective at doses quite inferior to the clinical dose level showing that the effect on endothelial stability might be of importance in its antithrombotic effect.

In the routine battery of models, sulfinpyrazone exerted a stabilizing effect on the endothelium after both citrate and hypotonic saline stimulus at the level of 0.5 mg/kg orally, in the arterial thrombosis model at the dose level of 1 to 2 mg/kg orally, and surprisingly, at the same dose level in the venous model (Figure 13). This high activity in the venous model is probably due to the relatively important contribution of platelets together with the vessel lesion in the model. Activity in the arterial model is practically the same, 1 and 6 h after the oral administration, casting some doubt on the alleged importance of metabolites based mainly on *in vitro* or *ex vivo* studies (Figure 14).

In general, sulfinpyrazone was effective in many models. We have seen that its antithrombotic effect, if its existence is accepted, might be based on the effect on platelet adhesion rather than on aggregation, on aggregation in the presence of a weak stimulus, on the inhibition of release (e.g., of serotonin), or on the handling of serotonin, in general. It may likewise be based on the effect on endothelial functions rather than on the effect on platelets.

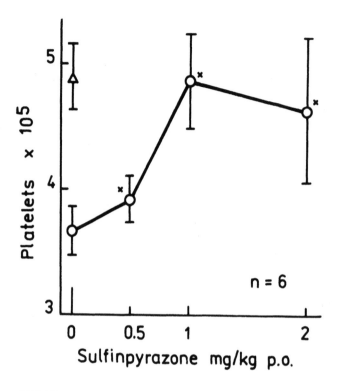

FIGURE 11.   Effect of oral sulfinpyrazone on platelet sequestration after the citrate challenge.

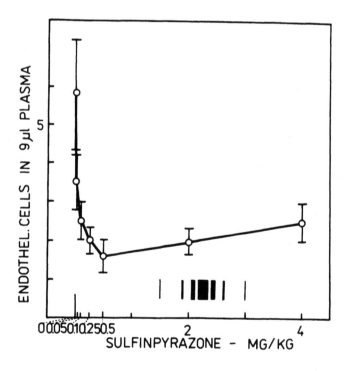

FIGURE 12.   Effect of oral sulfinpyrazone on endothelial stability after the i.v. citrate challenge.

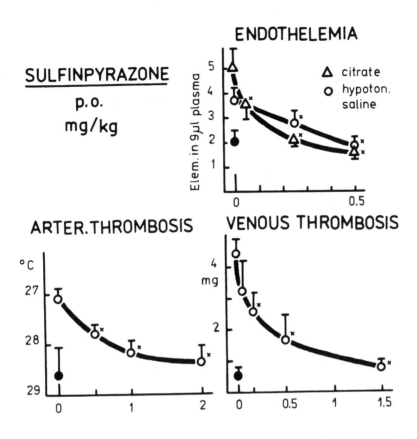

FIGURE 13.   Effect of oral sulfinpyrazone in the standard battery of models.

There exists apparently the multiplicity of effects mentioned already with other drugs. Provided we support a "monistic" theory we could forcibly attempt to reduce all these activities to one common for all situations, or we can simply accept that this multiplicity of effects is a matter of fact. The monistic theory could operate, for example, with the prostaglandin theory, but why then is the effect of aspirin so different? Or else we could suppose the existence of some vague mechanism such as a "membrane" effect caused by some physicochemical changes in the membrane properties. The drug unquestionably has many activities other than antithrombotic; it is a uricosuric, to some extent an antiphlogistic, it affects some immune reactions, arrhythmias, etc. For the time being, it may be concluded that the mechanism decisive for its antithrombotic activity is unknown, but that the interference with the interaction platelets-vessel wall or even with other surfaces may be important with both components influenced relatively more or less according to the actual situation.

IV. HEPARIN

Heparin is generally considered an anticoagulant. Testing anticoagulants seemed to pose no problem as their antithrombotic activity was often thought to be entirely reflected by their *in vitro* anticoagulant effect. This is not correct as the spectrum of heparin activities is obviously much broader.[187] Its indications overlap to some extent with those of antiplatelet agents, particularly if low dose heparin employed to prevent thrombotic phenomena even on the arterial side of circulation is taken into account. This is illustrated by the favorable results of a large Italian clinical study addressing methods of prevention of mycoardial infarction.[188] In this connection, it is important to distinguish two kinds of heparin use. One can be called "pharmacological" as very large doses have little in common with the presumed

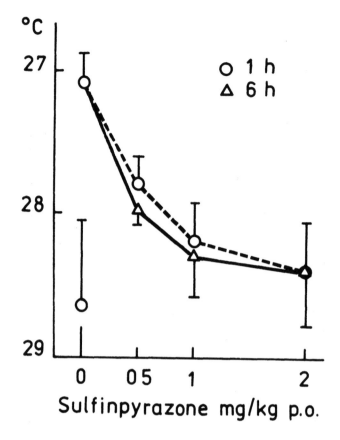

FIGURE 14.   Effect of sulfinpyrazone in the arterial model at two intervals after oral administration.

physiological functions of heparin, are closely associated with high blood levels of the agent, and consequently, can be monitored quite accurately using various *ex vivo* tests. The corresponding indications represent acute situations with the administration of the drug mostly in intravenous infusions and the aim of such treatment is to arrest the growth of already present thrombi and emboli and thus shift the dynamic equilibrium of thrombus producing and removing processes in favor of the latter. Meanwhile, the activation of thrombolysis by heparin and its derivatives is still a matter of controversy. The other group of heparin use is often of subacute or chronic character, is aimed at the prevention of thrombus initiation, and the doses are low or even ultra low. The route of administration is most often subcutaneous. The effect is probably localized much less in the blood than on the vascular surface and *ex vivo* tests could not be used reliably for its monitoring. In fact, no monitoring at all is often preferred. This application of heparin probably has much more in common with its physiological function and in the study of this kind of heparin effect animal models are indispensable particularly if some low molecular heparin derivatives, heparinoids, or combinations with other types of antithrombotics are investigated. This section is concerned mainly with this second type of heparin use, i.e., prevention of venous as well as arterial thrombosis.

Heparin is not a homogeneous drug. It is a mixture of molecules differing in chain length, and presumably, even in their exact composition. The recent interest in low molecular heparin derivatives has largely contributed to our knowledge of its most active components from particular points of view, e.g., inhibition of Xa factor. Of course, this is like breeding animals which while possessing some extra properties that might be useful for some special purposes, have lost much of their general utility and adaptability. Here again, isolated *in vitro* tests might easily supply misleading information. As pointed out by Jaques,[187] the total mixture of chains must be considered "the active principle" until proved on the contrary. While this ultimate proof would be clinical, animal models may supply most useful predictions.

Heparin disappears from the plasma after intravenous administration rapidly in an exponential way, and after high doses its presence may be demonstrated for 2 to 3 h. It is almost inactive alone and a manifestation of its activity is dependent on the presence of AT III and much less on heparin cofactor II. With high doses the unsaturable mechanism, mainly renal excretion, is of decisive importance for its elimination. With lower doses the saturable mechanism is preeminent. This is based on the binding of heparin to the vascular endothelium and the reticuloendothelial system.[189-193] Exogenous heparin replaces, at least partially, heparin monosulfate normally present on the endothelial surface in close association with AT III.[194] In this way exogenous heparin imparts an increased negative charge to the endothelial surface.[187] As the endothelium is also the site of action of adsorbed and activated blood-clotting factors, heparin may be at this active surface, also including platelets, incomparably more effective than in the blood and consequently, much lower concentrations are necessary.[195]

The question of heparin interaction with platelets is a very complex one. Under special artificial conditions heparin may inhibit platelet aggregation induced by collagen but, in general, tends to enhance aggregation and to potentiate the effects of many aggregating agents.[196,197] Most authors do not accept any antiaggregating activity of heparin unless a very high concentration has been reached. The aggregating activity was, at first, tentatively connected with admixtures in heparin preparations. This is probably not true. Though more recent studies comparing the effect of heparin with that of its low molecular derivatives mostly show some differences in favor of the latter, such differences are not substantial. Presumably the effect on platelet aggregation is somehow connected with the activity of heparin. Another question concerns the importance of *in vitro* findings which may be readily influenced by artificial conditions and even by species differences. Clinical observations of serious postheparin thrombocytopenias are rare. There could be some relation to low AT III level, immune reaction, etc. As a matter of fact, *in vitro* findings concerning the interaction of heparin with platelets do not need to be of any importance for the pathological interaction of platelets with the vessel wall. Under such conditions thrombin and factor Xa adsorbed on the endothelium and platelets may be of decisive importance for platelet adhesion and aggregation, and there is no question of effectiveness of heparin in the inhibition of the activity of these factors.[198] In artificial situations such as adhesion of platelets to isolated and everted vessels (e.g., Essien et al.[199]) these properties of heparin do not need to become manifested due to the antiheparin properties of more or less damaged biological materials. Heparin is, of course, mainly an anticoagulant. As such, it can also influence the stabilization of platelet thrombi by fibrin, and hence, the change from a reversible, basically defensive hemostatic process into the relatively irreversible actual thrombus formation.

Jaques pointed out the discrepancy of heparin effects *in vitro* and *in vivo* as manifested in the time latency of antithrombotic activity development in comparison with the anticoagulant one which is almost immediate. This discrepancy was also illustrated by the experimental and clinical antithrombotic effectiveness of ultra low doses while their *in vitro* effects were practically undemonstrable. Another example was repeatedly observed in the studies with LMW-heparin, heparinoids, and related mucopolysaccharides which may be ineffective *in vitro* while highly effective *in vivo* as antithrombotics (e.g., heparan monosulfate) and vice versa. This discrepancy further emphasizes the necessity to use animal models for testing heparin and heparin-like agents.

First studies of the antithrombotic effect of heparin in animals, mostly dogs, were of a particularly old date going back to the period before World War II. In 1937, Murray et al.[200]

for the first time used dog radial and saphenous veins for thrombus induction. A silk thread was inserted into the lumen with a needle and the vein was crushed over the thread with forceps. In some experiments sodium ricinoleate was injected into an occluded vein segment. Heparin had a good antithrombotic effect. Best[201] used a similar method involving a mechanical crushing in several animal species as well as occlusions of extracorporeal shunts in dogs.[202] Rabinowich and Pines[203] damaged rabbit veins mechanically, Reimann-Hunziker[204] by external application of ferric chloride and Moses[205] combined stasis with cotton thread stitches in dogs to demonstrate heparin effects. Loewe et al.[206,207] injured the jugular veins of rabbits mechanically, Kiesewetter and Shumaker[208] damaged veins as well as arteries in dogs by penetrating double silk sutures combined with clamps or by a sutured closure of transected vessels. All found heparin effective. Friedrich[209] found the heparinoid thrombocid effective in a varicocid-induced venous thrombosis in rabbits. In most of the above-mentioned studies, heparin was more or less effective but the dosage was relatively very high and often not sufficiently defined. Local damage was, as a rule, rather excessive. Improvement in sensitivity was achieved by a better design of the model in 1953 by Wessler[210] and in 1955 by Wessler and Morris[211] who combined venous stasis with an injection of serum or serum derivatives in dogs. Heparin was effective already at clinical therapeutic doses (0.23 mg/kg i.e., about 20 to 30 U/kg) but merely 60% of thrombi were prevented.

In other studies, about twofold prolongation of coagulation times was sufficient to prevent thrombus formation completely. In 1963 Jarret and Jaques,[212] using the venous thrombosis model of Murray, investigated the antithrombotic activity of the heparinoid G 31150 in dogs. In rats they used formol-methanol-induced lesions, and dog plasma after the injection of the tested agent was also used in rats. In the dose of 10 mg/kg the compound was highly effective. Borgström et al.[213] induced in 1959 a humoral defect with blunt blows by a padded hammer on the thigh muscles of rabbits often on the contralateral side of a cephalad ligature of their femoral veins. The injury was dosed by the number of blows and often 200 blows were used. Heparin was effective at a dose of 25 to 50 mg/kg (i.e., about 3000 U/kg). Blake et al.[214] preferred smaller animals (rats) for inducing a jugular vein injury by an external application of a formol-methanol solution. Heparin was only effective at a very high dose level (5000 to 10,000 U/kg). Williams and Carey,[215] Williams and Karaffa,[216] and Carey and Williams,[217] in a series of studies, investigated heparin effects in dogs with electrically induced thrombosis of jugular veins. Heparin was effective with clotting times *ex vivo* increased by a factor of 2.5. Zweifler[218] attained only a partial effect in the prevention of electrically induced thrombus growth in dogs with heparin administered subcutaneously or intravenously at doses of 90 to 200 mg/d. Allison and Lancaster[219] in their study of heat-damaged rabbit ear microcirculation and Zambouras et al.[220] with a severe lesion of dog veins by sodium morrhuate were unsuccessful with heparin just as Honour and Russell[221] using cortical or mesenteric microvessels (arterioles and venules) in rabbits, rats, and pigeons as well as various kinds of stimuli. Also unsuccessful were Jewell et al.[222] in rabbit ear vein thrombosis induced by monoethanolamine oleate. Fulton et al.[223] observed under similar conditions, even an enhancement of white body formation in rabbits. It is important to note that the ineffectiveness of heparin in the microcirculation thrombosis cannot be interpreted as proof of ineffectiveness of heparin on the arterial side of circulation, but rather a lack of effect on some prethrombotic or hemostatic reactions of platelets in a very special kind of the circulatory bed.

Ashwin observed in 1962 (see Chapter 1) a rebound enhancement of thrombosis in the rat jugular vein induced by external administration of formalin. This rebound occurred if heparin had been injected more than 4 h before thrombus induction. Hoak et al.[224] noted full prevention of thrombosis by heparin if coagulation times were longer than 60 min. York et al.[225] were again unsuccessful in the prevention of thrombosis in the hamster cheek pouch microcirculation. Mustard et al.[226] observed positive effects in the pig extracorporeal circulation and noted a rebound 4 h after the heparin injection. Hoak et al.[227] demonstrated that heparin was more effective than dicoumarol in a DIC model based on intravenous administration of fatty acids in dogs. Just-Viera and Yeager[228] using heparin (about 1500 to 2000 U/kg) prevented thrombosis in large canine veins with inserted catheters. Williams and Karaffa[216] used their model of electric current-induced venous thrombosis in dogs to compare thrombolysis after heparin and trypsin. They mentioned spontaneous thrombolysis occurring very frequently in dogs. Jorgensen et al.[229] followed the fate of thrombi in rabbits for several weeks and suspected a thrombolytic effect of heparin. They used either partially ligated arteries and veins with staphylococcal alpha-hemolysin injected into the vessel wall or tissue thromboplastin into the lumen, this time with a complete ligation. Heparin did not significantly prevent thrombus formation but the quality of thrombi was markedly influenced. Renaud[230] used his model of endotoxin thrombus induction in hyperlipemic rats. Heparin counteracted thrombosis when administered at very high doses. This is in contrast with the more recent studies of Müller-Berghaus and Hocke[231] who observed no effect of heparin in endotoxin thrombosis, whereas Theiss[232] confirmed the effect of heparin in endotoxin DIC in rats. Presumably, the quality of endotoxin plays a role, with some preparations leading to a more massive release of antiheparin activity from the endothelium and platelets. Hunt et al.[233] induced thrombosis by electric current in sheep arteries and veins. Heparin administered at a dose of 10,000 U i.v. every 8 h was an effective inhibitor, moreover, enhancing thrombolysis. The method was similar to that used by Zweifler[218] and Hoppenstein et al.[334] in dogs. The latter group concluded that heparin was effective irrespective of the route of administration (s.c. or i.v., 90 to 200 mg/d). In their experiments carried out in dogs, Rowsell et al.[235] studied platelet survival and found it prolonged after moderate heparin doses (50 U/kg). High doses (200 U/kg) were without effect and caused increased permeability. Reber[236] investigated the influence of heparin on electrically induced thrombi in rabbits. Heparin was effective, while in experiments with laser-induced thrombi in rabbits conducted by Arfors in 1968,[99] heparin (1200 U/kg) was without effect just as in the microcirculation studies of Didisheim[20] in rat intestinal loops with electric current as the stimulus. Fahlström et al.[237] in 1970 induced venous thrombosis in rats by combining stasis with a fracture trauma and intravenous tissue thromboplastin. Heparin was effective at doses of about 2000 U/kg. Turina in 1971[113] used an intracardiac device (metal probe) in dogs. Heparin was effective in preventing thrombi. No effect was observed on the survival of monkey cardiac allografts in presensitized dogs (1 mg/kg before and 4 mg/4 h after transplantation). Some improvement in renal allograft survival after heparin, particularly in combination with vasodilators, was observed by Colman et al.[239] Spilker and van Balken[27] demonstrated that heparin (5000 U/kg) was effective in the prevention of white body formation in the mesenteric and cortical microcirculation of five species after electric stimulation. Bourgain and Six[240] introduced a continuous registration method in the rat mesenterium using electric stimulation and heparin, at a dose of 2000 U/kg, was effective as a preventive agent. De Clerck et al.[241] described a modification of venous stasis thrombosis in the rat induced by the combination of stasis with an intravenous injection of ellagic acid. When administered at a relatively low dose of 10 and 20 U/kg i.v., heparin exerted a marked antithrombotic effect. Using heparin (1400 U/kg i.v.) Gertz et al.[242] protected the rabbit carotid artery against thrombotic occlusion after ischemic injury as demonstrated by electron microscopy.

Tkomikawa in 1975[38] observed an inhibitory effect of heparin at doses of about 300 U/kg in his model of lactic acid-induced DIC and Owen and Bowie[243] observed only a partial effect on thromboplastin-induced DIC in dogs. It was ineffective on fibrin monomer accumulation in rabbits.[244]

Heparin was effective in an extracorporeal model in dogs in the hands of Benis et al.[53] Barth in 1975[48] used rabbits for inducing stasis thrombi in jugular veins (Wessler's type) and found heparin most effective. Birek et al.[164] observed no effect of heparin during veno-

venous membrane oxygenator perfusion in sheep. On the other hand, Peipgras et al.[32] described a favorable effect of heparin as the only agent in cats with endarterectomized carotid arteries. Chiu et al.[245] investigated the relation of *in vitro* and *in vivo* activity of heparin using experimental venous thrombosis in rabbits. Radiofibrinogen accretion of thrombin plus stasis-induced jugular vein thrombosis was estimated. Heparin at a dose of 300 to 900 U/kg/10 h proved to be effective. Urizar et al. noted in 1979[246] the preventive effect in a DIC model in rats using a Liquoid induction. Adams and Mitchell[159] observed no effect of heparin at a relatively moderate dose in the cortical microcirculation of rabbits after a mechanical trauma. In the model of Seuter et al.[247] heparin was effective at doses of 1 to 3 mg/kg s.c. (i.e. about 200 to 600 U/kg). Thrombi were induced by the freezing technique in rat arteries. With venous thrombi about 150 U/kg s.c. were effective.[248] Kumada et al.[249] induced venous thrombosis in rats by inserting a stainless steel coil into the inferior vena cava of rats and heparin administered at a very high dose (500 to 1000 U/kg s.c.) was effective. Lavelle and McIomhair[250] induced venous thrombosis in rats by the insertion of a platinum wire into the vena cava with the addition, in some experiments, of ellagic acid or EACA administration. Heparin was effective with a good dose-effect relation. Reyers et al.[251] employed heparin in the prevention of arterial prosthesis occlusion in the rat abdominal aorta. Heparin was effective at a dose of 500 U/kg particularly if administered immediately before prosthesis insertion and in combination with an anti-rat antiserum. In the hands of Pangrazzi et al.[252,253] heparin was likewise effective in thrombus prevention after a one-sided cephalad ligature of the rat vena cava. Here the lesion was relatively mild and the necessary dose low (ca 75 U/kg). Performing experiments in dogs, Fedelles et al.[254] investigated the uptake of radiolabeled platelets in fresh venous thrombi. Heparin was effective at doses of 300 U/kg administered i.v. in bolus and followed by 90 U/kg/h infusions. Carter et al.[255] investigated the effect of a LMW-heparin in comparison with that of native heparin in rabbits on radiofibrinogen accretion to a thrombin-induced thrombus in an ear vein. Both substances proved to be equally effective. Smith and White[51] employed heparin to suppress the production of a mixed thrombus induced in A/V-shunts of bats by insertion of a cotton thread. Relatively low doses of 35 to 50 U/kg were effective. Collen et al.[256] prevented thrombus growth in rabbit jugular veins by 500 U/kg heparin s.c. as demonstrated by radiofibrinogen accretion. Doutremepuich et al. represented one of several groups over the past few years studying *in vivo* effects of LMW-heparins in comparison with native heparin. In their studies,[257-259] they used the Reyers model (single ligature of the inferior vena cava). According to their opinion, the molecular weight and anti-Xa activity cannot predict the *in vivo* effect. Both anti-IIa and anti-Xa activities seemed to be involved *in vivo*. This finding contradicts, to some extent, those reported by Bara et al.[260,261] who particularly stressed the necessity of anti-Xa activity. In general, a marked lack of correlation was noted between *in vitro* and *in vivo* activities in most such studies. Bianchini et al.[269] observed potentiation of stasis thrombosis by the hyperlipemia producing surface-active agent Tyloxapol in rats and LMW-heparin was very active as an antithrombotic. Ostergaard et al.[270] studied the effect of LMW-heparin in the prevention of jugular vein thrombosis in rabbits induced by ethoxysclerol. Its effectiveness was comparable to that of native heparin. Under similar conditions Mattson et al.[271] investigated LMW-heparin. Millet et al.[73] introduced a new venous thrombosis model associated with a relatively mild vascular trauma (distension of the rat vena cava by saline injection). Heparin was already effective at dose levels not demonstrating any anticoagulant activity *ex vivo*. Merton et al.[272,273] studied dermatan sulfate in comparison to native heparin in rabbit stasis thrombosis. While heparin at a dose of 150 μg/kg (ca 22 U/kg) inhibited thrombus formation completely, dermatan sulfate at the same dose (w/kg) was only partially effective. LMW-heparin was investigated by Reber et al.[274] in a veno-venous bypass for CO_2 removal in dogs. Standard heparin was more effective (300 U/kg followed by 100 U/kg/h). Shand et al.[275] studied the deposition of radiofibrinogen and labeled platelets in mechanically injured rabbit carotids. Heparin 250 U/kg i.v. did not and 670 U/kg did inhibit the depostion while leaving permeability changes unaffected. However, heparin prevented atherosclerosis-like proliferative changes in rat arteries damaged by chilling in the hands of Seuter et al.[276] Cyclic "thrombus" formation in the stenosed and mechanically damaged rabbit aorta was inhibited significantly by 800 U/kg heparin in the study of Kuhn et al.[277] In an experimental DIC model in the dog using tissue thromboplastin injection as a challenge,[278] heparin exerted some protective effect and manifested more than that of some tested heparinoids. Schmidt et al.[279] demonstrated an inhibitory effect of heparin (10 U/kg) on radiofibrinogen incorporation into a jugular venostatic thrombus in pigs and piglets. Heparin was more effective in adult animals probably reflecting an AT III deficiency in newborn animals. LMW-heparin potentiated thrombolysis in a rabbit jugular vein thrombosis model.[280,281] Bergqvist and Nilsson[282] demonstrated the possibility of combining LMW-heparin with DHE in ethoxysclerol plus stasis-induced rabbit jugular vein thrombosis and Fenichel et al.[283] compared LMW-heparin with standard heparin in a stasis thrombosis model in rabbits. On the weight basis the activity of both agents was similar. Heparinoid SP 54 was tested in a Wessler type rabbit venous thrombosis by Vassiliou at al.[284] The agent was effective just as in a previous study with cat venous thrombosis published by Bicher.[285]

When attempting to draw some comprehensive conclusions from the presented bulk of data, some points seem to be evident:

1. Little or no effect of heparin is seen in the microcirculation.
2. Less activity at least by one order of magnitude was observed in arterial thrombosis as compared with venous thrombosis while both were very dependent on the model design.
3. Heparin was mostly tested and was also quite effective in venous thrombosis models, but with severe trauma particularly if connected with a massive release of tissue thromboplastin and other antiheparin materials, it may be ineffective. On the other hand, only one dose was often tested and the models were, in general, not sufficeintly quantitative to detect a partial effect. For prevention purposes, full suppression of thrombus formation is probably not necessary. In some of the most sensitive tests (e.g., Wessler type of models), rather low doses of heparin were effective but this effect was often incomplete.
4. A lack of correlation between *in vitro* and *in vivo* effects was often observed particularly in the low dose range. Similarly, little *in vitro-in vivo* activity relations were observed between heparin and heparin derivatives.

Heparin was also tested in the author's laboratory in several types of models. Thus, heparin was used in the rat arterial model with thrombosis induced by electric current.[81] It was partially effective at a relatively high dose level of 300 U/kg and completely effective at a dose of 1000 U/kg i.v. (Figure 15). In a previously used model of venous thrombosis induced by the combination of stasis and a mild systemic endothelial lesion in rat mesenteric intestinal loops, heparin at a dose of 10 U/kg was significantly effective in the kaolin modification. Thrombus formation was completely inhibited at 100 U/kg (Figure 16).[286] In the platelet sequestration model reflecting the influence on platelet adhesion *in vivo* together with the effect on the endothelium and the interaction of both, two kinds of intravenous challenges were used: citrate (1.52%) and hypotonic saline (0.225% NaCl).[83] Heparin was about twice as effective with hypotonic saline than with citrate as a challenge, attaining a significant inhibition at 250 U/kg and complete inhibition at 1000 U/kg, respectively (Figure 17). This is in agreement with the results obtained in the endothelemia model where heparin was almost ten times more effective if hypotonic saline was used as a challenge in comparison with citrate, and still more effective in comparison with epinephrine as a challenge (Figure 37 in Chapter 3).[287] It is evident that not only the degree of endothelial perturbation, but

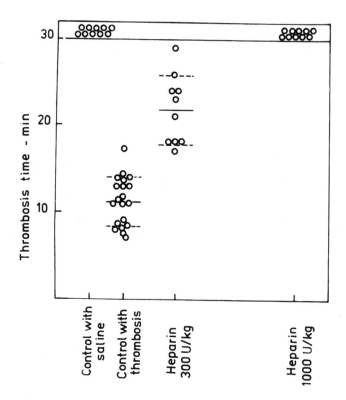

FIGURE 15.   Effect of heparin in the electrically induced thrombosis model.

also its quality is of importance for the sensitivity to heparin. Presumably, the quality is dependent on the release of antiheparin activity from tissues. The sensitivity of the endothelial test to the stabilizing effect was so high in the hypotonic saline modification that it was of some interest to investigate the activity of subcutaneous and oral administration of heparin (Figures 18, 19). Subcutaneous heparin is many times less effective than after intravenous administration also attaining much less complete maximum inhibition due probably to slow and insufficient release of the agent from the tissue. At a dose of 500 U/kg oral heparin was already significantly effective against the increased number of circulating elements after hypotonic saline. When tested in the standard battery of tests, heparin showed the highest effect in the venous model: the effective dose was less than 0.025 U/kg, while in the endothelemia model, the corresponding dose was about 0.05 U/kg.[139] Whether this stabilizing effect on the endothelium comes into play in the antithrombotic activity of heparin depends very much on the intensity and quality of the stimulus. Epinephrine as a stimulus seems to exert a particularly unfavorable influence in this respect (lesser effect of heparin under stress?). Arterial thrombosis was significantly inhibited at a dose level of 25 U/kg, which while being much less than in other models, is still within the relatively low clinical dose range (Figure 20).

It may be concluded that the battery of standard models used more recently was very sensitive to the heparin effect and that under the conditions of preventive administration the effect on the endothelium should be taken into account. This effect is balanced very finely with the adverse effect on platelets giving variable results according to details of experimental conditions.

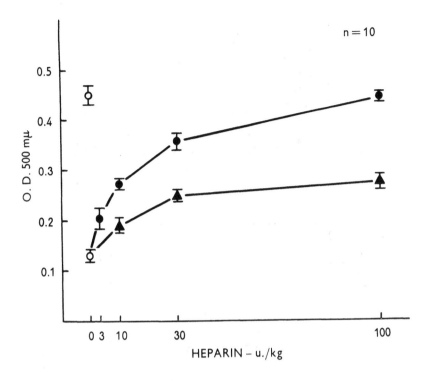

FIGURE 16. Effect of heparin in the mesenteric vessel venous thrombosis model (kaolin modification). Means ± S.E. Circles: heparin administered together with kaolin, triangles: both agents administered together.

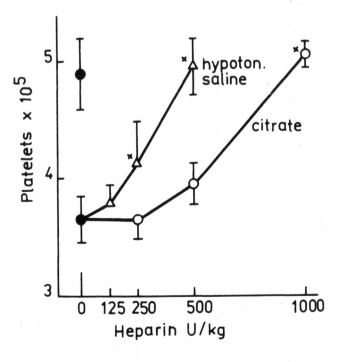

FIGURE 17. Effect of heparin on platelet sequestration after two challenges (citrate or hypotonic saline).

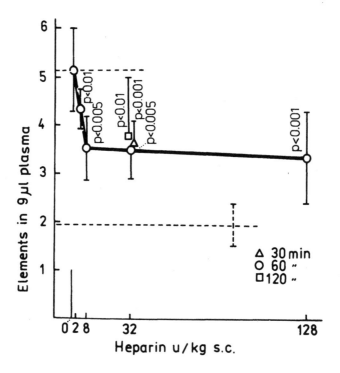

FIGURE 18.   Effect of s.c. heparin on endothelial stability after the hypotonic saline challenge.

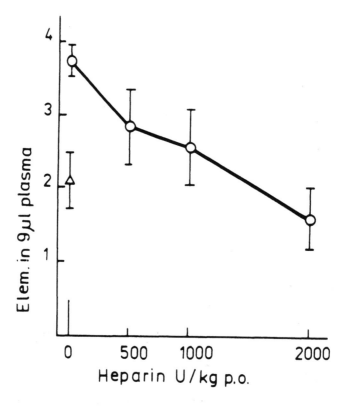

FIGURE 19.   Effect of oral heparin on endothelial stability after the hypotonic saline challenge.

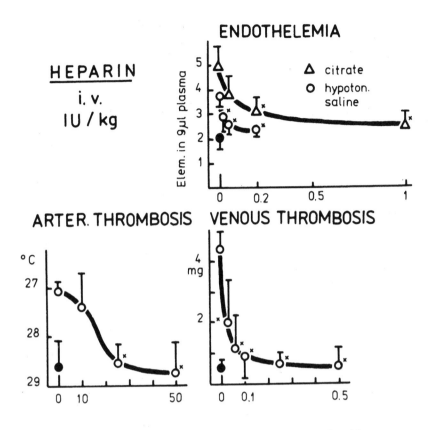

FIGURE 20.   Effect of i.v. heparin in the standard battery of models.

V. PENTOXIFYLLINE

Pentoxifylline was essentially developed as a hemorrheologically active drug suitable for the treatment of some peripheral vascular diseases. On the other hand, there exist many indications that it may also be a potential antithrombotic. Primarily, it should increase red blood cell deformability and consequently decrease the whole blood viscosity thus improving blood flow particularly in the microcirculation.

The drug is rapidly and extensively absorbed from the gastrointestinal tract in animals and in man. It is also rapidly metabolized with metabolites appearing in the urine. It is not bound to blood proteins and is uniformly distributed in the body without any accumulation.

Pentoxifylline has an antiaggregatory activity only at very high concentrations *in vitro*. At these concentrations, it might act by the inhibition of membrane-bound phosphodiesterase.[290] *Ex vivo* the drug is effective in therapeutic doses inhibiting both spontaneous, collagen, ADP, 5-HT, and epinephrine-induced aggregation and improving blood rheological properties.[291-297] It inhibits adhesion of platelets to the arterial wall in rabbits kept on a high cholesterol diet.[298] The effect on platelets is often interpreted by the release of prostacyclin from the vascular wall,[295,299-302] or by inhibition of thromboxane synthetase.[302]

In animal thrombosis models, pentoxifylline was generally effective. Thrombosis in arterioles of the rat mesenteric microcirculation induced by laser shots was significantly prevented by 10 mg/kg p.o. The quantification was carried out by counting necessary laser shots. The thrombus formation depressing effect lasted for about 3 h after a single dose.[303] White body formation induced by iontophoretic topical administration of ADP in the venules of the hamster cheek pouch was inhibited by the dose of 10 mg/kg i.p.[304] In an arachidonic acid-induced DIC in rats pentoxifylline decreased intravascular red cell aggregation and their

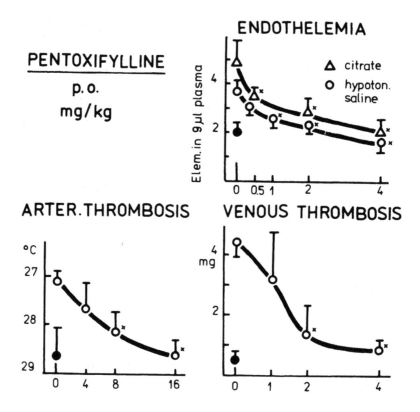

FIGURE 21.   Effect of pentoxifylline in the standard battery of models.

lysis but did not prevent mortality.[305] Puranapanda et al.[306] demonstrated the effect of pentoxifylline on erythrocyte deformability in a canine septic shock. The activation of fibrinolysis *in vivo* was described in some studies.[296,307,308]

To summarize, pentoxifylline is a powerful membrane active agent as demonstrated by its effect on erythrocyte deformability. As such it probably induced membrane reorganization in platelets and endothelial cells which is necessarily leading to changes in the balance of pro- and antithrombotic functions of these elements with these functions generally localized on their membranes. It is highly improbable that all the documented changes in PGI_2, TXA_2, tPA, PAI, fibrinogen, AT III, 5-HT, etc. as reported, e.g., by Angelkort,[309] with all of them in the favorable direction, could be specific at the same time. Thus, the inhibition of thrombus formation in animal models is probably the result of an indirect favorable membrane effect.

In the author's laboratory, pentoxifylline was investigated in the routine battery of standard tests (Figure 21). The results show that the drug was effective in all three tests. The inhibition of venous thrombosis was surprisingly achieved by doses lower than in arterial thrombosis. They were approximately equal to those effective in the endothelemia model (ca 2 mg/kg p.o.). In the arterial model the effective dose was 8 mg/kg p.o. This points to an effect directed more against the vascular wall rather than against platelets. At the same time, even the dose effective in the arterial model is still in the clinical range and shows that the drug may be used generally as an antithrombotic. Particularly interesting was the preventive effect against venous thrombosis which may be based on the regulatory role of endothelium in its pathogenesis (fibrinolysis, coagulation inhibitors).

VI. TICLOPIDINE

Ticlopidine, while not free of side effects, is a most interesting drug as it has little in common with other antithrombotics thus introducing a new and previously unknown aspect into the problem. It is a thienopyridine derivative quite rapidly absorbed after oral administration and also rapidly metabolized or eliminated mostly by feces.[310] Its effects in *ex vivo* platelet function tests develop in most species including man only after a lag period of at least several hours showing that either some metabolites are predominantly effective or the production of some factor(s) is indirectly influenced.[311] This is connected with a relatively prolonged effect after a single dose suggesting some irreversible change in platelets. No accumulation of the drug was observed. However, after intravenous administration the antithrombotic effect sets in quite rapidly. No effect on blood clotting was noted but the drug prolonged bleeding.[312] In contrast to *ex vivo* tests the activity *in vitro* is negligible and appears only after high concentrations.[313,314] The drug probably exerts no direct effect on the eicosanoid system,[315] nor the adenylate system.[312] *Ex vivo*, the primary aggregation in response to ADP is influenced in contrast to NSAID which affect only the secondary phase.[316-320] Simultaneously with ADP aggregation, the response to PAF is also affected.[321] There are many indications that the drug acts not only at the level of platelets but also of other cell membranes. According to the prevailing hypothesis, the drug acts by inhibiting the binding of fibrinogen and von Willebrand factor to exposed platelet glycoprotein IIb-IIIa.[322,323] A decrease in intra- and extracellular fibronectin was also described.[324] This might also be the explanation for some positive reports about the effects of ticlopidine in *ex vivo* adhesivity tests, e.g., glass bead platelet retention.[325] The enhancement of red blood cell deformability after ticlopidine is in accord with its supposed general membrane activity and may be of clinical significance.[326,327] Some authors noted ultrastructural changes in platelets[328] and mitochondria of other cells[329,330] after the drug administration due to metabolic changes.

In experiments with thrombosis models ticlopidine was often quite effective and occasionally even more so than other established antithrombotics. On the other hand, in some studies the drug was without any effect. Thus Vigdahl et al.[155] observed no effect (150 to 300 mg/kg p.o.) in rats with electric current-induced arterial thrombosis. It was fairly effective at a dose of 50 mg/kg p.o. daily in rats with a forceps crushed aorta as manifested by increased platelet survival and decreased platelet loss[161] and in those with a dental broach implanted into the abdominal aorta.[327] In dogs with a Dacron® graft implant, the effect was not significant.[161] Ashida et al.[331] observed a marked antithrombotic effect in rats with an AV-shunt already after 5 mg/kg p.o. while ASA was without any effect and dipyridamole only partially effective. Similarly, Kumada et al.[249] described a marked effect of ticlopidine (100 mg/kg p.o.) in rats with a steel wire coil inserted into the vena cava. ASA was again ineffective under the same conditions. Choe and Povalski[332] used rats again with electric current-induced thrombosis of the carotid artery and continuously registered flow changes by electromagnetic probe. Ticlopidine was effective at a dose of 30 mg/kg orally, inhibiting the early phase of thrombus formation but not the subsequent thrombus growth. ASA was again without an effect and dipyridamole was effective only at a dose of 150 mg/kg. Massad et al.[333] observed an antithrombotic effect of ticlopidine in electric current-induced carotid thrombosis in conscious rats and the drug was also effective in a rat model based on a carotid artery deendothelialization by air injury.[334] Kobayashi et al.[335] recorded a reduced size of stenosis-induced thrombi in the femoral arteries of rabbits. Furthermore, the drug was effective in laser-induced thrombosis in the mesenteric microcirculation of rats.[78] Smith and White[51,336] administered ticlopidine at a dose of 10 mg/kg i.v. and decreased thrombus growth (37% inhibition) in an AV-shunt of rats with an inserted cotton thread according to the method developed by Umetsu and Sanai[124] in 1978. Pumphrey et al.[337] observed a good antithrombotic effect of the drug in preserving artificial or autologous vein grafts implanted in the femoral artery of dogs. Accumulation of radiolabeled platelets was observed particularly in artificial prostheses and oral administration of ticlopidine (30 mg/kg/d for 2 d) was quite effective, more so than verapamil.

Surprisingly, ticlopidine was also effective in venous thrombosis in a rat model not substantially dependent on platelets,[338,339] i.e., Reyers' model, at doses of 100 to 200 mg/kg/d. Under similar conditions in the rat model of Millet et al.,[73] 200 mg/kg p.o. decreased thrombus weight by 59%.

Serious objections against the antithrombotic activity of ticlopidine were raised by Cattaneo et al.[340] While *ex vivo* effects of the drug on platelet functions and survival were confirmed, no effect was noted on platelet accumulation on the aortic wall of rats after an injury by an indwelling catheter or on thrombus formation around the catheter and the adjoining aortic surface after deendothelialization by balloon catheter in rabbits. The authors emphasized that in general, no inhibition of platelet accumulation was observed on an unmasked subendothelium and sought to explain the discrepancy with the results of other authors by the supposed local presence of larger amounts of thrombin in their own experiments. This conclusion was discussed by Escolar et al.[341] investigating the drug effect *ex vivo* using the Baumgartner method with everted arteries. They stressed that the main effect of ticlopidine is directed not on the interaction of platelets with the subendothelium where particularly glycoprotein Ib is involved, but on platelet to platelet interaction with glycoprotein IIb-IIIa playing the key role. The interaction of this glycoprotein at the membrane level with chief adhesive proteins, fibrinogen, fibronectin, and von Willebrand factor is probably the site of ticlopidine action leading to defective high shear stress-induced platelet to platelet interaction.

Another type of model was used by Tomikawa et al.,[342] i.e., lactic acid-induced DIC in rats. While ticlopidine was effective at a dose of 50 mg/kg p.o., ASA and dipyridamole were ineffective under the same conditions. Vigdahl et al.[155] used arachidonic acid-induced DIC and ticlopidine remained without any effect at doses of 150 to 300 mg/kg p.o. Lacaze et al.[343] observed an inhibition of Russell viper venom-induced DIC, Butler and White[344] noted a favorable effect of ticlopidine in ADP-induced DIC in rats, but not in DIC accompanying the Arthus reaction. Thörne et al.[345] studied pulmonary platelet sequestration after endotoxin.

Ashida et al.[346] published an interesting model simulating, to some extent, thromboangiitis obliterans in rats. For this purpose, he injected sodium laurate intraarterially. After 6 d, the paws of animals were gangrenous and became completely necrotic in 10 to 15 d. Ticlopidine at relatively low doses (ca 5 mg/kg) administered orally 3 h in advance and for several days after the challenge was quite effective, more so than ASA and dipyridamole. The authors concluded that rheological factors might be responsible besides the effect on platelet aggregate formation. The drug was also effective in hyperacute xenograft rejection[347] and arterial as well as vein graft preservation.[348,349]

To summarize, compared with other antiplatelet agents, ticlopidine acted in a different way in many respects. It predominantly influenced platelets and their primary aggregation. The process seemed not to be influenced by other mediators and what was actually affected was the terminal part of the process. In animal models, ticlopidine was frequently effective under conditions of excessive damage and with artificial surfaces while other agents no longer showed any effect.

In the author's laboratory, ticlopidine (Ticlid® Parcor) was tested in the usual routine battery of tests: the drug was highly effective in the endothelial test showing that this aspect cannot be neglected when seeking to interpret the drug action (Figure 22). Meanwhile there was some difference if the drug was given at single doses of 2.5 to 10 mg/kg orally 3 h before thrombus induction or at the same dose t.i.d. on the day before the experiment, the latter way of administration having been more effective. The drug was also effective in the venous and arterial models at a relatively low dose level.

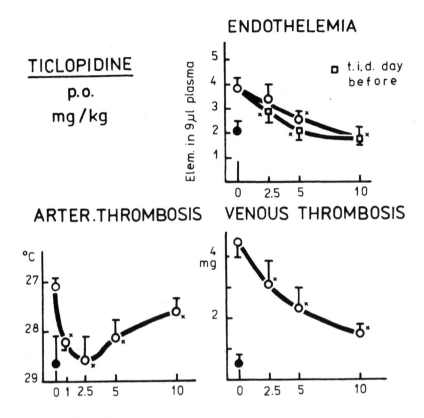

FIGURE 22. Effect of ticlopidine in the standard battery of models.

In conclusion, it is evident that the effect on the vessel wall, or more appropriately on the endothelium, is a contributing component in the overall antithrombotic effect of ticlopidine. This finding comes as no surprise supposing its general effect on cell membranes. On the other hand, the effect on platelets is probably predominant. The prolonged effect of the drug was confirmed. Ticlopidine is an effective antithrombotic even at a relatively low dose level and particularly in the arterial thrombosis model.

VII. NAFAZATROM

Nafazatrom enjoys a special status among other antithrombotic agents as its investigation using *in vivo* models was probably primary, whereas *in vitro* studies were secondary. It is characteristic for our still incomplete understanding of the mechanism of antithrombotic action, that these secondary attempts to explain the effects of nafazatrom were far from satisfactory.

After oral administration, nafazatrom is rapidly and almost completely absorbed. If administered intravenously, it is about ten times more effective, a fact indicating that extensive biotransformation already takes place during the first pass through the liver. It is possible that some early metabolites may be participating in its activity and the plasma concentrations of nafazatrom do not well reflect the effective concentrations at the membranes of endothelial cells as the probable main site of its action (Philipp et al.[350]).

Nafazatrom was effective after oral administration in freeze-induced thrombosis in rats, rabbits, and guinea pigs against both venous and arterial thrombosis.[247] As already mentioned, the method is relatively sensitive and ensures good quantification. The minimal effective dose in venous thrombosis in rats was 0.3 mg/kg orally, but only partial inhibition was attained. To achieve an effect lasting at least 4 to 6 h a dose of over 10 mg/kg was required.

In the arterial thrombosis model induced by freezing in the carotid artery of rats, the drug was effective again after the minimal dose of 0.3 mg/kg p.o. Almost complete suppression of thrombus formation was not achieved unless doses over 3 mg/kg were administered. In the rat iliac artery the necessary dose was 10 mg/kg. As already mentioned, intravenous administration of the drug was in general about ten times as effective as the oral administration. The minimal effective oral dose in rabbits was 1 mg/kg. Similar doses (1 to 10 mg/kg orally) were effective in guinea pigs.

Seuter et al.[351] used a modification of the method of Zekert and Gottlob[31] based on a severe lesion of the rabbit jugular vein by topical application of silver nitrate. About 50% reduction of thrombus weight was achieved after 3 mg/kg nafazatrom was administered orally.

Buchanan et al.[352] investigated the effect of nafazatrom in a venous thrombosis model in rabbits. Stasis due to the complete occlusion of a jugular vein segment for 30 min led after the release to accumulation of radiolabeled platelets and fibrinogen. Nafazatrom at a dose of 10 mg/kg orally was without effect on both parameters. On the other hand, in rabbits with polyethylene cannula-induced thrombosis, thrombus size again indicated by the accumulation of radiolabeled platelets, was decreased markedly by 3 mg/kg p.o., whereas platelet half-life was normalized only after a dose of 10 mg/kg.

Formation of thrombi induced in the coronary arteries of dogs and rats by electric current was inhibited by 1, and still more by 5 mg/kg orally administered nafazatrom. The consequences of thrombotic occlusion such as infarction and occurrence of arrhythmias, were also favorably influenced.[353,354] By contrast, *ex vivo* platelet aggregation was not affected. However, Shea et al.[355,356] observed an effect on both thrombus formation and *ex vivo* platelet aggregation under similar conditions.

Seuter et al.[247] noted increased thrombolysis in their venous thrombosis model in rats. Nafazatrom at a dose of 0.1 mg/kg was administered orally after thrombus induction. A similar decrease in thrombus weight was seen in an arterial model. These results have not been substantiated by any increase in the fibrinolytic activity in blood as reflected by tests carried out *in vitro* and *ex vivo*.

At least two types of microcirculation thrombosis models have been used for the evaluation of nafazatrom as an antithrombotic. Herrmann[357] and Herrmann and Seuter[358] observed the formation of white bodies in the arterioles of the hamster cheek pouch and heart transplants. The thrombi were formed by fluorescein isothiocyanate-dextran-injured platelets. The appearance of aggregates was delayed after the intraarterial administration of extra low doses of the drug. Laser-induced thrombosis in the veins of the rat mesenteric circulation was only influenced by 100 mg/kg of orally administered nafazatrom.[78]

The effect on microcirculatory thrombotic processes might have played some role in the increased survival of rats with a traumatic shock after nafazatrom doses corresponding to those effective in thrombosis models (0.5 to 2.0 mg/kg).[359] Similar considerations may be applicable to the influence of nafazatrom on myocardial ischemia and consequent arrhythmias. Administered at a dose of 5 to 10 mg/kg orally b.i.d. in dogs and rabbits, nafazatrom reduced the infarction size and the degree of necrosis after prolonged ischemia and reperfusion. This effect cannot be interpreted as mediated by the influence on hemodynamics or myocardial demands.[353,354] It is thought that the availability of endogenous prostacyclin is of particular importance in this effect.[360,361]

The unquestionable antithrombotic effectiveness of nafazatrom has not been explained satisfactorily by any *in vitro* tests. No effects on coagulation, fibrinolysis, and platelet functions were observed. However, some *ex vivo* effects were recorded on platelet aggregation and platelet survival was increased in rabbits with a cannula inserted into the carotid artery.[352] A similar *in vivo* effect on platelets was observed in connection with the investigation of the antimetastatic activity of nafazatrom.[362,363] Vermylen et al., pointed out that

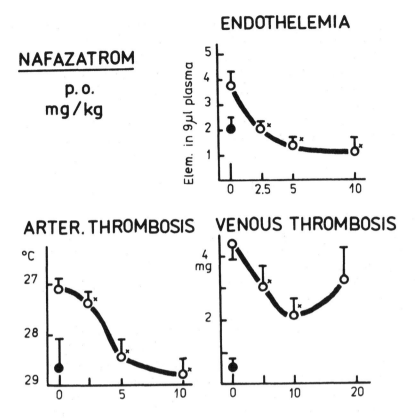

FIGURE 23. Effect of nafazatrom in the standard battery of models.

nafazatrom prevented the time-dependent decline of 6-ketoprostaglandin $F_{1\alpha}$ formation during chronic irritation of the rabbit jugular vein by the insertion of a nylon thread.[364] Their experiments together with some clinical studies in volunteers[365] suggested that nafazatrom triggers prostacyclin release or slows down its degradation by hydroxyprostaglandin dehydrogenase.[366] Nafazatrom has antioxidant properties, i.e., it might function as a scavenger of free oxygen radicals.[367] In this way, it could inhibit the activity of lipoxygenases.[368] On the other hand, a weakness inherent in all such theories is that the role of endogenous prostacyclin in the prevention of thrombosis is still disputable. It is quite possible that in the activity of nafazatrom other unknown mediators are involved.

The antithrombotic activity of nafazatrom was tested in the author's laboratory with the use of the standard battery of tests. Only oral administration was used (Figure 23). Nafazatrom was found to be effective in the endothelemia test. A dose of 2.5 mg/kg was already significantly effective and the curve probably shows that a dose of 1 mg/kg might be effective as well. The dose of 2.5 mg/kg was just significantly effective in the arterial thrombosis model. The drug was relatively less effective in the venous thrombosis model showing a narrow optimum dose of about 10 mg/kg and the inhibition attained 60% at most. In general, the results were not very different from those reported by Seuter et al.[351] In addition, they suggest that nafazatrom acts predominantly on endothelium.

The impression obtained from reports in the literature and from our own experiments can be summarized to say that the effect of nafazatrom on prostacyclin availability is probably not very specific. In an analogy to thromboxane production in platelets which probably represents a component of a general activation of defensive hemostatic function (in platelets and endothelium) the increase in prostacycline production and release might represent a nonspecific component of an activation of endothelial functions. It is perhaps in this sense that the increased thrombolytic activity reported by Seuter might be interpreted. Damage to endothelium is presumably associated with increased oxidative processes and vice versa, an increased oxidative potential may lead to further endothelial damage.[370] Consequently, the activation of endothelial defensive functions might be related to the shift of the oxido-reduction potential to the reduction side whose manifestations include the increased availability of prostacyclin.

Nafazatrom is an effective antithrombotic and an agent also interesting from the theoretical point of view. Unfortunately, it has not come on the market and its further research has been discontinued.

VIII. SULOCTIDIL

Suloctidil, a sulfur-containing aminoalcohol, was originally tested as an antispasmodic with special indications in the central nervous system. It was classified mostly as a loose member of the group of calcium antagonists having a variety of other pharmacological actions including effects on the energy and lipid metabolism.[371]

It is much more effective by the intravenous route than orally and is extensively metabolized in the body. However, an unchanged molecule seems to be the carrier of the main effect.

After the discovery of its antiplatelet effects, which are in fact quite weak *in vitro* and more readily observed *ex vivo*, many attempts have been made to explain its mechanism of action.[372] Thus, the peculiar effect on the ability of platelets to take up and retain serotonin could hardly be connected with its antithrombotic action.[374] It probably exerts no substantial effects on the eicosanoid system,[375] on adenosine uptake, etc. The most probable activity that could be connected with the antiplatelet effects is the strong membrane activity which may also be related to its calcium channel-blocking effects.[376,377] This strong membrane activity has been investigated *in vitro* as the effects on membrane phospholipids as well as *in vivo* as stabilization of erythrocyte membranes. It may also be related to the releasing effect on prostacyclin,[378] more prominent than in other membrane-active agents. Suloctidil produces a moderate bleeding tendency and is effective in decreasing viscosity. Oral toxicity is very low but is much higher with intravenous administration.[371] Oral suloctidil reduced spontaneous formation of circulating platelet aggregates in aged breeder rats.[379]

The drug has been tested quite extensively in thrombosis models with mostly positive results. Roba et al.[380,381] damaged the endothelium of canine femoral arteries by a proteolytic enzyme, and using suloctidil, significantly decreased the occurrence of thrombosis (5 mg/kg/d). Gurewich and Lipinski[118] evaluated suloctidil in rabbits with polyethylene tubing inserted into the carotid artery and with thrombi marked by radiolabeled fibrinogen. The drug at a dose of 50 mg/kg orally 2 h in advance was significantly effective, more so than ASA and dipyridamole when both were administered in a single dose. The same author also used an endotoxin model in rabbits with platelet decrease significantly inhibited.

Two other kinds of DIC models were used by Roba, induced by ADP in mice (suloctidil effective at a dose of 100 mg/kg p.o.) and by endotoxin in hyperlipemic rats. The score of lesions was decreased by 25 mg/kg/d p.o.

Roba et al.[382] tested suloctidil also in another rat model in cooperation with the author of the method, Bourgaine. Thrombi were induced in the mesenteric microcirculation by topical ADP administration and electric current. Thrombus formation was significantly reduced after 1 mg/kg i.v. and the existing thrombi, while not embolizing easily, did undergo a gradual fragmentation.

Oral administration of 3 mg/kg t.i.d. normalized platelet survival in baboons with prosthetic AV-shunts in experiments carried out by Harker et al. (see Roba[371]).

Tuma et al.[383] observed an inhibitory effect after 1 mg/kg on electric current-induced white body formation in the microcirculation of the bat wing.

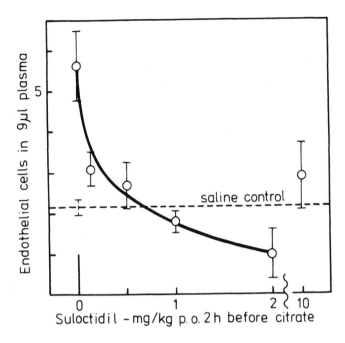

FIGURE 24. Effect of oral suloctidil on endothelial stability after the citrate challenge.

Vigdahl et al.[155] found suloctidil effective in inhibiting the formation of electric current-induced thrombi in rats, but only one very high oral dose (150 mg/kg) was used. In arachidonic acid-induced DIC, suloctidil administered at the same dose failed to exert any effect.

In another rat DIC model, de Gaetano et al.[384] demonstrated a protective effect of suloctidil (1 to 3 mg/kg i.v.) against platelet decreases after intravenous administration of collagen and ADP. The same effect was obtained if ADP was combined with dietary hyperlipemia. The drug was ineffective if administered orally (400 mg/kg) against endotoxin-induced DIC.

To summarize the literary data, suloctidil was extensively studied in various more or less adequate thrombosis models with generally positive results.

In the author's laboratory, suloctidil was tested in several models.[385] In the endothelial stability test, suloctidil was effective against a citrate challenge after oral administration of 2 mg/kg (Figure 24). With a much higher dosage, some tendency was observed to less favorable effects. In the platelet sequestration model using a citrate challenge suloctidil was quite effective at the same dose as in the endothelial test, i.e., 2 mg/kg p.o. (Figure 25). In the arterial thrombosis model with electric current thrombus induction the drug was not effective over the chosen range of doses (Figure 26). Of course, this cannot be interpreted as the lack of effect on arterial thrombosis as the vascular lesion was in excess, and consequently, the model was insufficiently sensitive to agents effective by influencing the vascular factor.

The results obtained in two previous models have shown that it is just this effect that might be of particular importance for the overall activity of the drug. The last test used was the venous thrombosis model combining stasis in the mesenteric vessels of an intestinal loop with the intravenous injection of several challenging agents (citrate, hypotonic saline, lactate, and epinephrine) (Figure 27). Suloctidil, 2 mg/kg p.o., was significantly effective against all these challenges.

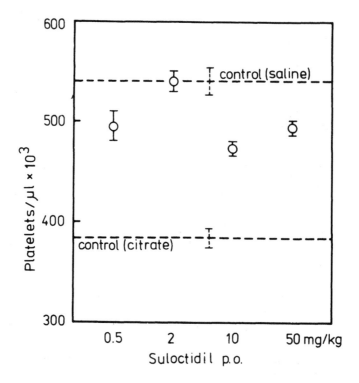

FIGURE 25.   Effect of oral suloctidil on platelet sequestration after the citrate challenge.

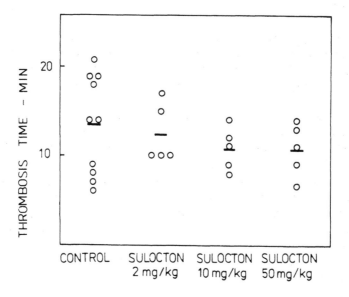

FIGURE 26.   Effect of i.v. suloctidil (Sulocton®) on electrically induced arterial thrombosis.

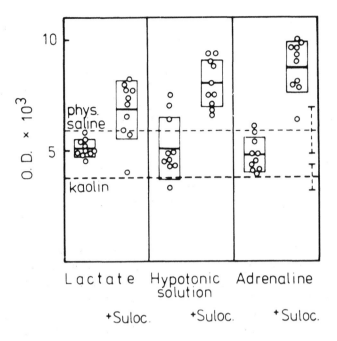

FIGURE 27.   Effect of suloctidil (2 mg/kg p.o.) in the mesenteric vessel venous thrombosis after several challenges.

It may be concluded that the drug is a potent antithrombotic with an important component acting on the vessel wall.

IX. DRUGS INTERACTING WITH THE EICOSANOID SYSTEM

The group of drugs interacting with the eicosanoid system can be tentatively classified as follows:

1.   Agents interacting with the platelet system
    a.   Inhibitors of TXA_2 synthesis (TXSI)
    b.   Antagonists of TXA_2 receptors (TXRA)
2.   Agents interacting with the tissue cell system (endothelium)
    a. PGI_2 (prostacyclin) and analogues
    b.   Stimulation of PGI_2 synthesis and release or inhibition of PGI_2 metabolism

This classification is rather vague and far from complete. There is much work going on in another direction of arachidonic acid metabolism, i.e., lipoxygenase route. Other agents influence the common portion of both the platelet and endothelial eicosanoid systems, i.e., release of arachidonic acid from membrane phospholipids, activity of various cyclo-oxygenases, etc. Various kinds of agents affecting one part of the system may possess in the same molecule, activities influencing other parts. Alternatively, various agents may be combined.

Selective inhibitors (1.a in the listing above) of TXA_2 synthesis (TXSI) are often imidazole or pyridine derivatives. Of these, the most tested was dazoxiben (UK 37, 248-01). The group includes UK 38,485, dazmegrel, OKY-1581, OKY-046, OKY-1555, CGS 13080, U-63557A, R-70416, etc. These agents effectively decrease the production of thromboxane A_2 in platelets as evidenced both *in vitro* and *ex vivo* by the decrease in the main metabolite TXB_2 in blood samples.[386,387] In some studies, threads were inserted into the jugular veins of rabbits or into extracorporeal circulations.[364,388] A concomitant increase of prostacyclin production was often observed as demonstrated by the increase in its main metabolite, 6-keto-PGF$_{1\ alpha}$. This is interpreted as the redirection of platelet cyclic endoperoxides to the endothelium providing the source of prostacyclin synthesis.[386,389,390] At the same time, the effects on metabolite levels are often unrelated to the action on aggregation.[391,392] Platelet aggregation *in vitro* and *ex vivo* is inhibited by TXSI after some stimuli such as arachidonic acid and much less or not at all, after collagen, ADP, epinephrine, thrombin, and PAF.[393,394] "Spontaneous" aggregation of rotated platelets is not inhibited[395] and obviously there exist species differences.[396] Often some schematism can be observed in this field. Thus platelets are not the only source of thromboxane,[397] cyclic endoperoxides are effective themselves and may be more important than TXA$_2$ as strong aggregants. In addition, they may switch off platelet adenylate cyclase.[398] The drugs may also exert effects different than those on the eicosanoid system as this group of drugs is particularly rich in pharmacological activities.[399]

Three groups of models have mainly been used in the evaluation of TXSI. Thus arachidonic acid was used producing DIC and sudden death in rabbits according to the method of Silver et al.[400] The method was used, e.g., by Puig-Parellada and Planas,[401] Lefer et al.,[402-404] Lindsay et al.,[39] and Randall et al.[405] The drugs were mostly effective, but the effect was relatively short-lived. Injection of arachidonic acid is, of course, a very artificial stimulus and may lead to many complex effects. Another method, selected again for its sensitivity to this group of drugs and a poor representative of natural thrombus formation, is cyclic flow reductions in stenosed canine coronary arteries. This method was introduced by Folts et al.,[72] and later was used by the Upjohn group of researchers.[406,407] It was then used by several other groups for testing TXSI and other antithrombotics.[408-412] The cyclic flow reduction is due to the transient formation of nonoccluding white bodies from platelets, rapidly detaching, and steadily embolizing into the periphery. On the other hand, thrombus is generally used to mean a relatively irreversible and mostly occluding mass persisting at one site for prolonged periods of time and leading to ischemic complications. Thrombus formation is determined by different processes setting in under special conditions after the primary platelet adhesion. It is possible that 5-HT, lipoxygenation products, etc., might be involved.[413] The primary process might be designated a compensated thrombotic tendency or *in vivo* platelet aggregation. It has something in common with the supposed compensated transient thrombi formation in the venous system, probably a frequent phenomenon but one rarely attaining the symptomatic level as the thrombi are rapidly lysed by the effective thrombolytic system. However, some authors speculate that similar platelet thrombi may participate in the development of arrhythmias and sudden death,[414] as well as in some TIAs. This might be true if the platelet emboli are sufficiently stable, depending on the presence of a vascular lesion. TXSI were, in general, effective in this type of model but it was questioned whether this was their direct effect or rather that of increased prostacyclin production.[408]

The third method frequently employed for TXSI testing was originally developed by the Michigan group[399,415-418] and used in various modifications (Randall and Wilding[419,420] in rabbits, van der Giessen and Zijlstra[421] in pigs). In principle, the vascular wall of a canine coronary was damaged by electric current and the gradual flow decrease was registered by a flowmeter. The model is probably more adequate than the former, but the vascular lesion is still severe. TXSI were practically ineffective in the study of van der Giessen, Hook, and Schumacher, and in other studies they were more or less partially effective. In most studies, simultaneous determinations of metabolites and *ex vivo* aggregation tests were carried out. Some differences in results might have been caused by different preparations. Thus OKY-1581 proved to be more effective than U-63557 A as an antithrombotic, but equally effective as a thromboxane synthesis inhibitor. This again led to the conclusion that the antithrombotic effect is due to increased prostacyclin production.[364]

In other models, no effect of TXSI was observed in the microcirculation of the hamster cheek pouch,[422] in an extracorporeal circulation,[388] on platelet survival in baboons with an AV-shunt,[66] and in a mechanically damaged rabbit central ear artery.[65] Massad et al.[333] noted no effect of dazmegrel and OKY-046 with electrically induced carotid artery thrombosis in conscious rats. No effect was found on thrombocytopenia after Arthus reaction and with cotton thread-induced thrombosis in a rat AV-shunt.[423] The agents were only partially effective on photochemically induced thrombi in the rat brain microcirculation.[424] Dazoxiben was effective in an electric current-induced thrombosis of the rabbit carotid artery as indicated by radiolabeled platelets,[419] in a venous silver nitrate-induced thrombosis in rabbits as indicated by prostaglandin metabolites,[425] in a cold compression-induced arterial thrombosis in rats,[426] and in arterial graft thrombus formation in sheep.[427] However, the same authors did not observe any effects in ethoxysclerol-induced jugular vein thrombosis in rabbits or in laser-induced thrombosis in the rabbit ear chamber. The negative results are in agreement with poor results in clinical practice.

Another group that originally held great promise are antagonists of platelet and vessel wall thromboxane receptors (TXRA) (1.b in the listing above) such as BM 13.177, a sulfonamide derivative,[428] SQ 28,668, R 68 070, and UK-37248.[402] Meanwhile, dazoxiben was claimed to also possess a similar additional activity. These agents are competitive inhibitors and the prolonged high levels in blood is a prerequisite for their *in vivo* effects. They may produce vascular spasms and even myocardial infarction.[429] On the other hand, they have been described to possess cardioprotective activity.[430] TXRA were particularly expected to be effective in combination with TXSI, and some *in vitro* and *ex vivo* experiments seemed to fulfill these expectations.[431,432] A marked antithrombotic effect was observed in conscious rats with electrically induced carotid artery thrombosis,[333] in pig coronary thrombosis,[421] and against silver nitrate-induced aortic thrombosis in rabbits, as well as arachidonic acid-induced DIC.[433]

The group of agents (2.a in the listing above) is based on the favorable effect of PGI_2 (epoprostenol, prostacyclin) against platelet aggregation by stimulating adenylate cyclase. This results in an increase of the powerful endogenous antiaggregant cAMP. Unfortunately, prostacyclin alone is chemically unstable, possesses a very short biological half-life, and has to be administered in infusions. In addition, tachyphylaxis develops rapidly and the drug may exert serious side effects. Therefore, a search was started for more stable analogues with a prolonged effect and devoid of side effects. Numerous drugs were tested, including a carbacyclin derivative, iloprost (ZK 36,374, Euprostil®), TRK-100, CG 4203, and CG 4305. The effort has only been partially successful since the agents are still unsuitable for prolonged thrombosis prevention and could be used as short-term antithrombotics only, e.g., in hemodialysis and cardiopulmonary bypass, often in place of heparin. Meanwhile, their main application is in indications other than antithrombotic.

Prostacyclin was shown to increase survival in rabbits after endotoxin,[434] to inhibit cyclic flow reductions in stenosed canine coronaries.[411,414] and thrombus formation in canine coronaries damaged by electric current.[435] The antiplatelet activity of ZK 36 375 was dissociated in cat myocardial ischemia from its cytoprotective effect, and the latter is often more emphasized.[436] The new analogue TRK-100 was effective against collagen-induced DIC and in extracorporeal circulation in rats.[57] The drugs may favorably influence red blood cell fluidity and adhesivity.[437] An anti-ischemic activity was demonstrated by Araki et al.,[438] Jugdutt et al.,[439] Ogletree et al.,[440] and Ubatuba et al.[441]

PGI_1 shares many positive effects with prostacyclin. It was effective in mechanically induced rabbit brain thrombosis[442] and in ADP-induced microthrombosis in the hamster cheek pouch if the drug was enclosed in lipid microspheres.[443] No effect was noted in laser-induced rabbit thrombosis.[99]

Many drugs have been shown (2.b in the listing above) to exert some effects on prostacyclin production, release and preservation but the relative importance of such findings is

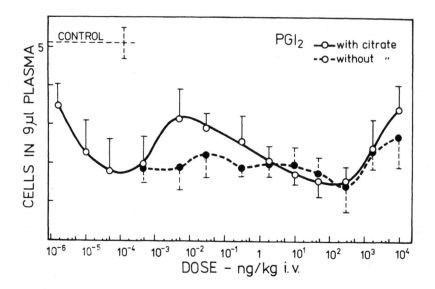

FIGURE 28.   Effect of PGI$_2$ on citrate-induced endothelemia in rats.

often questionable. Thus nafazatrom was reported to protect prostacyclin from oxidation, and prostacyclin effects were enhanced by suloctidil, anagrelide, and clofibrate. The first attempt to look for specific stimulators of prostacyclin release and synthesis was probably that of Boeynaems et al.[378] (SKF 525-A, proadifen).

Several eicosanoids were investigated in the author's laboratory in the endothelemia test.[444] Prostacyclin was effective against a citrate-induced endothelemia increase in rats at extremely low doses (10^{-3} ng/kg i.v.) (Figure 28). However, with the dose of 10^{-2} ng/kg this effect disappeared to show a second peak around 10^2 ng/kg and to vanish again at much higher doses. The agent alone, i.e., without the citrate challenge had no effect, but at a relatively high dose level of 10 ng/kg it had an unfavorable, destabilizing activity. Arachidonic acid likewise had a complicated dose-to-effect relation (Figure 29). Positively effective doses corresponded to those of prostacyclin, but adverse effects prevailed at doses around 10^2 ng/kg. Similar complicated dose-effect curves of exogenous arachidonic acid to platelet aggregating activity and TXB$_2$ production were observed in a higher concentration range by Tanoue et al.[392] This indicates the existence of a finely tuned balance of endogenous eicosanoid regulators, and all exogenous interventions may bring about a series of counter regulations influencing unfavorably and unpredictably the intended effect often resulting in an opposite response. The effective intervention is possible only with relatively high pharmacological doses exceeding by several orders of magnitude the levels of endogenous mediators.

Dazoxiben was also tested in the author's laboratory using the standard battery of models (Figure 30). The drug was relatively effective in all three models at a dose of about 1 mg/kg p.o. The inhibition of venous thrombosis was incomplete.

In conclusion, it has never been definitely proven that the eicosanoid system occupies a key or even an important position in the hemostatic[445] or antithrombotic functions *in vivo*.[88,446,447] It should also be kept in mind that the antithrombotic and hemostatic activities of eicosanoids are not necessarily their main function[448,449] and their use might be connected with many untold side effects.

X. ADRENOLYTICS

The fact that an increased level of catecholamines in the blood may somehow be related to the thrombotic tendency has been known for a long time. It obviously reflects the survival

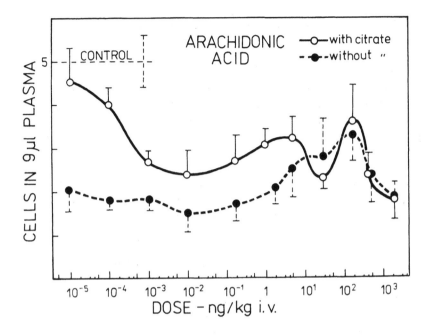

FIGURE 29.   Effect of arachidonic acid on citrate-induced endothelemia in rats.

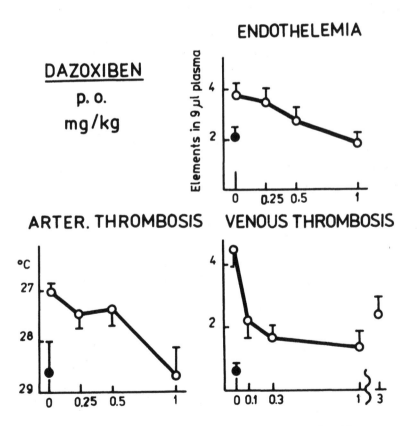

FIGURE 30.   Effect of dazoxiben in the standard battery of models.

value of a functional increase in hemostatic capacity under stressful situations. At the same time, the targets of the catecholamine effect may be manifold:

1. Vasoconstriction in special circulation areas together with the inotropic effect on the myocardium leading to hemodynamic changes and blood flow redistribution.
2. Direct injurious effects on the vascular wall, particularly endothelium.
3. Effects on blood clotting, fibrinolysis, and platelets.
4. Metabolic effects (lipomobilization, glycogenolysis, gluconeogenesis, etc.).

This still relatively simple and intelligible picture becomes rather complicated if the effect of catecholamines and their antagonists on platelets is solely considered. The schematism of adrenergic receptors, however useful in other fields, is not of much help in the case of platelets, particularly if the body of knowledge is still very fragmentary. Whichever way it is, any attempts at predictions of the clinical behavior of drugs based on such data seem to be very premature.

Epinephrine can serve as an inducer of platelet aggregation.[450] An indirect mechanism based on the potentiation of the activity of other mediators that may have been released already during platelet preparation was suggested.[451,452] As alpha-adrenergic blocking agents such as phentolamine are effective in blocking the proaggregatory effect of epinephrine, the presence of alpha-adrenergic receptors was suspected, and later alpha$_2$-receptors were found to be responsible.[453] Smith described the effect of beta-adrenolytics on platelet disaggregation.[454] Epinephrine inhibited the activity of adenylate cyclase and thus the increase of the endogenous antiaggregating agent, cAMP. It was suggested by Salzman[455] that the activity of catecholamines and their antagonists is connected mainly with this mediator, but this concept was later questioned as too simplified.[456] The effect of epinephrine is related to an influx of Ca^{2+} ions into the platelet.[457] On the surface of platelets, particularly rat platelets, there are also present beta$_2$-adrenergic receptors.[458] This might explain the lack of an aggregating effect of epinephrine in rats, the counteraction by a beta-adrenergic stimulation leading to an increase in cAMP concentration. In fact, inhibition of beta$_2$-receptors would release alpha$_2$-receptors causing, theoretically, a decreased cAMP production and an increased platelet aggregability.[459] Similar changes in platelet aggregability have been reported after the clinical administration of propranolol.[460] On the other hand, the warning against the use of nonselective beta-blocking agents on the basis of such *in vitro* and *ex vivo* findings, reflecting one aspect of their effects is not warranted. Whereas with the use of standard methods propranolol influenced platelet aggregation only at relatively high concentrations not attained after the clinical dosage, it was demonstrated by Greer et al.[461] to have an antiaggregating effect at much lower concentrations against collagen and ADP-induced aggregation if the whole blood method was used. Most beta-adrenergic blocking agents possess, in addition to the specific effect on platelet receptors, other effects which could be of importance. Most of them have a membrane stabilizing activity, and according to Campbell et al.,[462] inhibit the synthesis of thromboxane A$_2$ in platelets and may stimulate prostacyclin release.[463] The inhibition of thromboxane production may be related to the previously described inhibitory effect on phospholipase A$_2$.[464,465] They could also decrease the availability of calcium ions necessary for platelet aggregation.[466] It may be of interest to note here that platelet activation and secretion was observed in connection with emotional stress (PF 4 and beta-TG release) and this response was not inhibited by phenoxybenzamine or propranolol.[467]

The clinical success of beta-adrenolytics in secondary prevention of myocardial infarction as well as in other cardiovascular conditions gave rise to an impression that at least partially this favorable effect could have been accounted for by their antithrombotic activity.[468] Thus, abnormal platelet aggregability in patients with angina pectoris was normalized in the study of Frishman et al.[469]

A much more global approach to the problem of antithrombotic activity of adrenolytics was guaranteed by *in vivo* studies even though some confusion has remained. Epinephrine in combination with collagen was often used for the provocation of DIC.[119,470] Moriau et al.[471] investigated the effect of beta receptor stimulating and blocking agents on experimental DIC induced by thrombin infusions in rabbits. Stimulation of both beta and alpha receptors produced an increased mortality whereas a blockade of both resulted in an improvement in the survival and thrombus formation. As noted by the authors, this was in contrast with the results of some investigators and in agreement with others, the studies of McKay[472] and Müller-Berghaus[473] with alpha receptor stimulating and blocking agents serving as examples. Similar results were also obtained with propranolol by Berk.[474] Some reports advocating different opinions and describing a positive effect of isoproterenol and a lack of effect of adrenergic blockade concerned the endotoxin shock, which is of course, more than a DIC phenomenon as other effects of endotoxin may be involved.[475,476] It may be mentioned here that, in Vick's experiments, survival was improved by phenoxybenzamine not influencing the typical hypotension. Epinephrine alone produced latent DIC in dogs with activation not only of platelets, but also of blood clotting. This effect, at the same time, was dependent on the presence of the spleen.[477] Nowak and Markwardt[478] used thrombin in rats to produce DIC. Difenamine, i.e., an alpha$_1$-blocking agent, was most effective in the prevention of DIC consequences while yohimbine exerted adverse effects.

The contribution made by the studies of the group of Haft was impressive. They investigated the epinephrine-induced myocardial necrosis in dogs and rats and concluded that intravascular aggregation was an important contributing factor.[479] Furthermore, they observed a preventive effect of drugs inhibiting platelet function,[42,110] as well as of propranolol in the stress-induced platelet aggregation in the myocardial microcirculation.[480] They were able to induce intravascular platelet aggregation by various kinds of stress (cold and hot water, electric impulses) in rats most probably mediated by the release of catecholamines.[481] Hashimoto and Ogawa[181] observed a decrease in isoprenaline-induced myocardial necrosis by propranolol (2 and 10 mg/kg p.o. for 2 weeks), by high doses of sulfinpyrazone (100 mg/kg) but not by ASA. Folts and Bonebrake[482] observed an increased frequency of cyclic coronary flow reductions in stenosed canine coronary arteries after exposure to cigarette smoke or nicotine administration with a coincident increase in plasma epinephrine. The occurrence of such reversible platelet white bodies was reduced by phentolamine. Propranolol was also effective in the study of Hoak et al.,[483] in the prevention of acute myocardial necrosis after epinephrine in dogs. They ascribed the main deleterious effect to the elevated free fatty acid concentration in the plasma. It is possible that the antithrombotic component of the propranolol effect contributed to the favorable results obtained following its administration in myocardial recovery from ischemia in dog experiments of Bush et al.[484] and Reimer et al.[485] A potentiation of experimental thrombosis by epinephrine in an extracorporeal AV-shunt in pigs and rabbits was observed by Ozge et al.[486] and Rowsell et al.[487] Beta-adrenergic blockade in dogs with experimental thrombotic coronary artery occlusions decreased infarct size and improved the short-term survival if thrombolysis was combined with metoprolol.[488] Green et al.[489] observed a decrease in circulating platelet aggregates during the propranolol heart attack clinical trial. There even exists a possibility that propranolol may influence the development of experimental atherosclerosis.[490]

All these data supported the use of our models for testing adrenolytics as they particularly stress the role of endothelial function in thrombogenesis. Endothelial cells are known to possess both beta$_2$- and alpha$_2$-adrenergic receptors as well as receptors for propranolol.[491-493] In addition, they contain enzymes of catecholamine metabolism.[494,495] Epinephrine has been shown to injure endothelial cells under an electron microscope by Sunaga et al.[496] The influence of adrenolytics may be based on the membrane-stabilizing effects of some adrenomimetic and adrenolytic drugs.[497,498] An endothelial factor has been shown to inhibit

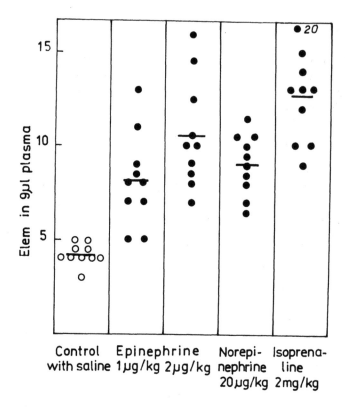

FIGURE 31.   Effect of i.v. administered catecholamines on endothelial stability.

the influx of calcium ions into the smooth muscles of the vessel wall, and in this way, an intact endothelium may modulate the alpha-adrenergic receptor stimulated contractions.[466]

Epinephrine was very effective in inducing endothelial sloughing with the subsequent increase in the number of circulating endothelial elements in the blood. Therefore it was used in some studies as a stimulus mostly at a dose of 1 μg/kg i.v. (Figure 31).[499] Norepinephrine and isoprenaline had similar effects when administered in pharmacological doses. In the platelet sequestration test, epinephrine again was fairly effective in decreasing the number of circulating platelets, but only in combination with citrate (Figure 32).[83] In this context, it might be useful to note that a significant increase in endothelial counts was observed in volunteers after a submaximal bicycle ergometer exercise, and also after mental stress caused by time-limited calculations (Figures 24, 25 in Chapter 3).[500] This may be interpreted as an effect of adrenergic activation. In the venous thrombosis model using stasis in an intestinal loop in rats, epinephrine exerted a significant enhancing effect on thrombus formation, while in the arterial thrombosis model using electric current for induction, no effect of epinephrine administered in several doses was registered (Figure 28 in Chapter 3). If adrenergic blocking agents were used in the endothelial model, the increased element counts after epinephrine were not influenced by propranolol or phentolamine (Figure 33).[499] On the other hand, the citrate potentiating effect of epinephrine was blocked by phentolamine and the effect of isoprenaline by propranolol, respectively, in the platelet sequestration model (Figure 34).[83]

Metipranolol, representing a mixed beta$_1$- and beta$_2$-blocking agent was used in the new standard battery of tests (Figure 35).[139] The drug was apparently effective in all three models showing a complex two-peak effect with increasing doses in both the arterial and venous model. The first peak, reflecting partial inhibition of thrombogenesis only, was seen after a similar dose in both models, i.e., 1 mg/kg orally, which corresponds to the usual clinical

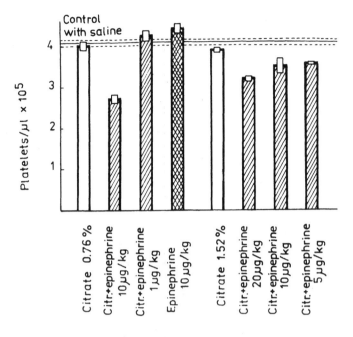

FIGURE 32. Effect of i.v. epinephrine alone and together with citrate (0.76 and 1.52%) on platelet sequestration.

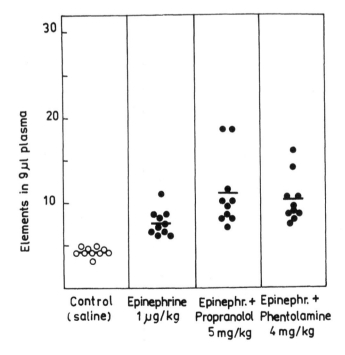

FIGURE 33. An attempt to inhibit the endothelial desquamation after epinephrine by adrenolytics.

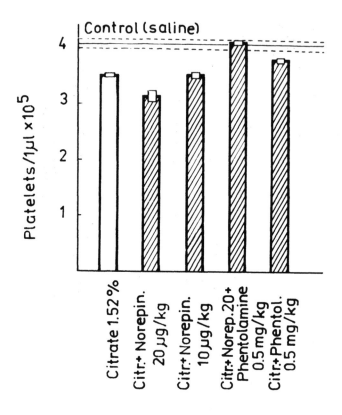

FIGURE 34.   Citrate-epinephrine synergism in the platelet sequestration test is inhibited by adrenolytics.

dosage. Endothelemia was inhibited at a lower dose level showing that the endothelial contribution is probably important in the overall antithrombotic effect. Metipranolol was not the only effective adrenolytic drug in the arterial model. While propranolol likewise proved to be effective with a maximum around 2 mg/kg orally (Figure 36), it failed to attain full suppression of thrombus formation. Practolol was not significantly effective showing some positive trend at a dose of 0.3 mg/kg p.o. (Figure 37). Prazosine showed a similar positive trend after 0.02 mg/kg (Figure 38) and yohimbine was partially, but significantly effective at doses of about 0.3 mg/kg (Figure 39).

It may be concluded that adrenolytics of a mixed $beta_1$ and $beta_2$ type were effective in the arterial thrombosis model just as those of the $alpha_2$ type. Practically no effect was observed with $alpha_1$ and $beta_1$ types. It is difficult to make any definite conclusions about the role of receptors as the drugs differed not only in their receptor specificity, but in other respects as well. By all means, more factors beside the effect on platelets are most probably involved, the endothelial function, and possibly, the vasoactivity, to name the most important ones. On the other hand, this effect of adrenolytics might be of importance, particularly if they are indicated in cardiovascular diseases often associated with thromboembolic phenomena, and in addition, often used simultaneously with established antithrombotics. Therefore the study of such combinations should be of particular interest, but this problem will be dealt with in detail in another chapter.

XI. CALCIUM CHANNEL BLOCKING AGENTS

It is well known that the influx of external calcium ions, as well as their mobilization from intracellular stores, plays a key role in all platelet functions.[501] It was therefore not

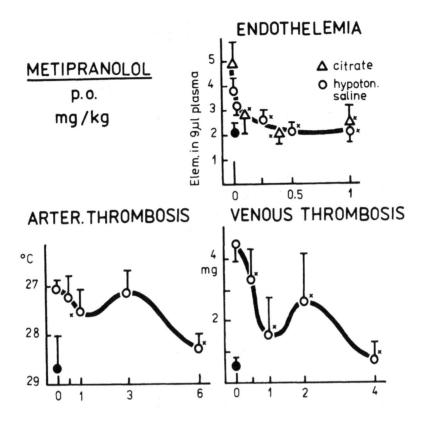

FIGURE 35. Effect of metipranolol in the standard battery of models.

very surprising that the inhibition of the slow inward calcium current by a group of drugs called by Fleckenstein in 1966[502,503] calcium antagonists was often investigated in connection with platelet functions. Ahn et al.[504] discovered an increased content of calcium ions in platelets of patients with cardiovascular diseases and noted its decrease after nifedipine administration. *In vitro*, the level of calcium ions in platelets was investigated mostly by indirect pharmacological methods,[505] but direct methods using indicators such as aequorin of Quin II have been increasingly used.[506] Some aggregating agents such as collagen increase calcium ions in platelets.[507] Baumgartner et al.[15] pointed out the necessity of calcium ions for platelet adhesion. The effect of calcium antagonists on platelet functions is probably mediated mainly by their influence on calcium ion influx and redistribution in platelets,[505,506] and possibly on PAF binding to a receptor closely associated with the calcium channel.[508] In fact, most studies with calcium antagonists assessed the effect on platelet aggregation.[509-512] The most tested agents, nifedipine, verapamil, and dilthiazem tended to usually inhibit, after some latency period, the aggregation induced by ADP, collagen, and occasionally by thrombin, epinephrine, arachidonic acid, thromboxane analogues, and PAF-acether (platelet activating factor). Particularly interesting was the antagonism against the calcium ionophore A 23187. Addition of calcium made the inhibitory effect reversible. On the other hand, the concentrations necessary to attain an inhibitory effect were, as a rule, quite high in comparison with those actually estimated after *in vivo* administration. Some authors noted an *ex vivo* effect at relatively low blood concentrations.[510,513] Disaggregation was enhanced by calcium antagonists in the studies of Horwitz and Ono with Kimura. Inhibition of the platelet release reaction and thromboxane generation together with an increased prostacyclin production were also recorded by Cremer[513] and Mehta et al.[514] Some differences between calcium antagonists became evident: all agents with the exception of

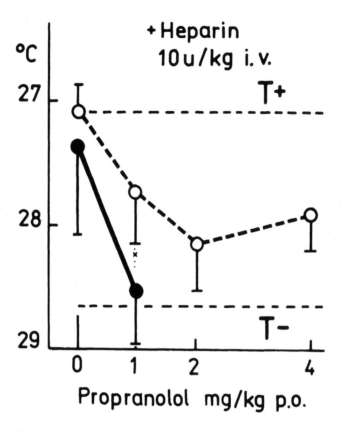

FIGURE 36.   Effect of oral propranolol in the arterial thrombosis model (broken line).

nifedipine have a membrane-stabilizing activity, verapamil possesses a marked $alpha_2$-adrenergic blocking component.[515] Some effect on the catecholamine content in nerve endings is known in prenylamine.[516] Dilthiazem seems to be particularly active as an inhibitor of PAF-induced aggregation.[508,511] *In vivo* administered verapamil decreased the counts of circulating platelet aggregates, increased as a rule, in patients with angina pectoris.[517] On the other hand, hemostasis was unaffected by calcium antagonists.[513]

A model of electric current-induced coronary artery thrombosis in conscious dogs was used for testing dilthiazem by Shea et al.[518] At the dose equal to that used clinically (0.75 mg/kg i.v.) dilthiazem had no effect on thrombus formation just as in *ex vivo* aggregation tests. The authors rightly pointed out that the search for antithrombotic agents using mostly *in vitro* and *ex vivo* platelet aggregation studies should also include *in vivo* thrombosis models. However, in their own model they administered only one dose and this was probably just under the effective level, particularly if a relatively severe lesion had been inflicted. Meanwhile, one of the main reasons for the use of animal models is the possibility to study the dose to effect relationship. Verapamil and nifedipine were administered by intravenous infusion as preventive agents in the study of Pumphrey et al.[126] The authors followed the thrombus development in artificial grafts interposed in femoral canine arteries as indicated by the deposition of radiolabeled platelets. The comparison with other studies is difficult, one dose having only been administered in infusions without giving the total dose. Despite that, both agents as well as dipyridamole were significantly effective. In the experimental studies of Henry et al.,[519] who tested nifedipine and Bush et al.,[484] who studied dilthiazem and propranolol, carried out in dogs with coronary occlusion, a marked cardioprotective effect was observed mediated mainly by their antiarrhythmic properties. Even though the

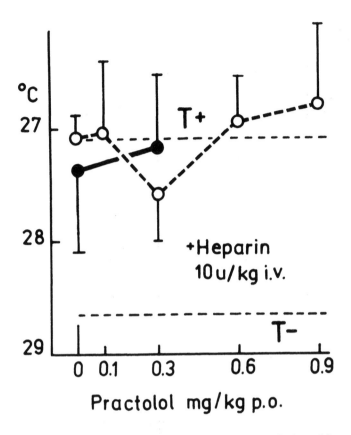

FIGURE 37. Effect of oral practolol in the arterial thrombosis model (broken line).

antithrombotic component of the favorable effect was not anticipated, it was not excluded either and is quite likely in the light of the well known role of microthrombi in the ischemic myocardium.[479,520]

A series of DIC models was used by Myers et al.[470] in rats and mice to compare verapamil and nifedipine with other calcium blockers and calmodulin antagonists. The stable thromboxane antagonist U 46619, arachidonate, and a combination of collagen with epinephrine were used for DIC induction and survival was used as an endpoint. Whereas verapamil remained without effect at doses of up to 0.5 mg/kg i.v., nifedipine was significantly effective as an antithrombotic at a dose of 0.2 mg/kg i.v., in a similar way in all the three modifications. Here of course, the author is well aware of the fact that DIC is not a very representative model of thrombosis and that the action on some sequelae of thrombosis leading to mortality might account for the favorable effect such as prevention of vasoconstriction and endothelial lesions. A similar method with DIC induced by arachidonic acid in rabbits was used by Okamatsu et al.[521] Verapamil, at a dose of 0.5 mg/kg i.v. had little effect as compared with nisoldipin 0.2 mg/kg i.v. Ortega et al.[522] observed in mice with a collagen plus epinephrine-induced DIC a high activity of nifedipine and no effect of dilthiazem.

In view of the presumed role of calcium ions in the pathogenesis of atherosclerosis, calcium antagonists have been tested in rabbits fed a hypercholesterolemic diet by Kramsch et al.[523] who used lanthanum, by Henry et al.[524] using nifedipin, Rouleau et al.[525] who studied verapamil, and by Willis et al.[526] who investigated nicardipine and nifedipine. The results were, in general, quite promising even though the doses had to be relatively high. Some negative results[527,528] were probably due to a low dosage.

In summary, calcium antagonists were often quite effective in *in vivo* studies, mostly when administered at a somewhat higher dose as compared with the usual clinical range.

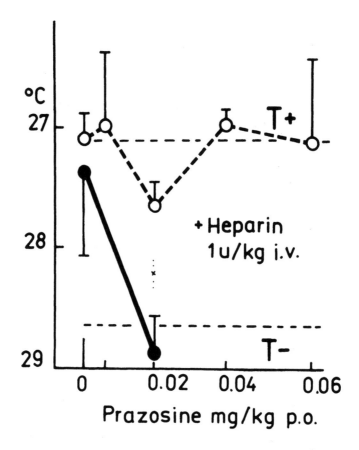

FIGURE 38.   Effect of oral prazosine in the arterial thrombosis model (broken line).

This favorable effect was not unexpected in view of the considerable involvement of calcium ions in all cellular activation processes.

Several calcium channel blocking agents were investigated in the author's laboratory using the test of endothelial stability.[529] Prenylamine, nifedipine, verapamil, and dilthiazem were effective in protecting rat endothelium against sloughing by intravenously injected citrate. Dilthiazem serves here as an example (Figure 40). The effective dosages did not greatly exceed the usual clinical dose range (Table 1). Only one representative of the group, prenylamine, was used in the complete standard battery of tests (Figure 41), showing that the drug was quite effective in all models, even though the effect on the venous thrombosis was partial at most. The activity in the arterial model was somewhat higher. In the latter model other drugs of the group were also tested (Figure 42 and Figure 8 and 9 in chapter 5). Both verapamil and nifedipine were significantly effective, but dilthiazem attained about 75% and verapamil merely about 50 to 60% inhibition. A survey of the approximate doses of the group significantly effective in the endothelial test and arterial thrombosis model, as compared with the clinical dose range, is shown in Table 1. The comparison shows that with verapamil and prenylamine the experimental doses were well within the range of clinical doses, while with nifedipine and dilthiazem they must be several times higher should an effect on arterial thrombosis be likely. The same concerns the effect of dilthiazem in the endothelial test. Still this does not mean that these agents are expected to be of no use in the prevention of arterial thrombosis: an increase in the clinical dose is possible and the main role of all calcium antagonists could be found in combinations with other agents. Lower doses may be sufficient under such conditions.

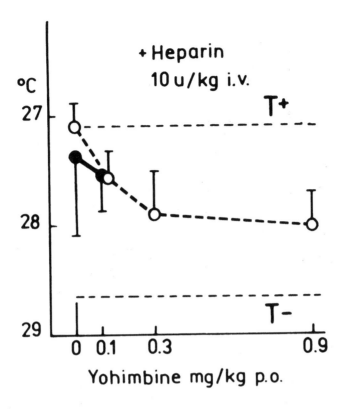

FIGURE 39.   Effect of oral yohimbine in the arterial thrombosis model
(broken line).

A very special class of calcium channel blocking agents with selective effect on the peripheral circulation includes flunarizine and similar agents (cinnarizine, lidoflazine).[530] As shown in Figure 43, flunarizine had a marked stabilizing effect on the endothelium against desquamation by citrate at doses of 0.1 mg/kg both after oral and intravenous administration. The effect of a single dose is relatively long lasting. Cinnarizine and lidoflazine exerted similar effects in the endothelial test at a somewhat higher dose level (Figure 44). At a dose of 0.1 mg/kg p.o. flunarizine also prevented endothelial sloughing after 50 mg/kg i.v. calcium chloride, and if given at a still lower dose of 0.03 mg/kg orally, it significantly prevented the platelet sequestration after intravenous citrate (Figures 45, 46). In venous thrombosis (intestinal loop of rats, intravenous lactate, and stasis) no significant effect was noted just as in the electrical arterial thrombosis model. Similarly no effects on DIC after i.v. injection of ADP, on *ex vivo* platelet aggregation, and on prostacyclin generation were observed. The drug exerted no effect on the bleeding time in rats. To summarize, this type of drug has a marked favorable effect on the endothelium without possessing an antithrombotic activity probably due to the lack of the platelet-inhibitory component.

XII. KETANSERIN

Ketanserin belongs to a large group of antiserotonin drugs, but while other agents have more or less mixed effects on serotonin receptors, ketanserin is a pure, selective, and specific inhibitor of only one kind of peripheral receptor (5-HT$_2$) and not of those present predominantly e.g., in the brain. Of course, this may be an oversimplification, since the differentiation of receptors goes probably much deeper and as yet all of them may not have been identified. Moreover, there exists a close interplay between adrenergic, histaminergic, and

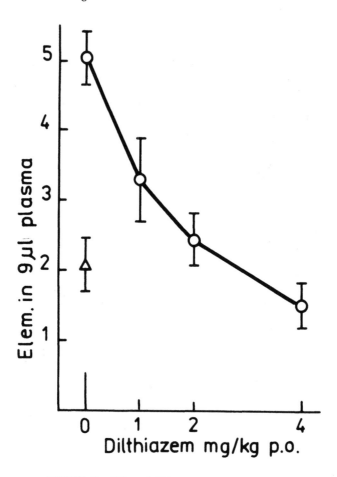

FIGURE 40.   Effect of dilthiazem on endothelial stability.

serotoninergic receptors. Most cardiovascular drugs share the activities on more than one type of receptors. Ketanserin has been included here as the main representative of the group because it is the 5-HT$_2$ receptors that seem to be in a particularly close relation to thrombogenesis, both directly and indirectly.[531] The drug is, therefore, of potential interest as an inhibitor of these processes.

However, the main rationale for its use as an antithrombotic is based on the supposed role of serotonin in thrombogenesis (Figure 47). Serotonin is the most abundant aggregating mediator in platelets of most species.[532-535] While in man it is only a weak mediator of primary and reversible platelet aggregation *in vitro*, it substantially amplifies the effect of other agents, i.e., epinephrine, ADP, and collagen.[535-537] It is released after platelet activation both *in vitro* and *in vivo* and may also influence, apart from platelets, vascular reactions accompanying and supporting thrombotic occlusions (vasospasm of both large and micro-circulation vessels, permeability increases). Not only the release of 5-HT from platelets but also the uptake or reuptake by platelets may be of importance in the thrombotic process.[538] Today, it is becoming increasingly evident that the character of this vascular response is closely dependent on endothelial integrity.[532,539] Serotonin for a long time was suspected to participate in this way in the severity of pulmonary embolism symptomatology and repeated attempts were made to influence it by antiserotonin agents.[540] In spite of some skeptical studies[541] the idea is still alive and has been recently supported by the favorable effects of ketanserin.[542] Earlier literature contains numerous conflicting reports on the effect of 5-HT on blood clotting and fibrinolysis. Benedict et al.[543] reported that the release of serotonin

TABLE 1
Comparison of Clinical and Experimental
Effective Doses of Calcium Channel Blocking
Agents

Generic name (mg/kg p.o.)	Endothelial model	Arterial thrombosis	Clinical single dose
Nifedipin	0.1	0.4	0.15
Verapamil	1.0	0.5	1.2
Dilthiazem	3.0	2.0	0.5
Carbocromen	0.5	—	2.0
Prenylamine	0.25	0.5	0.5

Note: — : not tested.

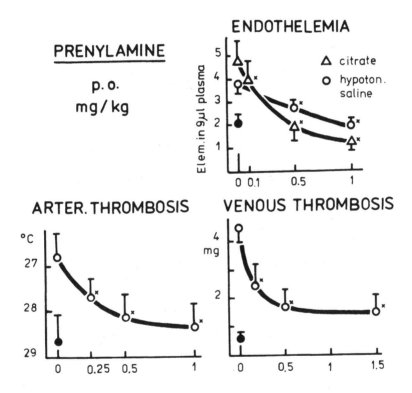

FIGURE 41.   Effect of prenylamine in the standard battery of tests.

is closely correlated with coronary occlusion in their dog model with electric current-induced thrombosis and Aiken noted a similar role of serotonin in the cyclic flow reduction model.

Ketanserin is absorbed relatively rapidly in the gut and remains quite unchanged in blood for many hours in rats, but is much more extensively metabolized in rabbits and in man to be eliminated in the urine (about 70%). In blood it is almost completely bound to proteins, particularly albumin.

Ketanserin is an effective inhibitor of *in vitro* platelet aggregation induced by 5-HT. It is also effective *ex vivo* and some doubts about its continuous effect have been explained by methodological factors.[545-548] It may cause some not very marked prolongation of bleeding[549] and prolongation of platelet survival time in rats.[550]

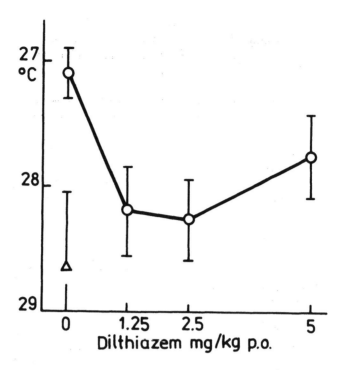

FIGURE 42.   Effect of oral dilthiazem in the arterial thrombosis model.

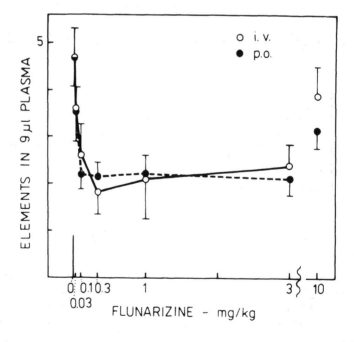

FIGURE 43.   Effect of i.v. and p.o. administered flunarizine on endo-thelial stability after the citrate challenge.

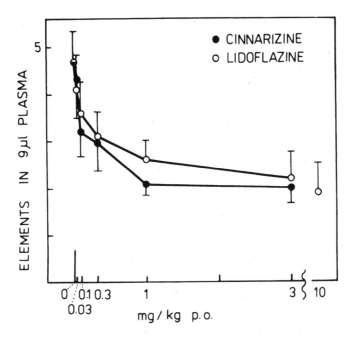

FIGURE 44. Effect of cinnarizine and lidoflazine on endothelial stability after the citrate challenge.

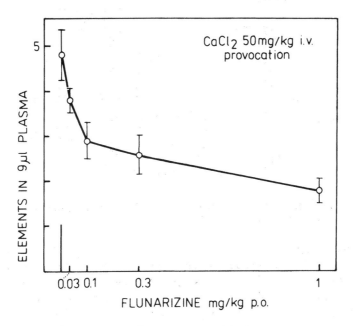

FIGURE 45. Effect of flunarizine on endothelial stability after the calcium chloride challenge.

In addition to the effects on platelets and vascular reactions, ketanserin and other anti-serotonins may favorably influence the rheological properties of blood, such as screen filtration pressure,[551] erythrocyte deformability, and whole blood viscosity,[552,553] but skeptical reports have been published.[554] There also exist papers suggesting an effect of antiserotonins on blood clotting.[555]

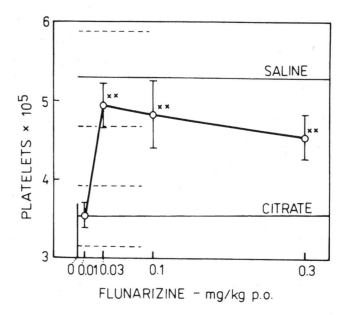

FIGURE 46.   Effect of flunarizine on platelet sequestration after the citrate challenge.

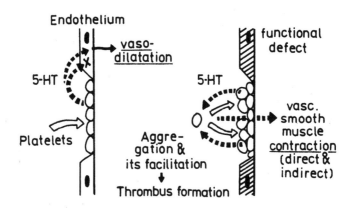

FIGURE 47.   Schematic diagram of serotonin effects on a normal and pathologically altered endothelium.

A very limited number of studies exists with ketanserin or other antiserotonins in thrombosis models. Some of these were not designed to explore the possible preventive effect of the drug, but rather the secondary consequences of an already existing thrombosis. Thus, Gautier et al.[556] used methysergide, BC 105, and some ergot derivatives as effective inhibitors of white body formation in the cerebral microcirculation of rabbits. Using ketanserin, Humphrey and Aiken[557] substantially decreased the transient platelet thrombus formation in stenosed canine coronary arteries (0.03 to 0.3 mg/kg i.v.). Bush et al.[558] prevented by i.v. ketanserin (0.25 to 0.5 mg/kg) the cyclic flow reductions due to transient platelet aggregate formation. In their further studies even much lower doses were effective.[559] Ashton et al.[560,561] in the same model confirmed the important role of 5-HT as a mediator and potentiating agent of other mediators of the phenomenon. They also confirmed the protective activity of ketanserin. De Clerck et al.[562] prevented by ketanserin the inhibitory effect of platelets on the development of collateral circulation in cats with an occluding thrombus in the aorta and noted improved perfusion. Kordenat and Kezdi[563] observed a protective effect of methysergide in an acute and chronic coronary thrombosis induced in dogs by the insertion of a thrombogenic wire via a catheter. A decreased accumulation of 5-HT in the myocardium and less severe necrotic changes were recorded. Sandler and Gerdin[564] observed a preventive effect of methysergide pretreatment on a thrombin-induced DIC and pulmonary edema in rats. Cyproheptadine inhibited the development of occlusive thrombi in injured peripheral canine arteries[30] and in primate AV-shunts.[54] Cyproheptadine likewise protected pigs against endotoxin DIC.[565] Der Agopian et al.[566] inhibited with nicergoline (presented as an alpha-blocking agent, also possessing antiserotonin activity) traumatic thrombosis in the cortical microcirculation of rabbits. Bolli et al.[567] noted inhibition of cyclic flow reductions in canine coronary arteries by the same agent. An interesting observation was a very specific antagonism of serotonin-induced platelet aggregation by 5-hydroxykynurenamide.[568] A preventive effect of BOL-148, chlorpromazine, and other drugs was observed against an *in vitro* ''thrombosis'' in the Chandler apparatus by Michal and Penglis[569] explained as an inhibition of 5-HT platelet uptake.

The studies with antiserotonins performed in the author's laboratory were stimulated by the finding that among several platelet aggregating and potential thrombosis promoting agents (ADP, thrombin, epinephrine, tannin, ellagic acid, epsilon-aminocaproic acid, and aprotinin) the only agent significantly shortening thrombosis times in electric current-induced arterial thrombosis in rats was serotonin[570] (Figures 41 and 42 in Chapter 3). On the contrary, lisuride effectively prolonged thrombosis times in the same model. Serotonin exerted a destabilizing effect on the endothelium and enhanced platelet sequestration particularly if combined with some other challenges (Figure 48).[499]

When ketanserin became available it was tested in the newly introduced standard battery of models (Figure 49). The arterial model included in this battery was in fact already based on the addition of exogenous serotonin.[138,571] Ketanserin was effective at approximate clinical doses in both thrombosis models, intravenous administration always being several times more effective than oral administration. In the venous thrombosis model the effect was never complete, attaining about 70% inhibition at the most. Interestingly, the drug was much less effective in the endothelial model, by approximately one order of magnitude, showing that the effect on the endothelium is probably of no importance for its overall antithrombotic action. The effects of ketanserin were compared with those of another antiserotonin, pizotifen (Figure 50). The drug was effective in a similar way, with arterial thrombosis relatively less and venous thrombosis more inhibited and with the same low activity in the endothelemia test. However, all effective dosages were much higher in relation to the clinical range making clinical use improbable. Other antiserotonins such as methiotepine and pipethiadene were also effective in the arterial model (Figures 51 and 52).

It may be concluded that ketanserin appears to be a promising agent for the prevention of thrombosis particularly on the arterial side. Compared with other antithrombotics, the effect on endothelial stability is negligible, showing that the main site of action is presumably localized on platelets. One objection that the effect in the arterial model was made possible by the administration of exogenous 5-HT, may be easily turned down by the fact that in the venous model the drug was effective, even though not completely, at approximately the same dose level and that another antiserotonin, lisuride was effective in electric current-induced arterial thrombosis. Thus, exogenous serotonin is not necessary to demonstrate the antithrombotic effect of antiserotonins.

XIII. BIOFLAVONOIDS

The selected representative of the bioflavonoid group, troxerutin, is a semisynthetic derivative of rutin (trihydroxyethylrutoside). The group can be more widely defined chem-

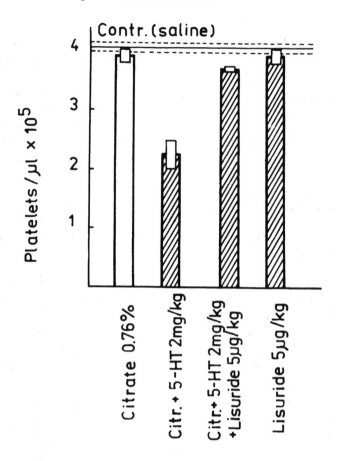

FIGURE 48.   Potentiation of the citrate effect on platelet sequestration by serotonin and its inhibition by lisuride.

ically as benzopyrones.[572] It includes coumarin derivatives (not identical with oral anticoagulants which are mostly 4-hydroxyderivatives of coumarin), flavone derivatives, such as (+)-catechin, cromoglycate, silymarin, hesperidin, quercetin, aescin, as well as some drugs which are chemically not benzopyrones but can be included from the pharmacological point of view, such as the two synthetic compounds, calcium dobesilate and ethymsylate.

Flavonoids are, in general, anti-inflammatory drugs with multiple activities. They are widely used clinically in Europe (not in the U.S.) in venous diseases, chronic inflammations of various kinds, high protein edemas, etc. While they are not established antithrombotics, these effects were suspected for a long time.

They are more or less readily absorbed in the gastrointestinal tract with semisynthetic derivatives absorbed better than natural compounds such as rutin. They are also rapidly eliminated from the blood mostly in feces, but blood levels do not tell much about their biological activity. They all bind easily to proteins, enter most tissues, and are metabolized by degradation to aglycons or by glucuronidation and excretion in urine. Their toxicity is very low.

Experimental studies with flavonoids, or more appropriately, benzopyrones mostly concerned edema formation and other models designed for testing anti-inflammatory activities. They were carried out mostly in Europe[573-575] and Australia.[572] Some important studies related to the problem of their effects on thrombogenesis originated in the U.S., where in spite of that, these drugs are not in use. Thus Robbins[576-580] investigated the effects of a series of flavonoids on red blood cell aggregation in animals as estimated by ESR, as well as in

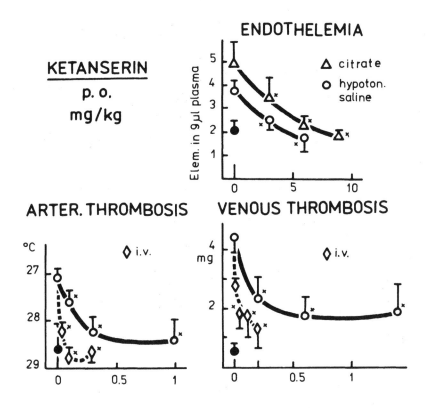

FIGURE 49.   Effects of ketanserin in the standard battery of models.

hospitalized patients both *in vitro* and *ex vivo*. Several authors investigated the effects of benzopyrones and related agents on platelet aggregation.[25,581-589] In general, platelet aggregation *in vitro* was only influenced by high drug concentrations or not at all, with the exception of collagen-induced aggregation, influenced by lower concentrations, but the possibility of direct binding to collagen should be kept in mind. They were effective both *in vitro* and *ex vivo*, and some differences were noted between various drugs of the group. The effects were doubted by Hoogendijk and Ten Cate.[590] Erythrocyte aggregation was almost always decreased,[591] and this effect was reflected also by the decrease in whole blood viscosity,[592] but this finding was not confirmed by Oughton and Barnes.[593] The effects on platelets, though not invariably confirmed, were interpreted as either the influence on phosphodiesterase with a resulting cAMP increase[594] or on the prostaglandin system such as increased prostacyclin synthetase activity.[595] More recently, Gryglewski et al.[596] suggested that flavonols (in contrast to flavanes) are effective by the free oxygen radical scavenger effect and by binding to platelets they could protect cyclo-oxygenase, prostacyclin synthetase, and EDRF, thus stimulating antithrombotic properties of the vessel wall. Other authors pointed to an effect on the lipoperoxidase system.[597] Thus esculetin and quercetin are particularly effective lipoxygenase inhibitors.[598] Flavonoids have repeatedly been described to exert a free oxygen scavenger effect.[599-601] Previously the inhibition of hyaluronidase was reported,[602,603] and remarkably enough, some increase in the coagulation factor XIII was noted.[604] Some shortening of blood clotting times was registered after several preparations. Most important for the effect of flavonoids seems to be the shifting of the oxidoreduction equilibria in endothelial cells and possibly in platelets to the reduced state, thus affecting various activation processes.

The possibility of using flavonoids as antithrombotics was suggested by Naegeli and Matis as early as 1957.[605] Several studies concerning similar problems were carried out by

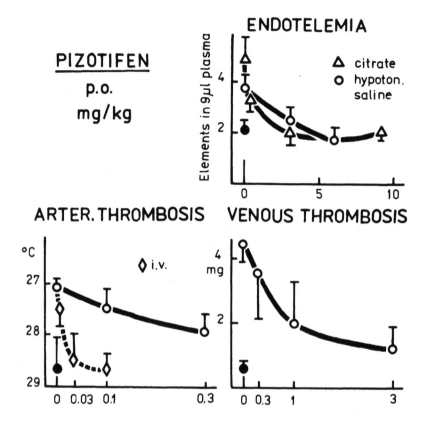

FIGURE 50.   Effects of pizotifen in the standard battery of models.

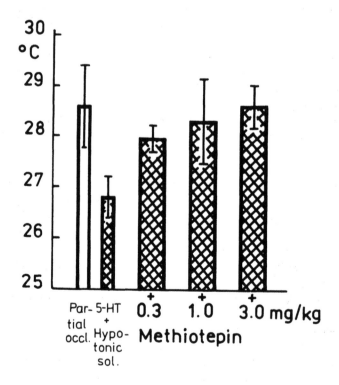

FIGURE 51.   Effect of oral methiotepine on arterial thrombosis.

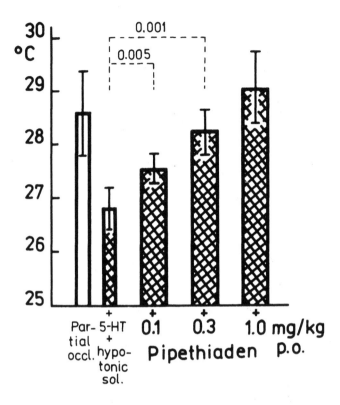

FIGURE 52.   Effect of oral pipethiadene on arterial thrombosis.

Földi and his group: Földi and Zoltán[606] have developed a model of thrombophlebitis in dogs by a paravenous injection of turpentine oil. The leg circumference was measured for the quantitation of edema. A flavonoid preparation (rutin with coumarin) was administered intramuscularly for 17 d and edema formation was significantly decreased. A similar study with a lower dose of the rutin component (25 mg/kg) and increased dose of coumarin (4 mg/kg) was even more effective.[608] The drug increased the content of glycoprotein in the leg tissue as compared with a thrombophlebitis control.[608] These studies concerned the consequences of thrombosis rather than thrombus formation. A somewhat different aspect was emphasized in the study of Mirkovitch et al.[609] Iliac canine veins were enveloped in a silicon rubber casing, and after several weeks the vessels were examined by phlebography for the degree of obstruction. A flavonoid preparation (mixture of hydroxyethylated rutosides) at a dose of 500 mg/kg/d intravenously prevented the obstruction. The casing damaged nutritional circulation of the vessel wall and the hematoma formation substantially influenced the obstruction. Niebes[603] observed in animals with thrombosis a decrease in pathologically increased glycosaminoglycan hydrolases in the wall after a flavonoid preparation (HR). These and similar enzymes are of lysosomal origin and flavonoids tend to increase lysosomal membrane stability. On the other hand, Casley-Smith and Gaffney[610] showed that flavonoids increase both the content of tissue macrophages and the level of proteolytic activity which they produce. Bergqvist et al.[611] investigated the activity of flavonoids in three models: hemostatic plug formation in the mesenteric microvessels of rabbits was the first one. Flavonoid (HR = hydroxyethylrutosides) at a dose of 500 mg/kg i.v. daily for 3 d prolonged bleeding. In laser-induced arteriolar thromboembolism of rabbit mesenteric microcirculation, HR had no effect at all after the same dose. On the other hand, some insignificant trend to a decreased thrombogenesis was observed in morrhuate-induced femoral vein thrombosis. In all three models only one very high dose was used. The authors justify the selection of

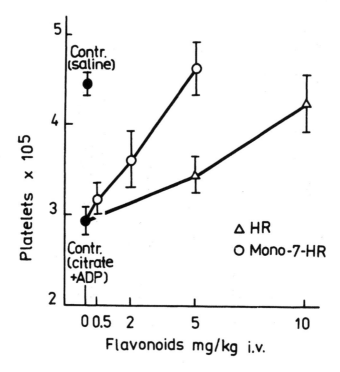

FIGURE 53.   Effect of intravenous HR (hydroxyethylated rutosides) and
mono-7-hydroxyethylrutoside on platelet sequestration.

this dose by the results of *in vitro* studies of Ten Cate et al.[584,585] with platelet aggregation. This is of course hardly acceptable, and as will be shown later, bioflavonoids probably have a much lower optimum dose with higher doses probably having adverse effects. The group of Sawyer[612] noted a more negative surface charge of canine carotid arteries after some flavonoids, with opposite effects on erythrocytes. They found a good correlation between the vascular surface charge and antithrombotic effects in electric current-induced thrombi in rat mesenteric vessels. The occlusion times were estimated and HR was effective at a dose of 50 mg/kg while catechin A was already similarly effective at the dose of 5 mg/kg. There was a trend to a marked dose optimum. Robbins[576] also used a DIC model based on ADP injections to rats. Hexamethylated flavonoid (nobiletine) displayed a high protective activity at a dose of 3.2 mg/kg i.v. The effect was even more pronounced than that of heparin. Klemm[613] registered on a film the thrombogenesis induced by ionizing radiation in the rabbit ear chamber and the preventive effect of HR (45 mg/kg i.m.). Michal and Giessinger[25] tested a functionally related drug, calcium dobesilate, in comparison with ASA on thrombus formation in the microcirculation of the hamster cheek pouch induced by ADP and electric current. Calcium dobesilate was effective, but the combination with ASA was better. Both the antithrombotic and oxygen-free radical scavenging effect could be used to explain a protective effect of HR (200 mg/kg i.v.) on ischemic canine myocardium.[614]

On the whole, benzopyrones were never systematically tested as antithrombotics. The existing studies used either unsuitable models or unsuitable doses. On the other hand, there exist sufficient indications that these kinds of drugs might be useful in this field and deserve further investigation.

In the author's laboratory troxerutin was tested in several models.[85,186] In the platelet sequestration test two agents were compared. Mono-7-HR was more effective than HR (designation for a mixture of hydroxyethylated rutosides with a prevailing trihydroxyethylated compound) (Figure 53). In the endothelemia model, troxerutin was fully effective at a dose 2 mg/kg which also represented a narrow dose optimum (Figure 54). Calcium dobesilate

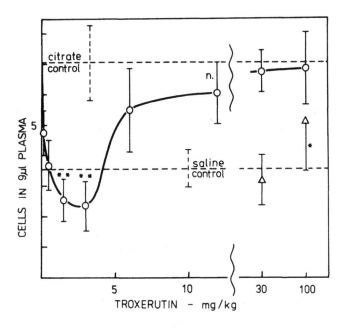

FIGURE 54. Effect of i.v. troxerutin on endothelial stability after the citrate challenge.

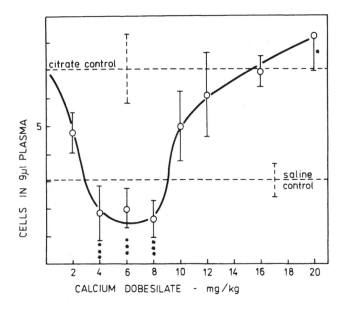

FIGURE 55. Effect of i.v. calcium dobesilate on endothelial stability after the citrate challenge.

which may be functionally included in the group had about 50% activity of troxerutin (Figure 55). The low effective dosage showed that the site of the pharmacological actions of these drugs is largely the endothelial lining, and flavonoids are among the most active agents in the endothelial model. It is interesting to note that their effectiveness is particularly marked if hydrogen peroxide is used as a challenge in the model, showing that the oxygen-free radical scavenger effect is prominent (Figure 56).[370] Silymarin and other agents mostly used

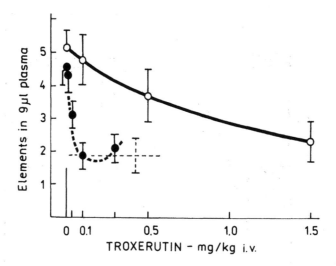

FIGURE 56.   Inhibitory effect of troxerutin on the endothelemia-increasing activity of hydrogen peroxide in comparison with that of citrate (broken line: hydrogen peroxide challenge, full line: citrate challenge).

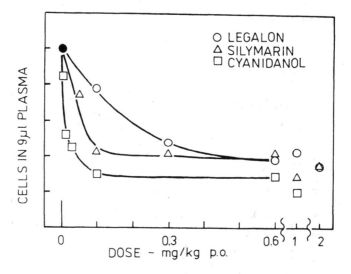

FIGURE 57.   Effect of oral silymarine, cyanidanole and Legalon® on endothelial stability after the citrate challenge.

to treat hepatic inflammations are also quite effective in the endothelemia model (Figure 57). In the next diagram, the ineffectiveness of HR over a wide dose range is shown in electric current-induced arterial thrombosis (Figure 58). This may be explained by the inability of agents predominantly inhibiting the vascular factor to manifest any activity under conditions of excessive lesions. In a model of venostatic thrombosis in the rat intestinal loops, HR alone had some activating effect on thrombus formation absent in mono-7-HR. This activating effect might be related to that of polyphenolic compounds such as tannin, ellagic acid, etc. Mono-7-HR also effectively inhibited the prothrombotic effect of papaverine, vasopressin, and epinephrine.

In the more recently introduced standard battery of models, troxerutin was effective both against citrate and hypotonic saline-induced endothelemia, but its action was several times

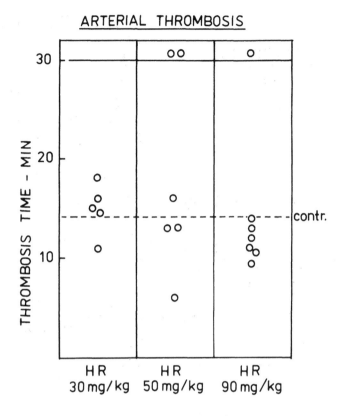

FIGURE 58.   Ineffectiveness of HR in the electrically induced arterial thrombosis.

less prominent in the latter modification (Figure 59).[138,139] The effective doses were under 1 mg/kg orally. In the arterial model the intravenous route of administration was by one order of magnitude more effective than the oral route, indicating some problems with resorption. Despite that, the drug was effective at the level of 20 mg/kg p.o., about four times the clinical single dose. On the other hand, in the venous model a dose as low as 2 mg/kg p.o. was significantly effective. This shows that the effect on platelets is probably not very prominent in the antithrombotic activity of troxerutin, and virtually all activity is probably aimed at preserving the functional integrity of the endothelium. Some studies[572] show that flavonoids might influence the structural calcium ion function in the properties of the cell membrane glycocalyx and intercellular matrix. The particularly strong effect in the citrate-induced modification of the endothelemia test points in the same direction. These drugs are not devoid of a possible application as antithrombotics by any means, especially if combined with other agents. They could be indicated in situations in which protection of the endothelium is of utmost importance and prolonged administration would pose no problem in view of their low toxicity.

XIV. CLOFIBRATE

Chlorophenoxy-isobutyrate or clofibrate was one of the first potential antithrombotics tested both experimentally nad clinically, but its main proposed use was as an antiathero-sclerotic, first in combination with androsterone (Atromid®) and later alone as Atromid-S. Following reports of some unfavorable side effects in a clinical trial designed to study primary prevention of ischemic heart disease, much of the interest in the drug subsided even though the cooperative study suggested the existence of an antithrombotic component of

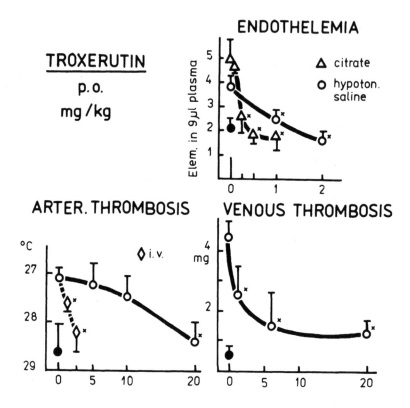

FIGURE 59.   Effects of troxerutin in the standard battery of models.

effect.[615] Meanwhile, clofibrate represents another interesting type of antithrombotic and as various analogues and related drugs are still looked for (etafibrate, bezafibrate, halofenate, etc.), it deserves our continuing attention.

The drug was investigated with, at that time, the most frequently used platelet function tests, i.e., stickiness to glass beads and other materials *in vitro* and *ex vivo*.[616-621] It was also found to be effective *ex vivo* (not *in vitro*) in platelet aggregation tests[619,622] and on platelet survival.[623-626] Similar results were obtained with halofenate.[627,628] A particularly interesting finding was the decrease in the fibrinogen and soluble fibrinogen complexes level in blood,[621] as well as the favorable effect in primate atherosclerosis.[490] All these effects seem to be independent of the lipid-lowering activity. Some inhibitory effects on lipid peroxidation were noted.[630]

Reports on the effects of clofibrate in animal thrombosis models were scarce. Roba et al.[380] investigated, among other antithrombotics, clofibrate in a mouse DIC model induced by intravenous ADP. The drug was effective at a dose of 100 mg/kg p.o., if given 1 h in advance. Sim et al.[631] used a combination of ADP and an electrical stimulus in the micro-circulation of the hamster cheek pouch. A preparation of etofylline clofibrate (4 to 8 mg/kg p.o.) was effective not only in the prevention of thrombosis, but also in enhancing thrombolysis.[632] This was explained by the effect on prostacyclin synthesis or synergism with the prostacyclin-induced vascular thrombolytic activity. On the other hand, this contrasts with the early studies of Chakrabarti et al.,[633] who found an antifibrinolytic activity in humans supposed to be due to the exhaustion of vascular activators. Haft et al.[634] and Wexler and Greenberg[635] observed an inhibitory effect on myocardial necrotic changes. Some of the more recent studies document the renewed interest in this group of drugs.

Clofibrate has never been tested in the author's laboratory in thrombosis models and has only been investigated in the endothelemia test using several challenging agents (Figure 60).

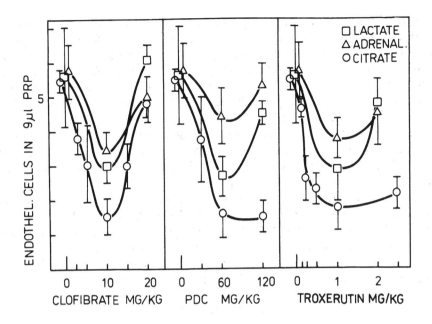

FIGURE 60. Comparison of effects of clofibrate, pyridinolcarbamate (PDC), and troxerutin on endothelemia after three challenges (lactate, epinephrine, citrate).

In comparison with two other vasotropic agents, i.e., pyridinolcarbamate and a bioflavonoid preparation, the drug was effective after oral administration to rats 2 h in advance against citrate, lactate, epinephrine, and nicotine-induced endothelemia increases at an equal dose of 10 mg/kg which is quite near to the single clinical dose of about 7 mg/kg. This effect was about six times stronger than after PDC, but the latter drug showed a greater specificity against nicotine and this specificity was still much more pronounced in the flavonoid preparation.

To summarize, clofibrate has unquestionably a stabilizing effect on the endothelium, an observation which may be of importance for its antithrombotic effect.

XV. ANAGRELIDE

Anagrelide is another theoretically interesting drug unrelated to other antiplatelet agents. It is chemically an imidazoquinazoline.[76,636,637] While studying the experimental data about the antithrombotic activity of this drug, one has the impression that it was discovered in a screening for *in vitro* antiaggregatory activity. This is already suggested by the name chosen for the drug. Anagrelide was *in vitro* very effective against aggregation induced by all agents. Particularly primary aggregation, and at a still lower concentration, the shape change was influenced. It turned out to be more potent than any other synthetic antithrombotic drug. A corresponding effectiveness was observed in several species even *ex vivo* after oral administration.[76,638] While *in vitro* the aggregation of human platelets was inhibited less than of platelets of other species, *ex vivo* the drug was more effective in man than in other species (0.25 to 5 mg/kg in animals and about 0.07 mg/kg p.o. in man).

The inhibition of biolaser-induced intravascular thrombosis in the microcirculation of the rabbit ear chamber required 1 to 5 mg/kg p.o. which is quite in agreement with the *ex vivo* aggregation studies. In electrically induced carotid artery thrombosis in dogs, the drug was markedly effective at a dose of 5 mg/kg p.o. It was supposed that the antithrombotic effect in man would run parallel with the antiaggregatory activity *ex vivo* and correspondingly low effective doses were expected. This presumption was not justified, and the agreement of effective doses in aggregation studies and very special animal models probably has to be looked upon as a happy coincidence. The drug was practically ineffective in ellagic acid-induced venous stasis thrombosis. However, at a dose of 8 mg/kg the drug exerted some potentiating effect on heparin 5 U/kg i.v. Anagrelide has some inhibitory effect on platelet aggregate formation in the canine hemorrhagic shock (0.2 to 5 mg/kg p.o.) and was partially effective in the rat endotoxin shock at a dose of 10 to 50 mg/kg p.o. It prolonged bleeding time but only at very high dosages.

The mechanism of action is not completely understood, but it was believed that the drug might act as a relatively strong inhibitor of phosphodiesterase probably acting on a subpool of low-K_m cAMP-phosphodiesterase. It is also a phospholipase A_2 inhibitor, not effective on cyclo-oxygenase or thromboxane synthetase.

The drug was unquestionably effective as an antiaggregant, and in some thrombosis models, as an antithrombotic. However, it may be asked whether a probably isolated effect on one platelet function only, i.e., aggregation, would be sufficient for a full-scale antithrombotic activity in a clinical setting. More recently, the drug has been found to decrease platelet production, a fact potentially limiting its use for short time periods. On the other hand, this relatively selective effect may be used in new kinds of indications.[639]

XVI. DEXTRAN

Dextran preparations serve, in general, as plasma volume expanders. They represent no uniform or homogeneous compound and various preparations differ particularly in the average molecular weight. Natural dextrans have a high molecular weight, while those used for therapeutic purposes are, in fact, partially degraded semisynthetic compounds. Standard preparations have a molecular weight of 70,000, but low molecular weight dextrans of about 40,000 are also often used and differ in some functional parameters.

The drug is administered parenterally in infusion and attains very high blood concentrations. It is broken down by dextranases in the body and about two thirds are excreted by the kidney. The plasma half-life is about 6 to 8 h. Maximum effects seem to be attained after an unexplained lag period.

Antithrombotic activity was expected particularly from the low molecular derivatives. The supposed mechanism of action was the formation of a film covering formed blood elements and probably also the endothelial surface ("coating"). In this way the drug may interfere with many functions associated with thrombogenesis which are known to be localized predominantly on such surfaces. It inhibits erythrocyte and platelet aggregation,[640] platelet adhesion,[641] interferes with blood clotting processes, and if fibrin forms, it has a modified character and is less resistant to thrombolysis.[642,643] The bleeding time may be prolonged simulating von Willebrand's disease.[644,645]

Dextran preparations were frequently tested in various thrombosis models over the years from 1957 to 1970, but rarely in more recent years. One of the first studies was carried out by Arendt et al.[646] and was based on the inhibition of platelet thrombus formation in the microcirculation of the hamster cheek pouch induced by local thrombin administration. Dextran of m.w. 75,000 not only slowed down thrombus formation, but also prolonged bleeding and increased capillary fragility. Borgström et al.[213] observed that low molecular (not high molecular) weight dextran was very effective in preventing venous thrombi in rabbits with a mechanical trauma inflicted to the thigh musculature. Ashwin and Jaques[647] confirmed the antithrombotic effect of dextran in rats with topical formalin-induced thrombi in jugular veins. Józsa et al.[648] did not observe any antithrombotic effect of dextran on thrombogenesis in the mesoappendix of rabbits induced by a thermocauter lesion. Ernst et al.,[649] on the other hand, used dextran to decrease the weights of electric current-induced thrombi in the femoral veins of dogs. Sawyer and Moncrieff[650] observed the inhibition of

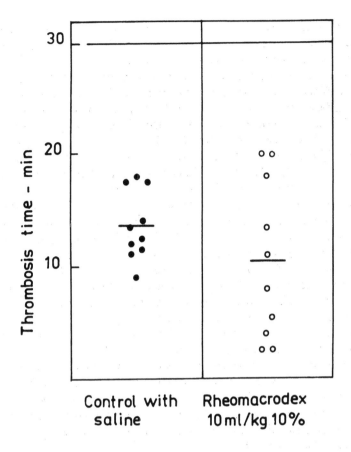

FIGURE 61. Lack of effect of low molecular dextran in the electrically induced arterial thrombosis.

propagation of thrombi induced in femoral veins by electric stimulation. Bryant et al.[651] confirmed an antithrombotic effect of several dextran preparations of different molecular weights in canine femoral arteries after arteriotomy and closure by silk sutures. However, no differences between preparations were observed. Just-Viera and Yeager[228] confirmed the effectiveness of dextran in the large canine veins into which polyethylene tubes had been introduced. Arfors et al.[99] inhibited successfully the formation of thrombi in rabbit ear chambers induced by laser shots. Interestingly enough, heparin was not effective under the same conditions. Mason et al.[54] tested successfully dextran, among other agents, to prevent thrombus formation in monkey AV-shunts. Aubert et al.[652] was particularly interested in antithrombotic properties of dextran-derived biomaterials.

Thus dextran preparations may have antithrombotic activity under various conditions, but their use would always be limited to acute situations such as prevention of postoperative thrombosis.[653]

In our hands, low molecular dextran (Rheomacrodex®) was not effective in the electrically induced arterial thrombosis (Figure 61). In view of the low sensitivity of the model this does not exclude an antithrombotic activity in arteries under suitable conditions.

XVII. ORAL ANTICOAGULANTS

The majority of presently used oral anticoagulants are derivatives of 4-hydroxycoumarine and a small portion may only be classified as indandione derivatives. The anticoagulant activity of these drugs is due to the competitive inhibition of vitamin K-dependent carboxylation of coagulation factor II, VII, IX, and X precursors. They need a latency period (18 to 72 h) before developing full effect. Their anticoagulant effectiveness was already discovered before World War II by Link and his group.

Most experimental evidence for their effectiveness as antithrombotics was published about 10 years after World War II and most of the first animal thrombosis models were designed just for testing these drugs. As a result, the models were often rather crude and not particularly adequate. The vascular lesions used were frequently very much in excess. Thus, electric current-induced thrombosis was employed in the studies of Williams and Elliot,[654] Carey and Williams,[217] and Reber.[655] Drastic chemical challenges were necessary in the models of Richards and Cortell,[656] Thill et al.,[657] Jansen and Tage-Hansen,[658] Kubik and Wright,[659] Wright and Kubik,[660] Jewell et al.,[661] Kamyia et al.,[662] and Blake et al.[21] Drastic mechanical trauma was used by Dale and Jaques,[663] Moses,[205] Kiesewetter and Shumaker,[208] Loewe et al.,[207] Rogers et al.,[664] and Borgström et al.[213] Intravascular thrombin injections were used by Holden et al.,[665] Wright et al.,[666] and Baeckeland,[667] especially to study the influence on recanalization processes. Stasis plus serum models were used in dogs by Wessler and Morris.[211,668] Saturated fatty acid injections were employed by Hoak et al.,[224,227] dietary induction by Davidson et al.,[669] and combined hyperlipemia with endotoxin injection by Renaud.[230] In most studies some partial preventive effect was observed particularly if very high doses were administered but often the effect was negligible.[217,219,221,654,655,661] Low doses led sometimes to enhanced thrombogenesis (Fulton et al.[223] in microcirculation, Murphy et al.[670] in extracorporeal circulation). Heparin was generally more effective and only exceptionally the reverse was true.[661] Microcirculation and arterial thrombi were influenced much less than those in large veins, but even under the latter conditions the effect was often incomplete. Some of these relatively unsuccessful prevention studies could be blamed on species differences as dosages higher than in man were necessary in many animals to attain the same clotting factor decreases, but mostly an unsuitable design of models inducing excessive trauma was responsible.

In the author's laboratory, indalitan given orally 48 h in advance was used as a representative of oral anticoagulants in rats.[81] While about 10% prothrombin complex level was attained by the drug alone or when combined with ASA (30 mg/kg 1 h before the blood collection), no effect was observed in the model of electric current-induced thrombosis in rats (Figures 62, 63). Meanwhile, this dose of ASA alone had no significant effect either. This shows the low sensitivity of such arterial models to oral anticoagulant effects.

Besides indandione derivatives, only 4-hydroxycoumarin derivatives are effective as anticoagulants. Coumarin, referred to in another section as one of the most effective benzopyrones, is therefore not effective as an anticoagulant. But is also the opposite true? That is, do oral anticoagulants show vasotropic or endotheloprotective activity typical of benzopyrones? In fact, they do exert such an effect which is practically immediate and should probably always be present even under clinical conditions (Figure 21 in Chapter 3).[385] On the other hand, the curve shows a typical optimum and the effective anticoagulant dose (as documented by *ex vivo* tests) already coincides with the ascending limb of the dose-to-effect curve, i.e., with an already endothelemia-increasing dose. This potentially unfavorable effect is particularly marked after repeated administration, i.e., has a cumulative nature (Figure 64). It can be remembered that an endothelial damage after therapeutic doses of warfarin was described by Kahn et al.[671] The endothelemia-increasing effect may be blocked by the concomitant administration of other endotheloprotective drugs, especially those possessing no marked optimum dose. Thus, prenylamine (0.5 mg/kg p.o.) completely inhibited the endothelemia-increasing effect of warfarin without influencing one-stage prothrombin time (Figures 65, 66). The favorable effect of added prenylamine was manifested also by the significant prevention of a hematocrit decrease after warfarin in rats, i.e., prenylamine may have a protective effect against capillary bleeding after coumarin anticoagulants.

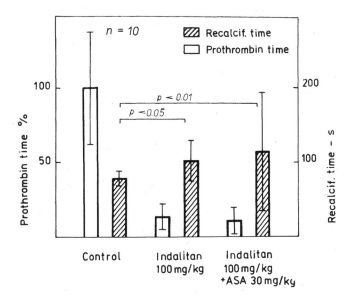

FIGURE 62. Effect of indalitan with and without ASA on coagulation parameters in rats.

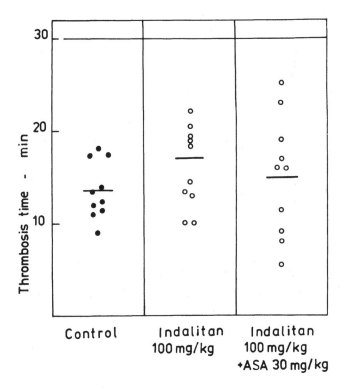

FIGURE 63. Effect of indalitan with and without ASA on electrically induced arterial thrombosis.

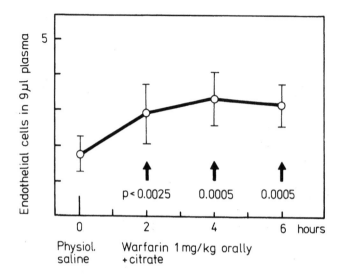

FIGURE 64.   Cumulative effect of warfarin on endothelemia.

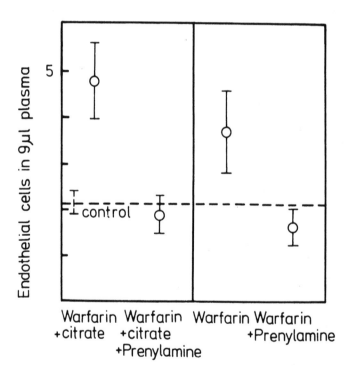

FIGURE 65.   Inhibitory effect of prenylamine on the endothelemia-increasing activity of warfarin.

XVIII. OTHER AGENTS

Many other agents or groups of agents have been tested as potential antithrombotics, mostly *in vitro*. Only a minority has reached a further stage, i.e., testing in animal models and it was only an exception that some agents were directly tested in this way.

One of the relatively well-tested groups is *thrombin inhibitors*, both natural (i.e., hirudin and other substances derived from blood-sucking animals) and synthetic. Many studies in

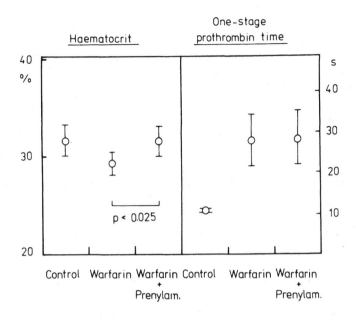

FIGURE 66. Protective effect of prenylamine against hematocrit decrease after warfarin treatment in rats with no simultaneous effect on Quick's time.

this field have been carried out by the Erfurt group.[672,673] Thus, hirudin was tested both in a thrombin-induced DIC model,[674] in the chemically injured rabbit jugular vein,[675] and rat stasis venous thrombosis.[676] Recombinant hirudin was tested against rat venous thrombosis induced by thromboplastin injection combined with stasis.[677] The main groups of synthetic inhibitors, benzamidine and arginine derivatives, were tested mostly in venous stasis thrombosis models in rats and rabbits,[678-684] and in carotid artery thrombosis in rats induced either by electric current or chemically.[678,685] In many studies the drugs were tested in DIC models using induction by thrombin, thromboplastin, endotoxin, snake venom, etc. Parenterally administered agents were, as a rule, quite effective,[686-689] just as in rabbit and dog AV-shunts.[681,690] As already mentioned, the drugs were administered only parenterally as bolus injections or infusions and the effect was relatively short-lived. Despite the high effectiveness and some advantages over heparin (e.g., independence of AT III levels), the impossibility of oral administration is presently the main obstacle to a wider clinical use today reserved to acute situations (hemodialysis, DIC).

A relatively large group includes some other nonsteroid anti-inflammatory drugs (NSAID), beside ASA. Many of them have been tested as potential antithrombotics. In general, they are known as competitive cyclo-oxygenase inhibitors, but other effects such as membrane-stabilizing activity and phosphodiesterase inhibition[691] are possible. However, their anti-inflammatory effects may be dissociated from the antithrombotic activity.[692] Indomethacin proved to be most effective in many models (Rosenblum and El-Sabban,[23,24] in mouse cortical microcirculation, Bourgain et al.,[26,86] rat mesenteric microcirculation, Cerskus et al.,[152] arachidonic acid-induced DIC, Vigdahl et al.,[155] a similar model and rat arterial electrically induced carotid thrombosis, and Kowey et al.,[414] dog coronary cyclic flow reductions). It was not effective in a carotid artery model and rat extracorporeal circulation.[693] Unfortunately, its "therapeutic window" is quite narrow.

Phenylbutazone was tested in several models such as in the rabbit ear chamber and laser-induced lesion,[40] canine AV-shunt,[681] against endotoxin shock,[150,694] and Arthus reaction,[695] with variable results.

Ibuprofen was effective in a DIC model designed by Nishizawa et al.[696] and Perlman et al.,[697] platelet deposition models of Gloviczki et al.[698] and Romson et al.,[699] and laser-induced thrombi in the rabbit ear chamber of Esquivel et al.[701] Indobufen was tested in an arterio-arterial microanastomosis in rats.[700] Fenoprofen was tested in an extracorporeal shunt model by Herrmann et al.[702]

A new type of NSAID is represented by benzydamine which differs from other agents in many respects and also possesses an oxygen-free radical scavenging activity. It prevented thrombosis after the insertion of a wire coil into the vena cava in rats.[703] The effects of another drug, suprofen, were reviewed by Todd et al.[704] It also inhibited mortality after arachidonic acid in rats.[705]

A special position among NSAID is occupied by ditazole[706] and related agents such as K 3920. According to de Gaetano et al.,[707,708] the drug shortened the bleeding time, did not influence platelet aggregation by ADP, but inhibited that by collagen. After 400 mg/kg p.o. it inhibited rabbit carotid artery thrombosis induced by electric current[709] and decreased thrombogenic properties of artificial surfaces in an *in vitro* study.[710] It also inhibited TXA_2 effects but not prostacyclin production.[711]

Two newly emerging groups of drugs have to be mentioned here. The first is inhibitors of platelet-activating factor, PAF. Even though main attention was paid to other roles of this mediator than in thrombogenesis (shock, allergic reactions, bronchial tonus control, etc.) some of its inhibitors (or rather, PAF receptor antagonists) such as BN 52021, BN 50 341, L-652731, triazolam, and alprazolam,[712,713] as well as kadsurenone[714] were not only tested on platelet function *in vitro*, but also in animal models. Etienne et al.[715] tested BN 50 341 in a model with electric current-induced carotid artery thrombosis in the rat. The drug was effective at doses of 50 mg/kg/h. In the mesenteric microcirculation, the drug was effective at a dose of 3 mg/kg i.v. against topical ADP administration.

The second group attracting increasing attention is lipoxygenase inhibitors. Lipoxygenase activity products have been shown to mediate thrombotic phenomena after endotoxin,[716] but some of them could also inhibit platelet aggregation.[717] Lipoxygenase inhibitor U-66,855 was effective against jugular vein thrombosis induced by stasis and surgical trauma in cats at a dose of 5 mg/kg i.v. Some authors suggested that leukocyte-produced leukotrienes participate in the pathogenesis of stasis thrombi.[718] An effective inhibitor of leukotriene biosynthesis is e.g., the antimycotic drug, ketoconazole.[719]

Several antibiotics were investigated for their *in vitro* effect on platelet functions because e.g., carbenicillin and penicillin at high doses tend to produce bleeding diathesis.[720-722] Similar effects were observed with chloramphenicol and cycloheximide,[723] but only carbenicillin was tested in a biomodel.[35] The dog artery was injured by pronase and doses of 250 to 750 mg/kg s.c. were quite effective in preventing thrombosis.

Antithrombotics that were among the first to be tested under clinical conditions in the prevention of venous thrombosis were antimalarics, particularly hydroxychloroquine.[724] Their activity was probably due to the inhibition of phospholipase A_2 activity, and thus, to a decrease in arachidonic acid availability. In contrast to this supposed mechanism of action directed chiefly against platelet functions, the drugs were effective in preventing postoperative venous thrombosis.[725] Studies in animal models were carried out with the chemically related quinazoline derivative BL-3459. At an oral dose of 150 mg/kg the drug was highly effective in arterial electric current-induced rat and dog thrombosis, prevented death after arachidonic acid and endotoxin DIC in mice, and inhibited laser-induced thrombosis in the microcirculation of the rabbit ear chamber.[155,636] The drug was also effective in rabbits with an AV anastomosis at a dose as low as 1 mg/kg i.p.[726]

In the endothelemia model hydroxychlorquine possessed a marked activity with an optimum at the dose approximately corresponding to the clinical range (Figure 67).

The organopreparation defibrotide (polydeoxyribonucleotide) was found effective against electrically induced thrombosis in dogs[727] and inhibited venous thrombosis probably by

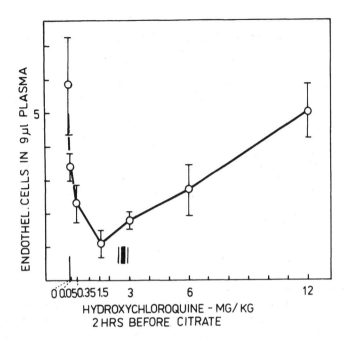

FIGURE 67. The effect of oral hydroxychloroquine on endothelemia in
rats after the citrate challenge.

supporting thrombolysis in rabbits.[728] The drug is more effective against thrombus removal than its formation.

Several monoaminooxydase inhibitors such as iproniazide were more or less effective in microcirculation thrombosis.[729,730]

Some new drugs were at a relatively early phase tested in animal models. Thus pyridazinone derivative C 85-3143 was tested in stenotic and freeze-injured carotids in rats, as well as in stenotic jugular veins of rabbits,[731] peptide derivative of factor X in the Wessler-type model of vein thrombosis in rabbits,[732] molsidomine and its metabolite SIN-1 in the rat mesenteric microcirculation,[733] as well as in silver nitrate-induced venous and arterial thrombosis in rabbits.[734] Diferuloyl methan (curcumin), isolated from the indian plant curcuma longa, was effective in a mouse DIC induced by intravenous collagen and epinephrine.[41] Born and Kovacs[97] successfully tested N-acetyl neuraminic acid in the microcirculation of rats and hamsters injured by laser shots. Herrmann et al.[735] observed a marked antithrombotic activity in hamster cheek pouch microthrombosis induced by the fluorescein-isothiocyanate method after the vasodilating agent naftidrofuryl (probably blocking 5-HT$_2$ receptors). Using the Hornstra method with the polyethylene loop in the carotid artery Lecker and Kumar[736] tested a new pyridazinone derivative. Ott and Smith[737] investigated a naphthyridine derivative in rats with a polyethylene tubing inserted into the carotid artery (Chan's method). The glycosaminoglycan sulodexide was successfully tested in electrically induced carotid artery thrombosis in rats.[738]

XIX. CONCLUSIONS

It is hoped that this survey has sufficiently documented the unsatisfactory situation in the use of animal models for testing antithrombotics. Often the models used had only a marginal relation to the natural process of thrombogenesis. Most probably, in many studies such models were only chosen deliberately which have shown in preliminary experiments sufficient sensitivity to the tested drug without respecting their representativeness. In other

TABLE 2
Comparison of Clinical and Experimental Effective Doses
of a Series of Drugs

Drugs (mg/kg p.o.)	Endothelial model	Arterial model	Venous model	Clinical single dose
Heparin	0.1 U/kg i.v.	10	0.25	ca 10
ASA	3	5°	10	7
Dipyridamole	0.2	4	1°	1
Sulfinpyrazone	0.5	1	1°	3
Prenylamine	0.5	0.5°	0.5°	0.5
Troxerutin	1.5	20°	10°	5
Ketanserin	4	0.5	0.6°	0.6
Pentoxifylline	2	8	2	6
Metipranolol	0.25	1—5	1—3	0.5—1

Note:°: incomplete inhibition.

studies the models were very sophisticated and required special equipment that would impress by the advanced technical level. Such tendencies, of course, decreased the reproducibility and were hardly desirable in attempts to design a standardized system of models. Meanwhile, no serious efforts at standardization were made. Methods suitable for such purposes should be as simple as possible limiting at the same time the human factor and making it possible to accumulate a large body of data. It may be argued that the criteria of models representativeness have never been sufficiently defined just as the whole concept of thrombogenesis is not very clear as yet. Consequently, the possible solution would seem to be drug testing in as many models of various types in different species as possible. However, this approach would only increase the present chaos. The current trend to reduce the number of biomodels in favor of *in vitro* testing would afford a very insufficient substitute even in the early screening phase of drug studies often leading to speculative approaches and revealing only one facet of the problem, inadequately founded by relevant facts. In principle, *in vivo* studies should not be based on *in vitro* ones, and rather the opposite should be true. An analogous situation exists with another type of model: mathematical models that can only provide such answers which have been entered implicitly into the computer as starting data. Unfortunately, unknown data still largely prevail. The presumptions on which many *in vitro* studies and similar theoretical models are based, are often extremely shaky.

Another trend which might have been noted in the survey was the general neglect of vascular factors even though today they are increasingly declared as important. The traditional stress on blood clotting was later replaced by platelet functions, but the vascular factors have not yet been included into the methodology in a routine way. While the methods introduced in this monograph may not be the best possible, they still represent the first attempt at an integrated and standardized methodology for the study of antithrombotics. The models of endothelemia, as well as both models of thrombosis, all share one concept and stress particularly the role of the vessel wall. They also use one stimulus, hypotonic saline injection, but it might be possible to obtain further information by comparing the effects of various other stimuli, e.g., citrate, epinephrine, hydrogen peroxide, calcium chloride, etc. Some interesting differences might have been noted e.g., with the endothelemia model in the presented data. By all means, the system is not considered a definitive solution and various modifications are possible and might be useful.

The comparison of effective doses in the new system of models with single clinical doses (in some potential antithrombotic drugs those used in other than antithrombotic indications) shows a very close correlation: the dosages are almost always within the same order of magnitude and often practically identical (Table 2). The following conclusions may be drawn from the comparison:

1. It is possible to design models showing approximately equal sensitivity to drugs in experimental animals and man.

2. Such models, while very simple, may be sufficiently quantitative to make possible dose-to-effect and combination studies.

3. It is also possible to compare, at least to some extent, the results obtained in all three models and to draw some conclusions about the prevailing mechanism of drug action, i.e., either the effect on platelets (relatively high activity in the arterial model and low in the endothelemia test) or on endothelium (high activity in all tests and particularly in the endothelemia test). A relatively high activity in the venous model in comparison with the other two points to an effect on the clotting and fibrinolytic system. If the effective dosage in the model is much higher than in the clinical practice and the clinical dose cannot be increased, the drug may be expected impractical for therapeutic purposes in antithrombotic indications.

REFERENCES

1. **Gibson, P. C.,** Aspirin in the treatment of vascular diseases, *Lancet,* 2, 1172, 1949.
2. **Bounameaux, Y. and van Cauwenberge, H.,** Action de la cortisone, de l'ACTH et du salicylate de soude sur les thrombocytes et la coagulation sanguine, *Sang,* 25, 889, 1954.
3. **Born, G. V. R.,** Quantitative investigations into the aggregation of blood platelets, *J. Physiol. (London),* 162, 67, 1962.
4. **O'Brien, J. R.,** Effect of salicylates on human platelets, *Lancet,* 1, 1431, 1968.
5. **O'Brien, J. R.,** Aspirin against arterial and venous thrombosis, *Lancet,* 1, 804, 1971.
6. **Weiss, H. J., Aledort, L. M., and Kochwa, S.,** The effect of salicylates on the hemostatic properties of platelets in man, *J. Clin. Invest.,* 47, 2169, 1968.
7. **Evans, G., Packham, M. A., Nishizawa, E. E., Mustard, J. R., and Murphy, E. A.,** The effect of acetylsalicylic acid on platelet function, *J. Exp. Med.,* 128, 877, 1968.
8. **Vane, J. R.,** Inhibition of prostaglandin synthesis as a mechanism of action of aspirin-like drugs, *Nature,* 231, 232, 1971.
9. **Smith, J. B. and Willis, A. L.,** Aspirin selectively inhibits prostaglandin production in human platelets, *Nature,* 231, 235, 1971.
10. **Moncada, S. and Vane, J. R.,** Pharmacology and endogenous roles of prostaglandin endoperoxides, thromboxane A_2 and prostacyclin, *Pharmacol. Rev.,* 30, 293, 1979.
11. **Atkinson, D. C. and Collier, H. O. J.,** Salicylates: molecular mechanism of therapeutic action, *Adv. Pharmacol. Chemother.,* 17, 234, 1980.
12. **Hoak, J. C.,** Mechanism of action: aspirin, *Thromb. Res.,* Suppl. 4, 47, 1983.
13. **Simrock, R., Spahn, H., Breddin, H. K., and Mutschler, E.,** Reversible Hemmung der Thrombozytenstimulation durch Azetylsalizylsäure und ihre Bedeutung für die antithrombotische Therapie, *Klin. Wochenschr.,* 61, 297, 1983.
14. **de Boer, A. C., Ping Han, Turpie, A. G. G., Butt, R., Gent, M., and Genton, E.,** Platelet tests and antiplatelet drugs in coronary artery disease, *Circulation,* 67, 500, 1983.
15. **Baumgartner, H. R.,** Effects of acetylsalicylic acid, sulfinpyrazone and dipyridamole on platelet adhesion and aggregation in flowing native and anticoagulated blood, *Haemostasis,* 8, 340, 1979.
16. **Davies, J. A. and Menys, V. C.,** Effect of sulphinpyrazone (SP), aspirin (ASA) and dipyridamole (DP) on platelet vessel wall interaction after oral administration to rabbits, presented at 7th Int. Congr. Thrombosis Haemostasis, Paris, 462 (Abstr.), 1979.
17. **O'Brien, J. R.,** Multiple therapy for multifactorial thrombosis, *Thromb. Haemost.,* 57, 232, 1987.
18. **O'Brien, J. R. and Butterfield, W. H. J.,** Aspirin in the prevention of thrombosis, *Am. Heart J.,* 86, 712, 1973.
19. **Seuter, F.,** Inhibition of platelet aggregation by acetylsalicyclic acid and other inhibitors, *Haemostasis,* 5, 85, 1976.
20. **Didisheim, P.,** Inhibition by dipyridamole of arterial thrombosis in rats, *Thromb. Diath. Haemorrh,* 20, 257, 1968.
21. **Honour, A. J., Hockaday, T. D. R., and Mann, J.,** The synergistic effect of aspirin and dipyridamole upon platelet thrombi in living blood vessels, *Br. J. Exp. Pathol.,* 58, 268, 1977.

22. **Rosenblum, W. I., El-Sabban, F., and Ellis, E. F.,** Acetylsalicylic acid and indomethacin enhance platelet aggregation in mouse mesenteric arterioles, *Am. J. Physiol.,* 239, H 220, 1980.

23. **Rosenblum, W. J. and El-Sabban, F.,** Platelet aggregation in the cerebral microcirculation. Effect of aspirin and other agents, *Circ. Res.,* 40, 320, 1977.

24. **Rosenblum, W. I., El-Sabban, F., and Ellis, E. F.,** Aspirin and indomethacin, nonsteroidal antiinflammatory agents alter the responses to microvascular injury in brain and mesentery, *Microvasc. Res.,* 20, 374, 1980.

25. **Michal, M. and Giessinger, N.,** Effect of calcium dobesilate and its interaction with aspirin on thrombus formation in vivo, *Thromb. Res.,* 40, 215, 1985.

26. **Bourgain, R. H.,** The effect of indomethacin and acetylsalicylic acid on in vivo induced white platelet arterial thrombus formation, *Thromb. Res.,* 12, 1079, 1978.

27. **Spilker, B. A., van Balken, H.,** Formation and embolization of thrombi after electrical stimulation. On the method and evaluation of drugs, *Thromb. Diath. Haemorrh.,* 30, 352, 1973.

28. **Bousser, M. G. and Lecrubier, C.,** Platelet aggregation and experimental thrombus formation. Effect of aspirin, *Presse Med.,* 2, 1687, 1973.

29. **Peterson, J. and Zucker, M. B.,** The effect of adenosine-monophosphate, arcaine and anti-inflammatory agents on thrombosis and platelet function in rabbits, *Thromb. Diath. Haemorrh.,* 23, 148, 1970.

30. **Danese, C. A. and Haimov, M.,** Inhibition of experimental arterial thrombosis in dogs with platelet-deaggregating agents, *Surgery,* 70, 927, 1971.

31. **Zekert, F. and Gottlob, R.,** Eine einfache experimentelle Methode zur quantitativen Bestimmung der antithrombotischen Wirkung von Thrombozytenaggregationshemmern, *Dtsch. Med. Wochenschr.,* 98, 1004, 1973.

32. **Piepgras, D. G., Sundt, T. M., and Didisheim, P.,** Effect of anticoagulants and inhibitors of platelet aggregation on thrombotic occlusion of endarterectomized cat carotid arteries, *Stroke,* 7, 248, 1976.

33. **Dyken, M. L., Campbell, R. L., Muller, J., Feuer, H., Horner, T., King, R., Kolar, O., Solow, E., and Jones, F. H.,** Effect of aspirin on experimentally injured arterial thrombosis during the healing phase, *Stroke,* 4, 387, 1973.

34. **Mayer, J. E. and Hammond, G. L.,** Dipyridamole and aspirin tested against an experimental model of thrombosis, *Ann. Surg.,* 178, 108, 1973.

35. **Lyman, B. T., Johnson, B. L., and White, J. G.,** Dose-dependent inhibition of experimental arterial thrombosis by carbencillin and ticarcillin, *Am. J. Pathol.,* 92, 473, 1978.

36. **Renaud, S. and Godu, J.,** Thrombosis prevention by acetylsalicylic acid in hyperlipemic rats, *Can. Med. Assoc. J.,* 103, 1037, 1970.

37. **Rüegg, M.,** Antithrombotic effects of sulfinpyrazone in animals: Influence on fibrinolysis and sodium arachidonate-induced pulmonary embolism, *Pharmacology,* 14, 522, 1976.

38. **Tomikawa, M.,** Pathophysiological studies on lactic acid-induced pulmonary thrombosis in rat I. Effect of heparin, acetylsalicylic acid, urokinase and tranexamic acid, *Thromb. Diath. Haemorrh.,* 34, 145, 1978.

39. **Lindsay, L. A., Olson, R. W., Sakam, Y., Ghai, R., and Smith, E.,** Dazoxiben, UK 38,485 and aspirin: duration of effect for preventing thrombotic sudden death in rabbits, *Thromb. Res.,* 43, 177, 1986.

40. **Fleming, J. S., Bierwagen, M. E., Losada, M., Campbell, J. A. L., King, S. P., and Pindell, M. H.,** The effect of three antiinflammatory agents on platelet aggregation in vitro and in vivo, *Arch. Int. Pharmacodyn. Ther.,* 186, 120, 1970.

41. **Srivastava, R., Dikshit, M., Srimal, R. C., and Dhawan, B. N.,** Anti-thrombotic effect of curcumin, *Thromb. Res.,* 40, 413, 1985.

42. **Haft, J. I., Geshengorn, K., Krantz, P. D., and Oestreicher, R.,** Effect of an antiplatelet agent (aspirin) on cardiac necrosis induced by epinephrine infusion, *Clin. Res.,* 19, 318, 1971.

43. **Mac Donald, A., Busch, G. J., Alexander, J. L., Pheteplace, E. A., Menzoian, J., and Murray, J. E.,** Heparin and aspirin in the treatment of hyperacute rejection of renal allografts in presensitized dogs, *Transplantation,* 9, 1, 1970.

44. **Chung-hsin Ts'ao,** Ultrastructural study of the effect of aspirin on in vitro platelet-collagen interaction and platelet adhesion to injured intima in the rabbit, *Am. J. Pathol.,* 59, 327, 1970.

45. **Sheppard, B. L.,** The effect of acetylsalicylic acid on platelet adhesion in the injured abdominal aorta, *Q. J. Exp. Physiol.,* 57, 319, 1972.

46. **Elcock, H. W. and Fredrickson, J. M.,** The effect of acetylsalicylic acid on thrombosis at microvenous anastomotic sites, *J. Laryngol. Otol.,* 86, 839, 1972.

47. **Marbet, G. A. and Duckert, F.,** Action of coagulation factors on experimental thrombogenesis and their changes after thrombosis, *Thromb. Diath. Haemorrh.,* 29, 619, 1973.

48. **Barth, P., Zimmermann, R., Zieboll, J., and Lange, D.,** The antithrombotic effect of acetylsalicylic acid, heparin and phenprocoumon in experimental thrombosis, *Thromb. Diath. Haemorrh.,* 34, 554, 1975.

49. **Graudins, J., Popp, G., and Düben, W.,** Thrombose-Prophylaxe beim Kavakatheter. Tierexperimentelle Untersuchungen mit Colfarit, *Zentralbl. Chir.,* 98, 280, 1973.

50. **Gurewich, V., Lipinski, B., and Wetmore, R.,** Inhibition of intravascular fibrin deposition by dipyridamole in experimental animals, *Blood,* 45, 569, 1975.

51. **Smith, J. R. and White, A. M.,** Fibrin, red cell and platelet interactions in an experimental model of thrombosis, *Br. J. Pharmacol.,* 77, 29, 1982.

52. **Friedman, E. A.,** Prevention of thrombosis by low dose aspirin in patients on hemodialysis, *N. Engl. J. Med.,* 302, 179, 1980.

53. **Benis, A. M., Nossel, H. L., Aledort, L. M., Koffsky, R. M., Stevenson, J. R., Leonard, E. F., Shiang, H., and Litwak, R. S.,** Extracorporeal model for study of factors affecting thrombus formation, *Thromb. Diath. Haemorrh.,* 34, 127, 1975.

54. **Mason, R. G., Zucker, W. H., Shinoda, B. H., and Mohammad, S. F.,** Effects of antithrombotic agents evaluated in a non-human primate vascular shunt model, *Am. J. Pathol.,* 83, 557, 1976.

55. **Dikshit, M., Srivastava, R., Kar, K., and Srimal, R. C.,** Antithrombotic effect of some platelet modifying drugs, *Thromb. Res.,* 46, 397, 1987.

56. **Paris, J., Fourmau, P., Granero, M., and Viens, C.,** Anti-thrombotic effect of very low doses of acetylsalicylic acid in rats, *Thromb. Res.,* 29, 313, 1983.

57. **Umetsu, T., Murata, T., Tanaka, Y., Osada, E., and Nishio, S.,** Antithrombotic effect of TRK-100, a novel, stable PGI_2 analogue, *Jpn. J. Pharmacol.,* 43, 81, 1987.

58. **Lewis, G. P., Lieberman, G. E., and Westwick, J.,** Adenosine diphosphatase, prostaglandins and aspirin, in *Acetylsalicylic Acid in Cerebral Ischemia and Coronary Heart Disease,* Breddin, K., Dorndorf, W., Loew, D., and Marx, R., Eds., Schattauer-Verlag, New York, 1978, 25.

59. **Philp, R. B.,** Experimental animal models of arterial thrombosis and the screening of platelet-inhibiting, antithrombotic drugs: a review, *Methods Find. Exp. Clin. Pharmacol.,* 1, 197, 1979.

60. **Cattaneo, M., Chahil, A., Somers, D., Kinlough-Rathbone, R. L., Packham, M. A., and Mustard, J. F.,** Effect of aspirin and sodium salicylate on thrombosis, fibrinolysis, prothrombin time, and platelet survival in rabbits with indwelling aortic catheter, *Blood,* 61, 353, 1983.

61. **Lavelle, S. M. and MacIomhair, M.,** The anti-thrombotic effect of Warfarin, dipyridamole and aspirin in the rat, 5th Int. Congr. Thrombosis Diathesis, Paris, 88 (Abstr.) 1975.

62. **Kelton, J. G., Hirsch, J., Carter, C. J., and Buchanan, M. R.,** Thrombogenic effect of high-dose aspirin in rabbits, *J. Clin. Invest.,* 62, 892, 1978.

63. **Dejana, E., Barbieri, B., and de Gaetano, G.,** "Aspirinated" platelets are hemostatic in thrombocytopenic rats with "nonaspirinated" vessel walls. Evidence from an exchange transfusion model, *Blood,* 56, 959, 1980.

64. **Zimmerman, R., Thiessen, M., Mörl, H., and Weckesser, G.,** The paradoxical thrombogenic effect of aspirin in experimental thrombosis, *Thromb. Res.,* 16, 843, 1979.

65. **Silver, M. J., Ingerman-Wojenski, C. M., Sedar, A. W., and Smith, M.,** Model system to study interaction of platelets with damaged arterial wall, *Exp. Mol. Pathol.,* 41, 141, 1984.

66. **Hanson, S. R., Harker, L. A., Björnsson, T. D.,** Effects of platelet-modifying drugs on arterial thromboembolism in baboons. Aspirin potentiates the antithrombotic actions of dipyridamole and sulfinpyrazone by mechanism(s) independent of platelet cyclooxygenase inhibition, *J. Clin. Invest.,* 75, 1591, 1985.

67. **Moschos, C. B., Lahiri, K., Lyons, M., Weisse, A. B., Olderwurtel, H. A., and Regan, T. J.,** Relationship of microcirculatory thrombosis to thrombus in the proximal coronary artery: effect of aspirin, dipyridamole and thrombolysis, *Am. Heart. J.,* 86, 61, 1973.

68. **Moschos, Ch. B., Lahiri, K., Peter, A., Jesrani, M. U., and Regan, T. J.,** Effect of aspirin upon experimental coronary and non-coronary thrombosis and arrhythmia, *Am. Heart. J.,* 84, 525, 1972.

69. **Levison, M. E., Carrizosa, J., Tanphaichitra, D., Schick, P. K., and Rubin, W.,** Effect of aspirin on thrombogenesis and on production of experimental aortic valvular streptococcus-viridans endocarditis in rabbits, *Blood,* 49, 645, 1977.

70. **Pick, R., Chediak, J., and Glick, G.,** Aspirin inhibits development of coronary atherosclerosis in cynomolgus monkeys (Macaca fascicularis) fed an atherogenic diet, *J. Clin. Invest.,* 63, 158, 1979.

71. **Clopath, P.,** The effect of acetylsalicylic acid (ASA) on the development of atherosclerotic lesions in miniature swine, *Br. J. Exp. Pathol.,* 61, 440, 1980.

72. **Folts, J. D., Crowell, E. B., and Rowe, G. G.,** Platelet aggregation in partially obstructed vessels and its elimination with aspirin, *Circulation,* 54, 365, 1976.

73. **Millet, J., Theveniaux, J., and Pascal, M.,** A new experimental model of venous thrombosis in rats involving partial stasis and slight endothelium alterations, *Thromb. Res.,* 45, 123, 1987.

74. **Reyers, I., Hennissen, A., Donati, M. B., Hornstra, G., and de Gaetano, G.,** Aspirin and the prevention of experimental arterial thrombosis: difficulty in establishing unequivocal effectiveness, *Thromb. Haemost.,* 54, 619, 1985.

75. **Reyers, I., Mussoni, L., Donati, M. B., and de Gaetano, G.,** Failure of aspirin at different doses to modify experimental thrombosis in rats, *Thromb. Res.,* 18, 669, 1980.

76. **Fleming, J. S. and Buyniski, J. P.,** A potent new inhibitor of platelet aggregation and experimental thrombosis, anagrelide (BL-4162 A), *Thromb. Res.,* 15, 373, 1979.

77. **Seiffge, D. and Weithmann, K. U.,** Surprising effects of the sequential administration of pentoxifylline and low dose acetylsalicylic acid on thrombus formation, *Thromb. Res.,* 46, 371, 1987.
78. **Weichert, W., Pauliks, V., and Breddin, H. K.,** Laser-induced thrombi in rat mesenteric vessels and antithrombotic drugs, *Haemostasis,* 13, 61, 1983.
79. **Meng, K. and O'Dea, K.,** The protective effect of acetylsalicylic acid on laser-induced venous thrombosis in the rat, *Naunyn Schmiedebergs Arch. Pharmacol.,* 283, 379, 1974.
80. **Meng, K., Seuter, F.,** Effect of acetylsalicylic acid on experimentally induced arterial thrombosis in rats, *Naunyn Schmiedebergs Arch. Pharmacol.,* 301, 115, 1977.
81. **Hladovec, J.,** The effect of some antithrombotic drugs on experimental arterial thrombosis, *Cor. Vasa,* 17, 66, 1975.
82. **Philp, R. B., Francey, I., and Warren, B. A.,** Comparison of antithrombotic activity of heparin, ASA, sulfinpyrazone and VK 744, in a rat model of arterial thrombosis, *Haemostasis,* 7, 282, 1978.
83. **Hladovec, J.,** Cement substance and platelet adhesion to the endothelial surface. Influence of several groups of drugs, *Physiol. Bohemoslov.,* 19, 425, 1970.
84. **Nordoy, A., Svensson, B., Schroeder, C., and Hoak, J. C.,** The inhibitory effect of aspirin on human endothelial cells, *Thromb. Haemost.,* 40, 103, 1978.
85. **Hladovec, J.,** Antithrombotic effects of some flavonoids alone and combined with acetylsalicylic acid, *Arzneimittelforschung,* 27, 1989, 1979.
86. **Bourgain, R. H., Andries, R., Braquet, P., and Deby, C.,** The effect of inhibition of endothelial cell cyclooxygenase on arterial thrombosis, *Prostaglandins,* 30, 915, 1985.
87. **Buchanan, M. R., Rischke, J. A., and Hirsh, J.,** Aspirin inhibits platelet function independent of the acetylation of cyclo-oxygenase, *Thromb. Res.,* 25, 363, 1982.
88. **de Gaetano, G., Cerletti, Ch., Dejana, E., and Vermylen, J.,** Current issues in thrombosis prevention with antiplatelet drugs, *Drugs,* 31, 512, 1986.
89. **Dejana, E., Cazenave, J.-P., Groves, H. M., Kinlough-Rathbone, R. L., Richardson, M., Packham, M. A., and Mustard, J. F.,** The effect of aspirin inhibition of PGI_2 production on platelet adherence to normal and damaged rabbit aorta, *Thromb. Res.,* 17, 453, 1980.
90. **Mills, D. G., Philp, R. B., and Hirst, M.,** The effects of some salicylate analogues on human blood platelets: I. Structure-activity relationships and the inhibition of platelet aggregation, *Life Sci.,* 14, 659, 1974.
91. **Buchanan, M. R., Butt, R. W., Magas, Z., Van Ryn, J., Hirsh, J., and Nazir, D. J.,** Endothelial cells produced lipoxygenase derived chemo-repellent which influences platelet/endothelial cell interaction — effect of aspirin and salicylate, *Thromb. Haemost.,* 53, 306, 1985.
92. **de Gaetano, G., Carriero, M. R., Cerletti, C., and Mussoni, L.,** Low dose aspirin does not prevent fibrinolytic response to venous occlusion, *Biochem. Pharmacol.,* 35, 3147, 1986.
93. **Collier, H. O. J.,** A pharmacological analysis of aspirin, *Adv. Pharmacol. Chemother.,* 7, 333, 1969.
94. **Irino, O., Saitoh, K., Okhubo, K., and Hashimoto, S.,** Inhibitory effect of sodium salicylate on ADP-induced platelet aggregation and on Ca^{2+} uptake into platelets, *Thromb. Res.,* 39, 369, 1985.
95. **Emmons, P. R., Harrison, M. J. G., Honour, A. J., and Mitchell, J. R. A.,** Effect of a pyrimido-pyrimidine derivative on thrombus formation in the rabbit, *Nature,* 208, 255, 1965.
96. **Born, G. V. R.,** Aggregation of blood platelets by adenosine diphosphate and its reversal, *Nature,* 194, 927, 1962.
97. **Born, G. V. R., Honour, A. J., and Mitchell, J. R. A.,** Inhibition by adenosine and 2-chloro-adenosine of the formation and embolization of platelet thrombi, *Nature,* 202, 761, 1965.
98. **Emmons, P. R., Harrison, M. J. G., Honour, A. J., and Mitchell, J. R. A.,** Effect of dipyridamole on human platelet behaviour, *Lancet,* 2, 603, 1965.
99. **Arfors, K.-E., Hint, H. C., and Dhall, D. P.,** Counteraction of platelet activity at sites of laser-induced endothelial trauma, *Br. Med. J.,* 4, 430, 1968.
100. **Philp, R. B. and Lemieux, V.,** Comparison of some effects of dipyridamole and adenosine on thrombus formation, platelet adhesiveness and blood pressure in rabbits and rats, *Nature,* 218, 1072, 1968.
101. **Didisheim, P., Owen, Ch. A., Jr., and Bowie, E. J. W.,** Effect of induced hypotension on thrombosis in the extracorporeal microcirculation of the rat, *J. Clin. Invest.,* 48, 21a, 1969.
102. **Didisheim, P., Bowie, E. J. W., and Owen, Ch. A.,** Inhibition of arterial thrombosis and platelet adhesiveness in the rat by intravenous 2,4,6-trimorpholinopyrimido-(5,4-d)-pyrimidine (RA 433), *Mayo Clin. Proc.,* 45, 51, 1970.
103. **Didisheim, P. and Owen, Ch. A.,** Prevention of experimental arterial thrombosis and platelet adhesiveness by 2,6-bis-(diethanolamino) 4-piperidino-pyrimido (5,4-d)-pyrimidine(RA 233), *Mayo Clin. Proc.,* 45, 695, 1970.
104. **Hassanein, A. A., Turpie, A. G. G., McNico, G. P., and Douglas, A. A.,** Effect of RA 233 on platelet function in vitro, *Br. Med. J.,* 2, 83, 1970.
105. **Elkeles, R. S., Hampton, J. R., Honour, A. J., Mitchell, J. R. A., and Prichard, I.,** Effect of a pyrimido-pyrimidine compound on platelet behaviour in vitro and in vivo, *Lancet,* 2, 751, 1968.

106. **Hampton, J. R., Harrison, M. J. G., Honour, A. J., Mitchell, J. R. A.,** Assessment of antithrombotic agents: effects of dipyridamole analogues on platelet behaviour, *Cardiovasc. Res.,* 6, 696, 1972.

107. **Honour, A. J. and Hockaday, T. D. R.,** Increased sensitivity of in vivo platelet aggregation after alloxan on streptozotocin, *Br. J. Exp. Pathol.,* 57, 1, 1976.

108. **Honour, A. J., Carter, R. D., and Mann, J. I.,** The effects of treatment with aspirin and an antithrombotic agent SH 1117 upon platelet thrombus formation in living blood vessels, *Br. J. Exp. Pathol.,* 58, 474, 1977.

109. **Cucuianu, M. P., Nishizawa, E. E., and Mustard, J. F.,** Effect of pyrimido-pyrimidine compounds on platelet function, *J. Lab. Clin. Med.,* 77, 958, 1971.

110. **Haft, J. I., Gershengorn, K., Kranz, P. D., and Oestreicher, R.,** Protection against epinephrine-induced myocardial necrosis by drugs that inhibit platelet aggregation, *Am. J. Cardiol.,* 30, 838, 1972.

111. **Watanabe, T., Shintani, F., Fu, L., Kato, K., and Koyama, S.,** Failure of dipyridamole (Persantin) in reducing the infarct size following experimental coronary occlusion, *Jpn. Heart J.,* 13, 512, 1972.

112. **Dragojevic, D., Hetzer, R., Corterier, H.,** Thromboembolie-Prophylaxe nach Herzklappenersatz in einem experimentellen Modell, *Thoraxchirurgie,* 20, 419, 1972.

113. **Turina, M., Bull, B., and Braunwald, N. S.,** Effect of dipyridamole on the accumulation of thrombotic deposit on an intracardiac prosthetic device. An experimental study, *Surgery,* 69, 445, 1971.

114. **O'Sullivan, F. F. and Vellar, J. D. A.,** Assessment of the efficacy of antiplatelet drugs in the prevention of experimental venous thrombosis in the rabbit, presented at 2nd Congr. Int. Soc. Thrombosis Haemostasis, Washington, 1972.

115. **Hasegawa, T., Matsumoto, H., Yamamoto, M., Fuse, K., Mizuno, A., and Saigusa, M.,** Prosthetic replacement of superior vena cava. Anti-platelet-adhesive drug influence, *Arch. Surg.,* 106, 848, 1973.

116. **Polterauer, P., Zekert, F., and Gottlob, R.,** Azetylsalizylsäure und Dipyridamole: Aggregationshemmung im Experiment am Kaninchen, *Vasa,* 4, 397, 1975.

117. **Yoshikawa, T., Murakami, M., Furukawa, Y., Takemura, S., and Kondo, M.,** Effect of dipyridamole on experimental disseminated intravascular coagulation in rats, *Thromb. Res.,* 29, 619, 1983.

118. **Gurewich, V. and Lipinski, B.,** Evaluation of antithrombotic properties of suloctidil in comparison with aspirin and dipyridamole, *Thromb. Res.,* 9, 101, 1976.

119. **Ortega, M. P.,** The antithrombotic in vivo effect of eterylate and dipyridamole in experimental thrombosis in mice, *Thromb. Res.,* 44, 555, 1986.

120. **Slabber, C. F., Theiss, W., and Beller, F. K.,** The prevention of endotoxin-induced glomerular fibrin deposition by pyrimido-pyrimidine compounds, *J. Med.,* 3, 341, 1972.

121. **Dikshit, M., Srivastava, R., Kar, K., and Srimal, R. C.,** Antithrombotic effect of some platelet modifying drugs, *Thromb. Res.,* 46, 397, 1987.

122. **Rosenblum, W. J. and El-Sabban, F.,** Effect of dipyridamole on platelet aggregation in cerebral microcirculation of the mouse, *Thromb. Res.,* 12, 181, 1977.

123. **Honour, A. J., Hockaday, T. D. R., and Mann, J. I.,** The reversibility by dipyridamole of the increased sensitivity of in vivo platelet aggregation in rabbits after alloxane, *Br. J. Exp. Pathol.,* 57, II15, 1976.

124. **Umetsu, T. and Sanai, K.,** Effect of 1-methyl-2-mercapto-5-(3-pyridil)imidazole (KC 6141), an antiaggregating compound on experimental thrombosis in rats, *Thromb. Haemost.,* 39, 74, 1978.

125. **Louie, S. and Gurewich, V.,** The antithrombotic effect of aspirin and dipyridamole in relation to prostaglandin synthesis, *Thromb. Res.,* 30, 323, 1983.

126. **Pumphrey, Ch. W., Fuster, V., Dewanjee, M. K., Chesebro, J. H., Vliestra, R. E., and Kaye, M. P.,** Comparison of the antithrombotic action of calcium antagonist drugs with dipyridamole in dogs, *Am. J. Cardiol.,* 51, 591, 1983.

127. **Groves, H. M., Kinlough-Rathbone, R. L., Cazenave, J.-P., Dejana, E., Richardson, M., and Mustard, J. F.,** Effect of dipyridamole and prostacyclin on rabbit platelet adherence in vitro and in vivo, *J. Lab. Clin. Med.,* 99, 548, 1982.

128. **Folts, J. D. and Smith, S. R.,** Dipyridamole alone and with low dose aspirin does not prevent acute platelet thrombus formation in stenosed dog coronary arteries, presented at 11th Int. Congr. Thrombosis Haemostasis, Brussels, 778 (Abstr.), 1987.

129. **Fuster, V., Dewanjee, M. K., Kaye, M. P., Josa, M., Metke, M. P., and Chesebro, J. H.,** Noninvasive radioisotopic technique for detection of platelet deposition in coronary artery bypass grafts in dogs and its reduction with platelet inhibitors, *Circulation,* 60, 1508, 1979.

130. **Rittenhouse, E. A., Hessel, E. A., Ito, C. S., and Merendino, K. A.,** Effect of dipyridamole on microaggregate formation in the pump oxygenator, *Ann. Surg.,* 175, 1, 1972.

131. **Becker, R. M., Smith, M. R., and Dobell, A. R.,** Effect of platelet inhibition on platelet phenomena in cardiopulmonary bypass in pigs, *Ann. Surg.,* 179, 52, 1974.

132. **Williams, I. M., Farmer, S., and Dixon, J.,** Effect of dipyridamole on retinal embolism associated with cardiopulmonary bypass surgery in the dog, *Graefes Arch. Clin. Exp. Ophthalmol.,* 189, 251, 1974.

133. **Coeugniet, E.,** Clinical and experimental effects of dipyridamole, *Thromb. Res.,* 7, 251, 1975.

134. **Harker, L. A., Ross, R., Slichter, S. J., and Scott, C. R.,** Homocystine-induced arteriosclerosis. The role of endothelial cell injury and platelet response in its genesis, *J. Clin. Invest.,* 58, 731, 1976.

135. **Harker, L. A., Slichter, S. J., Scott, C. R., and Ross, R.,** Homocystinemia. Vascular injury and arterial thrombosis, *N. Engl. J. Med.,* 291, 537, 1974.

136. **Friedman, R. J. and Burns, E. R.,** Role of platelets in the proliferative response of the injured artery, in *Progress in Hemostasis & Thrombosis,* Vol. 4, Spaet, T. H., Ed., Grune & Stratton, New York, 1978, 249.

137. **Dembińska-Kieć, A., Rücker, W., and Schönhofer, P. S.,** Effects of dipyridamole in experimental atherosclerosis. Action of PGI_2, platelet aggregation and atherosclerotic plaque formation, *Atherosclerosis,* 33, 315, 1979.

138. **Hladovec, J.,** The effect of antithrombotics in a new model of arterial thrombosis, *Thromb. Res.* 41, 665, 1986.

139. **Hladovec, J.,** Antithrombotics in view of thrombosis models, *Thromb. Res.,* 43, 545, 1986.

140. **Born, G. V. R.,** Adenosine diphosphate as a mediator of platelet aggregation in vivo: an editorial view, *Circulation,* 72, 741, 1985.

141. **Loeliger, E. A.,** Does dipyridamole have antithrombotic potential?, *Thromb. Haemost.,* 53, 437, 1985.

142. **FitzGerald, G. A.,** Dipyridamole, *N. Engl. J. Med.,* 316, 1247, 1987.

143. **Smythe, H. A., Ogryzlo, M. A., Murphy, E. A., and Mustard, J. F.,** The effect of sulphinpyrazone (Anturan) on platelet economy and blood coagulation in man, *Can. Med. Assoc. J.,* 92, 818, 1965.

144. **Steele, P., Rainwater, J., Vogel, R., and Genton, E.,** Platelet-suppressant therapy in patients with coronary artery disease, *JAMA,* 240, 228, 1978.

145. **Steele, P., Carrvel, J., Overfield, D., and Genton, E.,** Effect of sulfinpyrazone on platelet survival time in patients with transient cerebral ischemic attacks, *Stroke,* 8, 396, 1977.

146. **Steele, P. P., Weily, H. S., and Genton, E.,** Platelet survival and adhesiveness in recurrent venous thrombosis, *N. Engl. J. Med.,* 288, 1148, 1973.

147. **Kaegi, A., Pineo, G. F., Shimizu, A., Trivedi, H., and Hirsh, J.,** Arterio-venous-shunt thrombosis. Prevention by sulfinpyrazone, *N. Engl. J. Med.,* 290, 304, 1974.

148. **Kaegi, A., Pineo, G. F., Shimizu, A., Trivedi, H., Hirsh, J., and Gent, M.,** The role of sulfinpyrazone in the prevention of arterio-venous shunt thrombosis, *Circulation,* 52, 497, 1975.

149. **Mustard, J. F., Rowsell, H. C., Smythe, H. A., Senyi, A., and Murphy, E. A.,** The effect of sulfinpyrazone on platelet economy and thrombus formation in rabbits, *Blood,* 29, 859, 1967.

150. **Renaud, S. and Lecompte, F.,** Thrombosis prevention by coagulation and platelet aggregation inhibitors in hyperlipemic rats, *Thromb. Diath. Haemorrh.,* 24, 577, 1970.

151. **Evans, G. and Mustard, J. F.,** Inhibition of the platelet-surface reaction in endotoxin shock and the generalized Schwartzman reaction, *J. Clin. Invest.,* 47, 31a, 1968.

152. **Cerskus, A. L., Ali, M., Zamecnik, J., and McDonald, J. W. D.,** Effects of indomethacin and sulfinpyrazone on in vivo formation of thromboxane B_2 and prostaglandin D_2 during arachidonate infusion in rabbits, *Thromb. Res.,* 12, 549, 1978.

153. **Nishizawa, E. E., Williams, D. J., and Connell, C. L.,** Arachidonate induced aggregation of rat platelets may not require prostaglandin endoperoxides or thromboxane A_2, *Thromb. Res.,* 30, 289, 1983.

154. **Kohler, C., Wooding, W., and Ellenbogen, L.,** Intravenous arachidonate in the mouse: a model for the evaluation of antithrombotic drugs, *Thromb. Res.,* 9, 67, 1976.

155. **Vigdahl, R. L., Ferber, R. H., and Parrish, S. L.,** Evaluation of antiinflammatory and antithrombotic drugs in pulmonary and arterial thrombosis, *Thromb. Res.,* 16, 117, 1979.

156. **Duling, B. R., Berne, R. M., and Born, G. V. R.,** Microiontopheretic application of vasoactive agents to the microcirculation of the hamster cheek pouch, *Microvasc. Res.,* 1, 158, 1968.

157. **Lewis, G. P. and Westwick, J.,** The effect of sulphinpyrazone, sodium aspirin and oxprenolol on the formation of arterial platelet thrombi, *Br. J. Pharmacol.,* 55, 255 P, 1975.

158. **Wiedeman, M. P., Tuma, R. F., and Mayrovitz, H. N.,** Effects of vasoactive drugs on platelet aggregation in vivo and in vitro, *Thromb. Res.,* 15, 365, 1979.

159. **Adams, J. H. and Mitchell, J. R.,** The effect of agents which modify platelet behaviour and of magnesium ions on thrombus formation in vivo, *Thromb. Haemost.,* 42, 603, 1979.

160. **Hladovec, J.,** Experimental arterial thrombosis in rats with continuous registration, *Thromb. Diath. Haemorrh.,* 26, 407, 1971.

161. **Wilkinson, A. R., Hawker, R. J., and Hawker, L. M.,** The influence of antiplatelet drugs on platelet survival after aortic damage or implantation of a dacron arterial prosthesis, *Thromb. Res.,* 15, 181, 1979.

162. **Arfors, K.-E., Bergqvist, D., and Tangen, O.,** The effect of platelet function inhibitors on experimental venous thrombosis formation in rabbits, *Acta Chir. Scand.,* 141, 40, 1975.

163. **Pineo, G., Kaegi, A., Hirsh, J., Gent, M., and Moore, S.,** Antithrombotic effect of sulfinpyrazone in arterio-venous shunts, presented at 5th Int. Congr. Thrombosis Haemostasis, Paris, 422 (Abstr.), 1975.

164. **Birek, A., Duffin, J., Glynn, M. F. X., and Cooper, J. D.,** The effect of sulfinpyrazone on platelet and pulmonary responses to onset of membrane oxygenator perfusion, *Trans. Am. Soc. Artif. Intern. Organs,* 22, 94, 1976.

165. **Townsend, E. R., Duffin, J., Ali, M., McDonald, J. W. B., Thiesson, J. J., Masterson, J., Klement, P., and Cooper, J. D.,** Preservation of platelets during extracorporeal circulation in sheep: a comparison between aspirin and sulfinpyrazone, *Circ. Res.,* 49, 452, 1981.

166. **Harker, L. A., Harlan, J. M., and Ross, R.,** Effect of sulfinpyrazone on homocysteine-induced endothelial injury and atherosclerosis in baboons, *Circ. Res.,* 53, 531, 1983.

167. **Butler, K. D., Pay, G. F., and White, A. M.,** A comparison between sulphinpyrazone and other drugs on the thrombocytopenia of the Arthus reaction in the guinea pig, *Br. J. Pharmacol.,* 57, 441 P, 1976.

168. **Butler, K. D., Wallis, R. B., and White, A. M.,** A study of the relationship between ex vivo and in vivo effects of sulphinpyrazone in the guinea pig, *Haemostasis,* 8, 353, 1978.

169. **Butler, K. D. and White, A. M.,** Inhibition of the platelet involvement in the sublethal Forssman reaction by sulfphinpyrazone and not by aspirin, presented at Anturane®, an international symposium, Hamilton, 1979.

170. **Sharma, H. M., Moore, S., Merrick, H. W., and Smith, M. R.,** Platelets in early hyperacute allograft rejection in kidneys and their modification by sulfinpyrazone (Anturan) therapy, *Am. J. Pathol.,* 66, 445, 1972.

171. **Vaessen, L. M. B., Bonthuis, F., Hesse, C. J., and Lameijer, L. D. F.,** Effect of sulfinpyrazone (Anturan) on degree of vascular lesions and survival of cardiac allografts in rats, *Transplant. Proc.,* 9, 993, 1977.

172. **Jamieson, S., Burton, N., Shorthouse, R., Bieber, Ch., Bowden, R., Reitz, B., Oyer, P., Stinson, E., and Shumway, N.,** Platelets, sulfinpyrazone and organ graft rejection, presented at Anturane®, an international symposium, Hamilton, 1979.

173. **The Anturane® Reinfarction Trial Research Group,** Sulfinpyrazone in the prevention of sudden death after myocardial infarction, *N. Engl. J. Med.,* 302, 250, 1960.

174. **Moschos, C., Escobinas, A., Jorgensen, O., Jr., and Regan, T.,** Effect of sulfinpyrazone on survival following non-thrombotic coronary occlusion, *Am. J. Cardiol.,* 43, 372, 1979.

175. **Moschos, C., Escobinas, A., and Jorgensen, O.,** Effects of sulfinpyrazone on ischemic myocardium, presented at Anturane®, an international symposium, Hamilton, 1979.

176. **Povalski, H. J.,** Influence of sulfinpyrazone or aspirin on arrhythmias in the coronary occlusion-reperfusion dog model, presented at Anturane®, an international symposium, Hamilton, 1979.

177. **Kelliher, G. J., Dix, R. K., Laurence, T., and Jurkiewicz, N.,** Effect of sulfinpyrazone on ventricular arrhythmia after occlusion in cats, paper presented at Anturane®, an international symposium, Hamilton, 1979.

178. **Stäubli, R. C., Baur, H. R., Althaus, U., Pop, H. P., Wehrli, H. P., and Gurtner, H. P.,** Influence of sulfinpyrazone on infarct size, hemodynamics, and arrhythmia following coronary occlusion in the pig, *J. Cardiovasc. Pharmacol.,* 6, 829, 1984.

179. **Folts, J. D.,** Inhibition of platelet plugging in stenosed dog coronary arteries with sulfinpyrazone, presented at Anturane®, an international symposium, Hamilton, 1979.

180. **Beamish, R. E., Dhillan, K. S., Singal, P. K., and Dhalla, N. S.,** Protective effect of sulfinpyrazone against catecholamine metabolite adrenochrome-induced arrhythmias, *Am. Heart J.,* 102, 149, 1981.

181. **Hashimoto, H. and Ogawa, K.,** Effects of sulfinpyrazone, aspirin and propranolol on the isoproterenol-induced myocardial necrosis, *Jpn. Heart J.,* 22, 643, 1981.

182. **Innes, I. R. and Weisman, H.,** Reduction of severity of myocardial infarction by sulfinpyrazone, *Am. Heart J.,* 102, 153, 1981.

183. **Russell, D. C.,** Haemodynamic effects of sulfinpyrazone in experimental myocardial ischaemia, *Br. J. Pharmacol.,* 72, 5, 1981.

184. **Clopath, P. and Horsch, A. K.,** The effect of sulfinpyrazone on the development of atherosclerosis in various animal models, presented at Anturane®, an international symposium, Hamilton, 1979.

185. **Hladovec, J.,** Is the antithrombotic activity of "antiplatelet" drugs based on protection of endothelium?, *Thromb. Haemost.,* 41, 774, 1979.

186. **Hladovec, J.,** Vasotropic drugs — a survey based on a unifying concept of their mechanism of action, *Arzneimittelforschung,* 27, 1073, 1977.

187. **Jaques, L. B.,** Heparins-anionic polyelectrolyte drugs, *Pharmacol. Rev.,* 31, 99, 1980.

188. **Neri-Serneri, G. G., Rovelli, F., Gentini, G. F., Pirelli, S., Carnovali, M., and Fortini, A.,** Effectiveness of low-dose heparin in prevention of myocardial reinfarction, *Lancet,* 1, 937, 1987.

189. **Hiebert, L. M. and Jaques, L. B.,** Heparin uptake on endothelium, *Artery,* 2, 26, 1976.

190. **Mahadoo, J., Hiebert, L., and Jaques, L. B.,** Vascular sequestration of heparin, *Thromb. Res.,* 12, 79, 1977.

191. **Glimelius, B., Busch, Ch., and Höök, M.,** Binding of heparin on the surface of cultured human endothelial cells, *Thromb. Res.,* 12, 773, 1978.

192. **Barzu, T., Molho, P., Tobelem, G., Petitou, M., and Caen, J. P.,** Binding of heparin and low molecular weight heparin fragments to human vascular endothelial cells in culture, *Nouv. Rev. Fr. Hematol.,* 26, 243, 1984.

193. **Psuja, P., Drouet, L., and Zawilska, K.,** Binding of heparin to human endothelial cell monolayers and extracellular matrix in culture, *Thromb. Res.,* 47, 469, 1987.

194. **Kraemer, P. M.,** Heparin releases heparan sulfate from the cell surface, *Biochem. Biophys. Res. Commun.,* 78, 1334, 1977.

195. **Miletich, J. P., Jackson, C. M. and Majerus, P. W.,** Properties of the factor Xa binding site on human platelets, *J. Biol. Chem.,* 253, 6908, 1978.

196. **Zucker, M. B.,** Effect of heparin on platelet function, *Thromb. Diath. Haemorrh.,* 33, 63, 1974.

197. **Salzman, E. W., Rosenberg, R. D., Smith, M. H., Lindon, J. N., and Favreau, L.,** Effect of heparin and heparin fractions on platelet aggregation, *J. Clin. Invest.,* 65, 64, 1980.

198. **Wessler, S., Ward, K., and Ho, C.,** Studies on intravascular coagulation III. The pathogenesis of serum-induced venous thrombosis, *J. Clin. Invest.,* 34, 647, 1955.

199. **Essien, E. M., Cazenave, J.-P., Moore, S., and Mustard, J. F.,** Effect of heparin and thrombin on platelet adherence to the surface of rabbit aorta, *Thromb. Res.,* 13, 69, 1978.

200. **Murray, D. W. G., Jaques, M. A., Perrett, T. S., and Best, C. H.,** Heparin and the thrombosis of veins following injury, *Surgery,* 2, 163, 1937.

201. **Best, C. H.,** Heparin and thrombosis, *Br. Med. J.,* 2, 977, 1938.

202. **Solandt, D. Y. and Best, C. H.,** Time-relations of heparin action on blood clotting and platelet agglutination, *Lancet,* 1, 1042, 1940.

203. **Rabinovitch, J. and Pines, B.,** The effect of heparin on experimentally produced venous thrombosis, *Surgery,* 14, 669, 1943.

204. **Reimann-Hunziker, G.,** Über experimentelle Thrombose und ihre Behandlung mit Heparin, *Schweiz. Med. Wochenschr.,* 74, 66, 1944.

205. **Moser, C.,** Effect of heparin and dicoumarol on thrombosis induced in the presence of venous stasis, *Proc. Soc. Exp. Biol. Med.,* 59, 25, 1945.

206. **Loewe, L., Hirsch, E., and Grayzel, D. M.,** The action of heparin on experimental venous thrombosis, *Surgery,* 22, 746, 1947.

207. **Loewe, L., Hirsch, E., Grayzel, D. M. and Kashdan, F.,** Experimental study of the comparative action of heparin and dicoumarol on the in vivo clot, *J. Lab. Clin. Med.,* 33, 721, 1948.

208. **Kiesewetter, W. B. and Shumaker, H. B., Jr.,** An experimental study of the comparative efficacy of heparin and dicumarol in the prevention of arterial and venous thrombosis, *Surg. Gynecol. Obstet.,* 86, 687, 1948.

209. **Friedrich, H. W.,** Experimenteller Beitrag zur Thrombocidbehandlung der Thrombose, *Arztl. Wochenschrift.,* 5, 178, 1950.

210. **Wessler, S.,** Experimentally produced phlebotherombosis in the study of thromboembolism, *J. Clin. Invest.,* 32, 610, 1953.

211. **Wessler, S. and Morris, L. E.,** Studies in intravascular coagulation IV. The effect of heparin and dicumarol on serum-induced venous thrombosis, *Circulation,* 12, 553, 1955.

212. **Jarrett, C. L. and Jaques, L. B.,** The antithrombosis activity of heparinoid G 31150, *Thromb. Haemost.,* 10, 431, 1963.

213. **Borgström, S., Gelin, L.-E., and Zederfeldt, B.,** The formation of vein thrombi following tissue injury: an experimental study in rabbits, *Acta Chir. Scand.,* Suppl. 247, 1, 1959.

214. **Blake, O. R., Ashwin, J. G., and Jaques, L. B.,** An assay for the antithrombic activity of anticoagulants, *J. Clin. Pathol.,* 12, 118, 1959.

215. **Williams, R. D. and Carey, L. C.,** Studies in the production of ''standard'' venous thrombosis, *Ann. Surg.,* 149, 381, 1959.

216. **Williams, R. D. and Karaffa, F.,** Protection from thrombosis in large veins, *Surg. Gynecol. Obstet.,* 121, 79, 1965.

217. **Carey, L. C. and Williams, R. D.,** Comparative effects of dicoumarol, tromexan, and heparin on thrombus propagation, *Ann. Surg.,* 152, 919, 1960.

218. **Zweifler, A. J.,** Standardized technique for the study of thrombus growth: effect of heparin therapy, *J. Lab. Clin. Med.,* 60, 254, 1962.

219. **Allison, F., Jr. and Lancaster, M. G.,** Studies on the pathogenesis of acute inflammation. III. The failure of anticoagulants to prevent the leucocytic sticking reaction and the formation of small thrombi in rabbit ear chambers damaged by heat, *J. Exp. Med.,* 114, 535, 1961.

220. **Zambouras, D. A., Anezyris, P., and Kalakonas, P.,** La cortisone et l'héparine dans les thrombophlébites expérimentales. Etude comparative de leur action, *Presse Med.,* 69, 1134, 1961.

221. **Honour, A. J. and Ross Russell, W. R.,** Experimental platelet embolism, *Br. J. Exp. Pathol.,* 43, 350, 1962.

222. **Jewell, P., Pilkington, T., and Robinson, B.,** Heparin and ethylbiscoumacetate in prevention of experimental venous thrombosis, *Br. Med. J.,* 1, 1013, 1954.

223. **Fulton, S. P., Akers, R. P., and Lutz, B. R.,** White thrombo-embolism and vascular fragility in the hamster cheek pouch after anticoagulants, *Blood,* 8, 140, 1953.

224. **Hoak, J. C., Connor, W. E., and Warner, E. D.,** Antithrombotic effects of Warfarin and heparin, *Circulation,* 25, 657, 1962.

225. **York, I. M., Rogers, W. I., and Kensler, C. J.,** The production of thrombi and emboli in the hamster cheek pouch by phthalanilides and related compounds, *J. Pharmacol. Exp. Ther.,* 141, 36, 1963.

226. **Mustard, J. F., Murphy, E. A., Downie, H. G., and Rowsell, H. C.,** Heparin and thrombus formation: early suppression and late enhancement, *Br. J. Haematol.,* 9, 548, 1963.

227. **Hoak, J. C., Connor, W. E., Eckstein, J. W., and Warner, E. D.,** Fatty acid-induced thrombosis and death: mechanism and prevention, *J. Lab. Clin. Med.,* 63, 791, 1964.

228. **Just-Viera, J. O. and Yeager, G. H.,** Protection from thrombosis in large veins, *Surg. Gynecol. Obstet.,* 118, 354, 1964.

229. **Jorgensen, L.,** Experimental platelet and coagulation thrombi: A histological study of arterial and venous thrombi of varying age in untreated and heparinized rabbits, *Acta Pathol. Microbiol. Immunol. Scand.,* 62, 189, 1964.

230. **Renaud, S.,** Anticoagulants in the prevention of endotoxin-induced phlebothrombosis in the rat, *J. Lab. Clin. Med.,* 66, 253, 1965.

231. **Müller-Berghaus, G. and Hocke, M.,** Effect of endotoxin on the formation of microthrombi from circulating fibrin monomer complexes in the absence of thrombin generation, *Thromb. Res.,* 1, 541, 1972.

232. **Theiss, W., Heyes, H., and Müller, G.,** Therapeutic approaches to experimental endotoxin-induced disseminated intravascular coagulation, presented at 4th Int. Congr. Thrombosis Haemostasis, Vienna, 303 (Abstr.), 1973.

233. **Hunt, P. S., Reeve, T. S., and Hollings, R. M.,** A ''standard'' experimental thrombus: observations on its production, pathology, response to heparin and thrombectomy, *Surgery,* 59, 812, 1966.

234. **Hoppenstein, R., Clark, R. L., and Clifton, E. E.,** Experimental arterial thrombi: formation and lysis, *J. Surg. Res.,* 2, 382, 1962.

235. **Rowsell, H. C., Glynn, M. F., Mustard, J. F., and Murphy, E. A.,** Effect of heparin on platelet economy in dogs, *Am. J. Physiol.,* 213, 915, 1967.

236. **Reber, K.,** Versuche zur Beeinflussung der Thrombozytenadhäsivität in vivo, *Thromb. Diath. Haemorrh.,* Suppl. 24, 35, 1967.

237. **Fahlström, G., Öhman, U., and Magnusson, P. H.,** Intramuscular heparin prophylaxis in experimental thrombosis in rats, *Acta Chir. Scand.,* 136, 489, 1970.

238. **Kahn, D. R., Dufek, J. H., Oberman, H. A., Beck, M. L., Brec, M., Kirsh, M. M., Moores, W. Y., and Prior, M.,** The effect of heparin and dipyridamole on chronic vascular lesions in monkey cardiac allografts, *J. Thorac. Cardiovasc. Surg.,* 63, 720, 1972.

239. **Colman, R. W., Habal, M., Hollenberg, N. K., Birtch, A. G., and Busch, G. J.,** Hyperacute renal allograft rejection in the primate. Therapeutic limitations of antiplatelet agents alone and combined with heparin, *Am. J. Pathol.,* 82, 25, 1976.

240. **Bourgain, R. H. and Six, F.,** A continuous registration method in experimental arterial thrombosis in the rat, *Thromb. Res.,* 4, 599, 1974.

241. **De Clerck, F., Goosens, J., Vermylen, J., Hornstra, G., and Reneman, R. S.,** Modification of venous stasis thrombosis in the rat by platelet-active drugs and by heparin, *Arch. Int. Pharmacodyn. Ther.,* 222, 233, 1976.

242. **Gertz, S. D., Rennels, M. L., and Nelson, E.,** Endothelial cell ischemic injury: protective effect of heparin or aspirin assessed by scanning electron microscopy, *Stroke,* 6, 357, 1975.

243. **Owen, Ch. A. and Bowie, E. J. W.,** Effect of heparin on chronically induced intravascular coagulation in dogs, *Am. J. Physiol.,* 229, 449, 1975.

244. **Lipinski, B. and Gurewich, V.,** The effect of heparin and dipyridamole on the deposition of fibrin-like material in rabbits infused with soluble fibrin monomer or fibrinogen, *Thromb. Res.,* 5, 343, 1974.

245. **Chiu, H. M., Hirsh, J., Yung, W. L., Regoeczi, E., and Gent, M.,** Relationship between the anticoagulant and antithrombotic effects of heparin in experimental venous thrombosis, *Blood,* 49, 171, 1977.

246. **Urizar, R. E., Dodds, W. J., Roth, M., Rohloff, J., Zdeb, M., and Largent, J.,** Disseminated intravascular coagulation induced by liquoid in the rat, IV. Modification of the Shwartzman reaction by ancrod and cobra venom factor, *Lab. Invest.,* 40, 645, 1979.

247. **Seuter, F., Busse, W. D., Meng, K., Hoffmeister, F., Möller, E., and Horstmann, H.,** Antithrombotic activity of BAY g 6575, *Arzneimittelforschung,* 29, 54, 1979.

248. **Meng, K.,** Tierexperimentelle Thrombose und Behandlung mit Acetylsalicylsäure, *Med. Welt,* 27, 1359, 1976.

249. **Kumada, R., Ishihara, M., Ogawa, H., and Abiko, Y.,** Experimental model of venous thrombosis in rats and effect of some agents, *Thromb. Res.,* 18, 189, 1980.

250. **Lavelle, S. M. and McIomhair, M.,** The quantitative reduction by heparin of intravenous thrombosis in normal and hypercoagulated animals, *Ir. J. Med. Sci.,* 149, 266, 1980.

251. **Reyers, I., Mussoni, L., Donati, M. B., and deGaetano, G.,** Severe thrombocytopenia delays but does not prevent the occlusion of an arterial prosthesis in the rat, *Thromb. Haemost.,* 46, 558, 1981.

252. **Pangrazzi, J., Abbadini, M., Zametta, M., Naggi, A., Torri, G., Casu, B., and Donati, M. B.**, Antithrombotic and bleeding effect of a low molecular weight heparin fraction, *Biochem. Pharmacol.*, 34, 3305, 1985.

253. **Pangrazzi, J., Reyers, I., Valenti, I., Naggi, A., Torri, G., Casu, B., and Donati, M. B.**, Antithrombotic mechanisms of a low molecular weight (LMW) heparin: more than anticoagulation, presented at 9th Int. Congr. Thrombosis Haemostasis, Stockholm, 564 (Abstr.), 1983.

254. **Fedelles, P. F., Moser, K. M., Moser, K. S., Konopka, R., and Hartman, M. T.**, Indium-111-labeled platelets — effect of heparin on uptake by venous thrombi and relationship to the activated partial thromboplastin time, *Circulation*, 66, 632, 1982.

255. **Carter, C. J., Kelton, J. G., Hirsh, J., Cerskus, A., Saretus, A. V., and Gent, M.**, The relationship between the hemorrhagic and antithrombotic properties of low molecular weight heparin in rabbits, *Blood*, 59, 1239, 1982.

256. **Collen, D., Stassen, J. M., and Verstraete, M.**, Thrombolysis with human extrinsic (tissue-type) plasminogen activator in rabbits with experimental jugular vein thrombosis. Effect of molecular form and dose of activator, age of the thrombus, and route of administration, *J. Clin. Invest.*, 71, 368, 1983.

257. **Doutremepuich, C., Gestreau, J. L., Maury, M. O., Quilchini, R., Boisseau, M. R., Toulemonde, F., and Vairel, E. G.**, Experimental venous thrombosis in rats treated with heparin and a low molecular weight heparin fraction, *Haemostasis*, 13, 109, 1983.

258. **Doutremepuich, C., Bousquet, F., and Toulemonde, F.**, Are molecular weight and anti-Xa activity sufficient to predict the antithrombotic power of heparin fractions?, *Thromb. Res.*, 44, 709, 1986.

259. **Doutremepuich, C., de Seze, O., Castrioto, T., Pereira, F., Doutremepuich, F., and Toulemonde, F.**, Treatment of experimental venous stasis model in rats by heparin and a very low molecular weight heparin fragment. Relationship to plasmatic heparin activity, presented at 11th Int. Congr. Thrombosis Haemostasis, Brussels, 2051 (Abstr.), 1987.

260. **Bara, L., Billaud, E., Kher, A., and Samama, M.**, Increased anti-Xa bioavailability for a low molecular weight heparin (PK 10169) compared with unfractionated heparin, *Semin. Thromb. Hemost.*, 11, 316, 1985.

261. **Bara, L., Trillou, M., Mardigniau, J., and Samama, M.**, Comparison of antithrombotic activity of two heparin fragments PK 10169 (mol. wt. 5,000) and EMT 680 (mol. wt. 2,500) and unfractionated heparin in a rabbit experimental thrombosis model: relative importance of systemic anti-Xa and anti-IIa activities, *Nouv. Rev. Fr. Hematol.*, 28, 355, 1986.

262. **Bianchini, P., Osima, B., Parma, B., Nader, H. B., and Dietrich, C. P.**, Lack of correlation between "in vitro" and "in vivo" antithrombotic activity of heparin fractions and related compounds. Heparan sulfate as an antithrombotic agents "in vivo", *Thromb. Res.*, 40, 597, 1985.

263. **Walenga, J. M., Petitou, M., Lormeau, J. C., Samama, M., Fareed, J., and Choay, J.**, Antithrombotic activity of a synthetic heparin pentasaccharide in a rabbit stasis thrombosis model using different thrombogenic challenges, *Thromb. Res.*, 46, 187, 1987.

264. **Walenga, J. M., Fareed, J., Petitou, M., Samama, M., Lormeau, J. C., and Choay, J.**, Intravenous antithrombotic activity of a synthetic heparin pentasaccharide in a human serum induced stasis thrombosis model, *Thromb. Res.*, 43, 243, 1986.

265. **Thomas, D. P., Merton, R. E., Barrowcliffe, T. W., Thunberg, L., and Lindahl, U.**, Effects of heparin oligosaccharides with high affinity for antithrombin III in experimental venous thrombosis, *Thromb. Haemost.*, 47, 244, 1982.

266. **Buchanan, M. R., Boneu, B., Ofosu, F., and Hirsh, J.**, The relative importance of thrombin inhibition and factor Xa inhibition to the antithrombotic effects of heparin, *Blood*, 65, 198, 1985.

267. **Meuleman, D. G., Hobbelan, P. M. J., von Dedern, G., and Moelker, H. C. T.**, A novel antithrombotic heparinoid (Org 10172) devoid of bleeding inducing capacity. A survey of its pharmacological properties in experimental animal models, *Thromb. Res.*, 27, 353, 1982.

268. **Hirsh, J.**, In vivo effects of low molecular heparins on experimental thrombosis and bleeding, *Haemostasis*, 16, 82, 1986.

269. **Bianchini, P., Parma, B., and Osima, B.**, Inhibition of tyloxapol (Triton WR 1339) enhanced venous thrombosis by low molecular weight heparin (OP 2123), *Thromb. Res.*, Suppl. 6, 94, 1986.

270. **Ostergaard, P. B., Nilsson, B., Bergqvist, V., Hedner, U., and Pedersen, P. C.**, The effect of low molecular weight heparin on experimental thrombosis and haemostasis, *Thromb. Res.*, 45, 739, 1987.

271. **Mattsson, Ch., Holmer, E., Uthne, T., Hoylaerts, M., and Collen, D.**, Antithrombotic effect of a high affinity heparin fragment covalently coupled to antithrombin III, presented at 9th Int. Congr. Thrombosis Haemostasis, Stockholm, 695 (Abstr.), 1983.

272. **Merton, R. E., Barrowcliffe, T. W., and Thomas, D. P.**, A comparison of dermatan sulphate and heparin as antithrombotic drugs, presented at 11th Int. Congr. Thrombosis Haemostasis, 134 (Abstr.), 1987.

273. **Merton, R. E. and Thomas, D. P.**, Experimental studies on the relative efficacy of dermatan sulphate and heparin as antithrombotic agents, *Thromb. Haemost.*, 58, 839, 1987.

274. **Reber, G., de Moerloose, Ph., Sinclair, M., Schweizer, A., Gardaz, J. P., and Bouvier, C. A.,** Low molecular weight heparin, standard heparin and ancrod as anticoagulant for extracorporeal membrane lung CO_2 removal in dogs, presented at 11th Int. Congr. Thrombosis Haemostasis, Brussels, 287 (Abstr.), 1987.

275. **Shand, R. A., Butler, K. D., and Davies, J. A.,** Heparin anticoagulation and its effects on arterial thrombus formation in the rabbit, presented at 11th Int. Congr. Thrombosis Haemostasis, Brussels, 374 (Abstr.), 1987.

276. **Seuter, F., Sohnius, H., Wohlfeil, St., and Voigt, W. H.,** Injury-induced atherosclerosis in rats, and its suppression by heparin, presented at 9th Int. Congr. Thrombosis Haemostasis, Stockholm, 1200 (Abstr.), 1983.

277. **Kuhn, M., Müller, T. H., and Eisert, W. G.,** Cyclic thrombus formation in rabbit aorta: a new model of acute arterial thrombosis, presented at 11th Int. Congr. Thrombosis Haemostasis, Brussels, 375 (Abstr.), 1987.

278. **Marbet, G. A., Zbinden, B., Satiropas, P., and Duckert, F.,** Tissue thromboplastin-induced reversible DIC as an in vivo model of thrombus generation and inhibition, presented at 11th Int. Congr. Thrombosis Haemostasis, Brussels, 379 (Abstr.), 1987.

279. **Schmidt, B., Buchanan, M. R., Ofosu, F., Brooker, L. A., and Andrew, M.,** Antithrombotic properties of heparin in a neonatal model of thrombin-induced venous stasis thrombosis, presented at 11th Int. Congr. Thrombosis Haemostasis, Brussels, 809 (Abstr.), 1987.

280. **Juhan-Vague, I., Stassen, J. M., Alessi, M. C., Kieckens, L., and Collen, D.,** Effect of different heparins on thrombolysis with t-PA and scu-PA in rabbits with experimental thrombosis, presented at 11th Int. Congr. Thrombosis Haemostasis, Brussels, 993 (Abstr.), 1987.

281. **Stassen, J. M., Juhan-Vague, I., Alessi, M. C., De Cock, F., and Collen, D.,** Potentiation by heparin fragments of thrombolysis induced with human tissue-type plasminogen activator or human single-chain urokinase-type plasminogen activator, *Thromb. Haemost.,* 58, 947, 1987.

282. **Bergqvist, D. and Nilsson, B.,** The influence of low molecular weight heparin in combination with dihydroergotamine on experimental thrombosis and haemostasis, *Thromb. Haemost.,* 58, 893, 1987.

283. **Fenichel, R. L., Carmint, W., Small, B., and Willis, J.,** Comparison of the antithrombotic, anticlotting and antiplatelet aggregatory activities of low molecular weight RD heparin with heparin, presented at 11th Int. Congr. Thrombosis Haemostasis, Brussels, 2055 (Abstr.), 1987.

284. **Vassiliou, I., Wölfl, I., Haas, S., Stemberger, A., and Blümel, G.,** The effect of heparin and polysulfate polysaccharide (SP 54), presented at 9th Int. Congr. Thrombosis Haemostasis, Stockholm, 1515 (Abstr.), 1983.

285. **Bicher, H. I.,** Antithrombotic effect of an heparin-like substance (SP 54) preventing red cell and platelet aggregation, *Arzneimittelforschung,* 20, 379, 1970.

286. **Hladovec, J.,** A quantitative model of venous stasis thrombosis in rats, *Physiol. Bohemoslov.,* 24, 551, 1975.

287. **Hladovec, J.,** The effect of heparin on endothelial stability, *Thromb. Res.,* 35, 347, 1984.

288. **Ward, A. and Clissold, S. P.,** Pentoxifylline. A review of its pharmacodynamic and pharmacokinetic properties, and its therapeutic efficacy, *Drugs,* 34, 50, 1987.

289. **Schröer, R. H.,** Antithrombotic potential of pentoxifylline, a hemorheologically active drug, *Angiology,* 36, 387, 1985.

290. **Stefanovich, V.,** The biochemical mechanism of action of pentoxifylline, *Pharmatherapeutica,* 2 (Suppl. 1), 5, 1978.

291. **Angelkort, B.,** Coagulation phenomena and blood fluidity in peripheral occlusive arterial disease. Study with pentoxifylline, in *Disorders of Blood Flow, New Therapeutic Aspects,* Manrique, R. V. and Müller, R., Eds., Excepta Medica, Amsterdam, 1981, 68.

292. **Müller, R. and Lehrach, F.,** Haemorheological role of platelet aggregation and hypercoagulability in microcirculation: therapeutical approach with pentoxifylline, *Pharmatherapeutica,* 2, 372, 1980.

293. **Kostka-Trbkowa, E., Dembinska-Kiec, A., Grodzinska, L., Bieron, K., and Gryglewski, R. J.,** Beneficial results of pentoxifylline (Trental) therapy in arteriosclerosis obliterans: possible mechanism of action, *Curr. Med. Res. Opin.,* 9, 407, 1985.

294. **Ott, E., Fazekas, F., and Lechner, H.,** Haemorheological effects of pentoxifylline in disturbed blood flow behavior in patients with cerebrovascular disease, *Eur. Neurol.,* 22 (Suppl. 1), 105, 1983.

295. **Poggesi, L., Scarti, L., Boddi, M., Masotti, G., and Serneri, G. G. N.,** Pentoxifylline treatment in patients with occlusive peripheral arterial disease. Circulatory changes and effects on prostaglandin synthesis, *Angiology,* 36, 628, 1985.

296. **Strano, A., Davi, G., Avellone, G., Novo, S., and Pinto, A.,** Double-blind, crossover study of the clinical effects of pentoxifylline in patients with occlusive arterial disease of the lower limbs, *Angiology,* 35, 439, 1984.

297. **Aznar, J., Villa, P., Valles, J., Santo, M. T., Vaya, A., Martinéz-Saler, V., and Yaya, R.,** The effect of dipyridamole and pentoxifylline on prostacyclin generation and platelet aggregation in patients with diffuse cerebrovascular insufficiency, *Thromb. Res.* Suppl. 6, 142, 1986.

298. **Zinzadse, K. I., Gulischwilli, L. N., Tavchelidse, T. D., and Vorobjov, O. J.,** The effect of pentoxyfylline on the blood flow properties in experimental atherosclerosis in rabbits, *Pharmatherapeutica,* 2, 118, 1978.

299. **Weithmann, K. U.,** Reduced platelet aggregation by pentoxifylline stimulated prostacyclin release, *Vasa,* 10, 249, 1981.

300. **Matzky, R., Darius, H., and Schrör, K.,** The release of prostacyclin (PGI$_2$) by pentoxifylline from human vascular tissue, *Arzneimittelforschung,* 32, 1315, 1982.

301. **Sinzinger, H.,** Pentoxifylline enhances formation of prostacyclin from rat vascular and renal tissue, *Prostaglandins Leukotrienes Med.,* 12, 217, 1983.

302. **Pohanka, E. and Sinzinger, H.,** Effect of single pentoxifylline administration on platelet sensitivity, plasma factor activity, plasma-6-oxo-PGF$_{1alfa}$ and thromboxane B$_2$ in healthy volunteers, *Prostaglandins Leukotrienes Med.,* 22, 191, 1986.

303. **Weichert, W. and Breddin, H. K.,** Antithrombotic effects of acetylsalicylic acid (ASA) and pentoxifylline in laser-induced thrombosis in rat mesenteric vessels, *Vasa,* 14, 280, 1985.

304. **Michal, M. and Giessinger, N.,** The effect of pentoxifylline on thrombus formation in vivo, presented at 9th Int. Congr. of Pharmacology, London, 565 (Abstr.), 1984.

305. **Sherement'ev, Yu. A., Shtykhno, Yu. M., Udovichenko, V. I., and Levin, G. Ya.,** Effect of acetylsalicylic acid and pentoxifylline (Trental) on intravascular erythrocyte aggregation stimulated by arachidonic acid, *Biul. Eksp. Biol. Med.,* 90, 1187, 1980.

306. **Puranapanda, V., Hinshaw, L. B., O'Rear, E. A., Chang, A. C. K., and Whitsett, T. L.,** Erythrocyte deformability in canine septic shock and the efficacy of pentoxifylline and a leukotriene antagonist, *Proc. Soc. Exp. Biol. Med.,* 185, 206, 1987.

307. **Ambrus, C. M., Ambrus, J. L., Gastpar, H., Sharma, S. D., and Suhow, B.,** The role of fibrinolysis in the therapy of peripheral vascular disease, *Angiology,* 35, 436, 1984.

308. **Di Perri, T., Carandente, O., Vittoria, A., Guerrini, M., and Messa, G. L.,** Studies of the clinical pharmacology and therapeutic efficacy of pentoxifylline in peripheral arterial disease, *Angiology,* 35, 427, 1984.

309. **Angelkort, B.,** Thrombozytenfunktion, plasmatische Blutgerinnung und Fibrinolyse bei chronisch arterieller Verschlusskrankheit, *Med. Welt,* 30, 1239, 1979.

310. **Bruno, J. J. and Molony, B. A.,** Ticlopidine, in *New Drug Annual: Cardiovascular Drugs,* Scriabine, A., Ed., Raven Press, New York, 1983, 295.

311. **Picard-Fraire, C.,** Ticlopidine hydrochloride: relationship between dose, kinetics, plasma concentration and effect on platelet function, *Thromb. Res.,* Suppl. 4, 119, 1983.

312. **Bruno, J. J.,** The mechanism of action of ticlopidine, *Thromb. Res.,* Suppl. 4, 59, 1983.

313. **Johnson, M., Walton, P. L., Cotton, R. C., and Strachan, C. J. L.,** Pharmacological evaluation of ticlopidine, a novel inhibitor of platelet function, *Thromb. Haemost.,* 38, 64, 1977.

314. **Ashida, S. and Abiko, Y.,** Inhibition of platelet aggregation by a new agent, ticlopidine, *Thromb. Haemost.,* 40, 542, 1979.

315. **Lagarde, M., Ghazi, I., and Dechavanne, M.,** Effect of ticlopidine on arachidonic acid metabolism in platelet phospholipids in vitro, *Biochem. Pharmacol.,* 30, 1463, 1981.

316. **Thebault, J. J., Blatrix, C. E., Blanchard, J. F., and Panak, E. A.,** Effects of ticlopidine, a new platelet aggregation inhibitor in man, *Clin. Pharmacol. Ther.,* 18, 485, 1975.

317. **Conard, J., Lecrubier, C., Scarabin, P. Y., Horellon, M. H., Samama, M., and Bousser, M. G.,** Effects of long term administration of ticlopidine on platelet function and hemostatic variables, *Thromb. Res.,* 20, 143, 1980.

318. **Kirstein, P., Jogestrand, T., Johnsson, T. L., and Olsson, A. G.,** Antiaggregation, physiological and clinical effects of ticlopidine in subjects with peripheral atherosclerosis, *Atherosclerosis,* 36, 471, 1980.

319. **Ellis, D. J., Roc, R. L., Bruno, J. J., Carnston, B. J., and McSpaden, M. M.,** The effects of ticlopidine hydrochloride on bleeding time and platelet function in man, *Thromb. Haemost.,* 46, 1973, 1981.

320. **Davi, G., Pinto, A., and Francavilla, G.,** Inhibition of platelet function by ticlopidine in arteriosclerosis obliterans of the low limbs, *Thromb. Res.,* 40, 275, 1985.

321. **Odiot, J., Benveniste, J., and Delabassee, D.,** Inhibition par la ticlopidine de l'aggrégation des plaquettes humaines stimulées par "le platelet activating factor" (PAF acether), presented at 6th Congr. Mediterranean Thromboembolism, Monte-Carlo, 259 (Abstr.), 1980.

322. **Dunn, F., Soria, C., Soria, J.,** Effet de l'administration de ticlopidine sur la fixation du fibrinogène au niveau des plaquettes, *Nouv. Rev. Fr. Hematol.,* 25, 132, 1983.

323. **Di Minno, G., Cerbone, A. M., Mattioli, P. L., Iovine, C., and Mancini, M.,** Functionally thrombasthenic state in normal platelets following the administration of ticlopidine, *J. Clin. Invest.,* 75, 328, 1985.

324. **Piovella, F., Ricetti, M. M., Almasio, P., Samaden, A., Semino, G., and Ascari, E.,** The effect of ticlopidine on human endothelial cells in culture, *Thromb. Res.,* 33, 323, 1984.

325. **Paleirac, G., Meynadier, J., Guilhow, J. U., and Castaigne, J. P.,** Comparison of the platelet inhibiting properties of ticlopidine and dipyridamole, *Mediterr. Med.*, 2, 77, 1979.

326. **Ono, S., Ashida, S., and Abiko, Y.,** Hemorheological effect of ticlopidine in rats, *Thromb. Haemost.*, 46, 173, 1981.

327. **Ferrand, J. C., Aubert, D., Lacaze, B., Pepin, O., and Thebault, J. J.,** In vivo activity of ticlopidine, a new drug with platelet aggregation inhibiting, antisludge and antithrombotic properties, *Thromb. Diath. Haemorrh.*, 34, 342, 1975.

328. **Le Menn, R.,** Ultrastructure of blood platelet aggregates: effect of an inhibitor, ticlopidine, *Biol. Cell.*, 43, 179, 1982.

329. **Abou-Khalil, S., Abou-Khalil, W. H., and Yunis, A. A.,** Swelling mitochondria by the platelet-antiaggregating agent ticlopidine, *Biochem. Pharmacol.*, 35, 1849, 1986.

330. **Leblondel, G. and Allain, P.,** Effect of an inhibitor of platelet aggregation, ticlopidine on energy transduction of rat liver mitochondria, *Biochem. Pharmacol.*, 27, 2099, 1978.

331. **Ashida, S. I., Sakumo, K., and Abiko, Y.,** Antithrombotic effects of ticlopidine, acetylsalicylic acid and dipyridamole in vascular shunt model in rats, *Thromb. Res.*, 17, 663, 1980.

332. **Choe, D. T. and Povalski, H. J.,** Effects of sulfinpyrazone, dipyridamole, aspirin and indomethacin on initiation and growth rate of experimental arterial thrombosis in the rat, *Fed. Proc.*, 40, 772, 1981.

333. **Massad, L., Plotkine, M., Capdeville, C., and Boulu, R. G.,** Electrically induced arterial thrombosis in the conscious rat, *Thromb. Res.*, 48, 1, 1987.

334. **Vallee, E., Maffrand, J. P., Bernat, A., Delebassee, D., and Tissinier, A.,** Ticlopidine as an experimental antithrombotic agent, *Agents Actions*, Suppl. 50—59, 15, 1984.

335. **Kobayashi, N., Takada, M., Tanaka, H., Gonmori, H., and Maekawa, T.,** The effect of ticlopidine on experimentally induced arterial thrombosis of rabbits, *Blood Vessels*, 11, 164, 1980.

336. **Smith, J. R. and White, A. M.,** Fibrin, red cell and platelet interactions in an experimental model of thrombosis, *Br. J. Pharmacol.*, 73, 219 P, 1981.

337. **Pumphrey, C. W., Fuster, V., Dewanjee, M. K., Murphy, K. P., Vlietstra, R. E., and Kaye, M. P.,** A new in vivo model of arterial thrombosis. The effect of administration of ticlopidine and verapamil in dogs, *Thromb. Res.*, 28, 663, 1982.

338. **Bernat, A., Maffrand, J. P., Tissinier, A., and Vallée, E.,** Antithrombotic activity of ticlopidine in a platelet independent model of venous thrombosis in the rat, *Haemostasis*, 12, 138, 1982.

339. **Bernat, A., Vallée, E., Maffrand, J. P., and Roncucci, R.,** Antithrombotic effect of ticlopidine in a platelet-independent model of venous thrombosis, *Thromb. Res.*, 37, 279, 1985.

340. **Cattaneo, M., Winocour, P. D., Somers, D. A., Groves, H. M., Kinlough-Rathbone, R. L., Packham, M. A., and Mustard, J. F.,** Effect of ticlopidine on platelet aggregation, adherence to damaged vessels, thrombus formation and platelet survival, *Thromb. Res.*, 37, 20, 1985.

341. **Escolar, G., Bastida, E., Castillo, R., and Ordinas, A.,** Ticlopidine inhibits platelet thrombus formation studied in a flowing system, *Thromb. Res.*, 45, 561, 1987.

342. **Tomikawa, M., Ashida, S. I., Kakihata, K., and Abiko, Y.,** Anti-thrombotic action of ticlopidine, a new platelet aggregation inhibitor, *Thromb. Res.*, 12, 1157, 1978.

343. **Lacaze, B., Ferrand, C., and Pepin, O.,** Induction of DIC by Russell's viper venom in the rat. Preventive and curative action of ticlopidine, *Thromb. Haemost.*, 42, 75, 1979.

344. **Butler, K. D. and White, A. M.,** Inhibition of thrombocytopenic episodes caused by the Arthus reaction, the sublethal Forssman reaction and adenosine diphosphate, *Artery*, 8, 457, 1980.

345. **Thörne, L. J., Jönsson, B. A., Norgren, L., and Strand, S. E.,** Effect of ticlopidine and PGE on endotoxin-induced pulmonary platelet sequestration in vivo, *Circ. Shock*, 20, 61, 1986.

346. **Ashida, S., Ishihara, M., Ogawa, H., and Abiko, Y.,** Protective effect of ticlopidine on experimentally induced peripheral arterial occlusive disease in rats, *Thromb. Res.*, 18, 55, 1980.

347. **Green, C. J., Kemp, E., and Kemp, G.,** Effect of cyclosporin A, ticlopidine hydrochloride and cobra venom factor on the hyperacute rejection of discordant renal xenografts, *Invest. Cell. Pathol.*, 3, 415, 1980.

348. **Hashimoto, M., Tanabe, T., Honma, H., Moriyama, Y., Shinsoto, M., Sakamoto, K., Takeoka, T., Aoki, H., and Sugie, S.,** Effects of ticlopidine, an inhibitor of platelet aggregation and aspirin in arteriole substitution, *Blood Vessels*, 11, 170, 1980.

349. **Murphy, K. P., Dewanjee, M. K., Furster, V., Didisheim, P., and Kaye, M. P.,** Effect of ticlopidine on platelet deposition on Gore-Tex and autologous vein grafts, *Thromb. Haemost.*, 46, 175, 1981.

350. **Philipp, E., Ritter, W., and Patzschke, K.,** The relationship between dose pharmacokinetics, plasma-concentrations and antithrombotic effects of nafazatrom, *Thromb. Res.*, Suppl. 4, 129, 1983.

351. **Seuter, F., Fiedler, V. B., and Philipp, E.,** Nafazatrom, in *New Cardiovascular Drugs*, Scriabine, A., Ed., Raven Press, New York, 1986, 163.

352. **Buchanan, M. R., Blajchman, M., and Hirsh, J.,** Inhibition of arterial thrombosis and platelet function by nafazatrom, *Thromb. Res.*, 28, 157, 1982.

353. **Fiedler, V. B.,** The effects of oral nafazatrom (= Bay g 6575) on canine coronary artery thrombosis and myocardial ischemia, *Basic Res. Cardiol.*, 78, 266, 1983.

354. **Fiedler, V. B.,** Reduction of myocardial infarction and dysrhythmic activity by nafazatrom in the conscious rat, *Eur. J. Pharmacol.,* 88, 263, 1983.

355. **Shea, M. J., Driscoll, E. M., Romson, J. L., Pitt, B., and Lucchesi, B. R.,** The beneficial effects of nafazatrom (Bay G 6575) on experimental coronary thrombosis, *Am. Heart J.,* 107, 629, 1983.

356. **Shea, M. J., Murtagh, J. J., Jolly, S. R., Abrams, G. D., Pitt, B., and Lucchesi, B. R.,** Beneficial effect of nafazatrom on ischemic reperfused myocardium, *Eur. J. Pharmacol.,* 102, 63, 1984.

357. **Herrmann, K. S.,** Antiaggregatory efficacy and its time-course after applications of acetylsalicylic acid, prostacyclin and nafazatrom in vivo, *Arch. Int. Pharmacodyn. Ther.,* 272, 150, 1984.

358. **Herrmann, K. S. and Seuter, F.,** Platelet aggregation in arterioles of the hamster cheek pouch and in heart transplants: Its tissue-dependent influencibility by acetylsalicylic acid and nafazatrom, *Haemostasis,* 14, 281, 1984.

359. **Lefer, A. M. and Messenger, M.,** Protective actions of nafazatrom in traumatic shock, *Arzneimittelforschung,* 32, 1089, 1982.

360. **Deckmyn, H., Gresele, P., Arnout, J., Todisco, A., and Vermylen, J.,** Prolonging prostacyclin production by nafazatrom or dipyridamole, *Lancet,* 2, 410, 1984.

361. **Coker, S. J. and Parratt, J. R.,** The effects of nafazatrom on arrhythmias and prostanoid release during coronary artery occlusion and reperfusion in anaesthetized greyhounds, *J. Mol. Cell. Cardiol.,* 16, 43, 1984.

362. **Ambrus, J. L., Ambrus, C. M., Gastpar, H., and Williams, P.,** Study of platelet aggregation in vivo. IX. Effect of nafazatrom on in vivo platelet aggregation and spontaneous tumor metastasis, *J. Med.,* 13, 35, 1982.

363. **Gastpar, H.,** Platelet aggregation and cancer metastasis, *Ann. Chir. Gynecol.,* 71, 142, 1982.

364. **Deckmyn, H., Van Houtte, E., Verstraete, M., and Vermylen, J.,** Manipulation of the local thromboxane and prostacyclin balance in vivo by the antithrombotic compounds dazoxiben, acetylsalicylic acid and nafazatrom, *Biochem. Pharmacol.,* 32, 2757, 1983.

365. **Vermylen, J., Chamone, D. A. F., and Verstraete, M.,** Stimulation of prostacyclin release from vessel wall by BAY g 6575, an antithrombotic compound, *Lancet,* 1, 518, 1979.

366. **Wong, P. Y. K., Chao, P. H. W., and McGiff, J. C.,** Nafazatrom(BAY,G 6575), an antithrombotic and antimetastatic agent, inhibits 15-hydroxy-prostaglandin dehydrogenase, *J. Pharmacol. Exp. Ther.,* 223, 757, 1982.

367. **Sevilla, M. D., Neta, P., and Marnett, L. J.,** Reaction of the antithrombotic and antimetastatic agent, nafazatrom, with oxidizing radicals, *Biochem. Biophys. Res. Commun.,* 115, 800, 1983.

368. **Busse, W. D., Mardin, M., Gruetzmann, R., Dunn, J. K., Theodorou, M., Sloane, B. F., and Honn, K. V.,** Nafazatrom (BAY G 6575), an inhibitor of cellular lipoxygenase activity, *Fed. Proc.,* 41, 1717, 1982.

369. **Strasser, T., Fischer, S., and Weber, P. C.,** Inhibition of leukotriene B_4 formation in human neutrophils after oral nafazatrom (BAY G 6575), *Biochem. Pharmacol.,* 34, 1891, 1985.

370. **Hladovec, J.,** Protective effect of oxygen-derived free radical scavengers on the endothelium in vivo, *Physiol. Bohemoslov.,* 35, 97, 1986.

371. **Roba, J., Calderon, P., Cavalier, R., Defreyn, G., Gorissen, H., Saerens, E., and Lambelin, G.,** Suloctidil, in *New Cardiovascular Drugs,* Scriabine, A., Ed., Raven Press, New York, 1986, 185.

372. **Mürer, E. H., Niewiarowski, S., and Stewart, G. J.,** Effect of suloctidil (1(4-isopropylthiophenyl)-2-n-octyl aminopropanol) on human platelets in vitro, *Biochem. Pharmacol.,* 28, 471, 1979.

373. **de Gaetano, G., Roncaglioni, M. C., Miragliotta, G., Wielosz, M., and Garrattini, S.,** In vivo effect of suloctidil on ^{14}C-5-hydroxytryptamine uptake and liberation in rat platelets, *Pharmacol. Res. Commun.,* 9, 315, 1977.

374. **Mills, D. C. B. and Macfarlane, D. E.,** Depletion of platelet amine storage granules by the antithrombotic agent, suloctidil, *Thromb. Haemost.,* 38, 1010, 1977.

375. **Bucchi, F., Cerletti, C., and de Gaetano, G.,** Inhibition of platelet thromboxane generation by suloctidil in man, *Haemostasis,* 16, 362, 1986.

376. **Roba, J., Claeys, M., van Roet, R., Opstal, W., and Lambelin, G.,** Erythrocyte membrane as a target for antithrombotic agents, in *Adaptability of Vascular Wall,* Reiniš, Z., Pokorný, J., Linhart, J., Hild, R., and Schirger, A., Eds., Springer-Verlag, Berlin, 1980, 96.

377. **Calderon, P., van Dorsser, W., von Szendrai, G. K., de Mey, J. G., and Roba, J.,** In vitro vasorelaxing activity of suloctidil, *Arch. Int. Pharmacodyn. Ther.,* 284, 101, 1986.

378. **Boeynaems, J. M., Demolle, D., and Van Coevorden, A.,** Stimulation of vascular prostacyclin by SKF 525-A (Proadifen) and related compounds, *Biochem. Pharmacol.,* 36, 1637, 1987.

379. **Stelzer, M. R., Burne, T. S., and Saunders, N.,** In vivo effect of suloctidil as an antiplatelet agent, *Thromb. Haemost.,* 41, 465, 1979.

380. **Roba, J., Claeys, M., and Lambelin, G.,** Antiplatelet and antithrombogenic effect of suloctidil, *Eur. J. Pharmacol.,* 37, 265, 1976.

381. **Roba, J., Defreyn, G., and Biagi, G.**, Antithrombotic activity of suloctidil, *Thromb. Res.*, Suppl. 4, 53, 1983.

382. **Roba, J., Bourgain, R., Andries, R., Claeys, A., Van Opstal, W., and Lambelin, G.**, Antagonism by suloctidil of arterial thrombus formation in rats, *Thromb. Res.*, 9, 585, 1976.

383. **Tuma, R. F., Wiedeman, M. P., and Mayrovitz, H. N.**, Microvascular responses to suloctidil, *Physiologist*, 19, 394, 1976.

384. **de Gaetano, G. and Cavenaghi, A. E.**, Effect of suloctidil on bleeding time and in vivo platelet aggregation in rats, *Thromb. Res.*, 10, 525, 1977.

385. **Hladovec, J. and Přerovský, I.**, Experimental prevention of venous thrombosis, *Czech. Med.*, 3, 11, 1980.

386. **Vermylen, J., Defreyn, G., Carreras, L. O., Machin, S. J., Schaeren, J. V., and Verstraete, M.**, Thromboxane synthetase inhibition as antithrombotic strategy, *Lancet*, 1, 1073, 1981.

387. **Randall, M. J.**, Selective inhibition of thromboxane synthesis with dazoxiben in animals and man, *Thromb. Res.*, Suppl. 4, 81, 1983.

388. **Goldman, M., Hall, C. Hawker, R. J., and McCollum, C. N.**, presented at 9th Int. Congr. Thrombosis Haemostasis, Stockholm, 690 (Abstr.), 1983.

389. **Bertelé, V., Falanga, A., Roncaglioni, M. C., Cerletti, C., and de Gaetano, G.**, Thromboxane synthetase inhibition results in increased platelet sensitivity to prostacyclin, *Thromb. Haemost.*, 47, 294, 1982.

390. **Parry, M. J., Randall, M. J., Tyler, H. M., Myhre, E., Dale, J., and Thaulow, E.**, Selective inhibition of thromboxane synthetase by dazoxiben increases prostacyclin production by leucocytes in angina patients and healthy volunteers, *Lancet*, 2, 164, 1982.

391. **Bertelé, V., Cerletti, Ch., Schieppati, A., di Minno, G., and de Gaetano, G.**, Inhibition of thromboxane synthetase does not necessarily prevent platelet aggregation, *Lancet*, 1, 1057, 1981.

392. **Tanoue, K., Yamaguchi, A., Sakakibara, C., Ariga, S., Ikeda, M., Yamamoto, N., Suzuki, H., and Yamazaki, H.**, Relative importance of thromboxane A_2 production in various types of human platelet aggregation, presented at 9th Int. Congr. Thrombosis Haemostasis, Stockholm, 908 (Abstr.), 1983.

393. **Belch, J. J. F., Saniabadi, A. R., McLaughlin, K., and Forbes, C. D.**, Platelet changes after a saturated fat meal and their prevention by Dazmegrel, a thromboxane synthetase inhibitor, *Lipids*, 22, 159, 1987.

394. **Monge, A., Erro, A., Parrada, P., Font, M., Aldana, I., Rocha, E., and Fernandez-Alvarez, E.**, Effects of 2-indolecarbohydrazides on thromboxane synthetase activity and on in vitro and ex vivo blood platelet aggregation. New selective inhibitors, *Arzneimittelforschung*, 36, 1184, 1986.

395. **Steinhauer, H. B., Lubrich, I., Günter, B., and Schollmeyer, P.**, Response of human platelets to inhibitors of thromboxane synthetase, *Clin. Hemorheol.*, 3, 1, 1983.

396. **Gentry, P. A. and Bondy, G. S.**, The aggregation of bovine platelets is not dependent on thromboxane B_2 production, presented at 11th Int. Congr. Thrombosis Haemostosis, Brussels, 1701 (Abstr.), 1987.

397. **Saldeen, P. and Saldeen, T.**, Thromboxane production by pathological vessels and its possible contribution to the development of thrombosis, presented at 11th Int. Congr. Thrombosis Haemostasis, Brussels, 581 (Abstr.), 1987.

398. **Lewis, P., Tyler, H. M. (Eds.)**, Dazoxiben. Clinical prospects for a thromboxane synthesis inhibitor, *Br. J. Clin. Pharmacol.*, 15, 1 S, 1983.

399. **Simpson, P. L., Smith, Ch. B., Jr., Rosenthal, G., and Lucchesi, B. R.**, Reduction in the incidence of thrombosis by the thromboxane synthetase inhibitor CGS 13080 in a canine model of coronary artery injury, *J. Pharmacol. Exp. Ther.*, 238, 497, 1986.

400. **Silver, M. J., Hoch, W., Kocsis, J. J., Ingerman, C. M., and Smith, J. B.**, Arachidonic acid causes sudden death in rabbits, *Science*, 183, 1085, 1974.

401. **Puig-Parellada and Planas, J. M.**, Action of selective inhibitor of thromboxane synthetase on experimental thrombosis induced by arachidonic acid in rabbits, *Lancet*, 2, 40, 1977.

402. **Lefer, A. M., Okamatsu, S., Smith, E. F., III., and Smith, J. B.**, Beneficial effects of a new thromboxane synthetase inhibitor in arachidonate-induced sudden death, *Thromb. Res.*, 23, 265, 1981.

403. **Lefer, A. M., Burke, S. E., and Smith, J. B.**, Role of thromboxanes and prostacyclin endoperoxides in the pathogenesis of eicosanoid-induced sudden death, *Thromb. Res.*, 32, 311, 1983.

404. **Lefer, D. J., Mentley, R. K., and Lefer, A. M.**, Protective effects of a new specific thromboxane antagonist in arachidonate-induced sudden death, *Arch. Int. Pharmacodyn. Ther.*, 287, 89, 1987.

405. **Randall, M. J., Parry, M. J., Hawkeswood, E., Cross, P. E., and Dickinson, R. P.**, UK-37,248, a novel, selective thromboxane synthetase inhibitor with platelet anti-aggregatory and antithrombotic activity, *Thromb. Res.*, 23, 145, 1981.

406. **Aiken, J. W., Shebuski, R. J., Miller, O. V., and Gorman, R. R.**, Endogenous prostacyclin contributes to the efficacy of a thromboxane synthetase inhibitor for preventing coronary artery thrombosis, *J. Pharmacol. Exp. Ther.*, 219, 299, 1981.

407. **Gorman, R. R., Johnson, R. A., Spilman, C. H., and Aiken, J. W.**, Inhibition of platelet thromboxane A_2 synthase activity by sodium 5-(3'-pyridinyl) methylbenzofuran-2-carboxylate, *Prostaglandins*, 26, 325, 1983.

408. **Tada, M., Esumi, K., Yamagishi, M., Kuzuya, T., Matsuda, H., Abe, H., Uchida, Y., and Murao, S.**, Reduction of prostacyclin synthesis as a possible cause of transient flow reduction in a partially constricted canine coronary artery, *J. Mol. Cell. Cardiol.*, 16, 1137, 1984.

409. **Bush, L. R., Campbell, W. B., Buja, L. M., Tilton, G. D., and Willerson, J. T.**, Effects of the selective thromboxane synthetase inhibitor dazoxiben on variations in cyclic blood flow in stenosed canine coronary arteries, *Circulation*, 69, 1161, 1984.

410. **Schmitz, J. M., Apprill, P. G., Buja, L. M., Bush, L. R., Campbell, W. B., and Willerson, J. T.**, The effect of the platelet activating factor (PAF) on coronary blood flow and platelet aggregation, *Fed. Proc.*, 43, 933, 1984.

411. **Prosdocimi, M., Tessari, R., Finesso, M., Zatta, A., Gorio, A., Dejana, E., Languino, L. R., Del Maschio, A., and de Gaetano, G.**, Coronary artery stenosis in the dog. Intravascular platelet aggregation, 6-keto-PGF$_{1\,alfa}$ and TXB$_2$ determinations, presented at 9th Int. Congr. Thrombosis Haemostasis, Stockholm, 689 (Abstr.), 1983.

412. **Folts, J. D. and Smith, S. R.**, Dipyridamole alone and with a low dose aspirin does not prevent acute platelet thrombus formation in stenosed dog coronary arteries, presented at 11th Int. Congr. Thrombosis Haemostasis, Brussels, 778 (Abstr.), 1987.

413. **Kloeze, J.**, Prostaglandins and platelet aggregation in vivo. Part II. Influence of PGE$_1$ and PGF$_{1\,alfa}$ on platelet thrombus formation induced by an electric stimulus in veins on the rat brain surface, *Thromb. Diath. Haemorrh.*, 23, 293, 1970.

414. **Kowey, P. R., Verrier, R. L., Lown, B., and Handin, R. I.**, Influence of intracoronary platelet aggregation on ventricular electrical properties during partial coronary artery stenosis, *Am. J. Cardiol.*, 51, 596, 1983.

415. **Romson, J., Haack, D., and Lucchesi, B. R.**, Electrical induction of coronary artery thrombosis in the ambulatory canine: a model for in vivo evaluation of antithrombotic agents, *Thromb. Res.*, 17, 841, 1980.

416. **Schumacher, W. A. and Lucchesi, B. R.**, Effect of the thromboxane synthetase inhibitor UK-37,248 (Dazoxiben) upon platelet aggregation, coronary artery thrombosis and vascular reactivity, *J. Pharmacol. Exp. Ther.*, 227, 790, 1983.

417. **Shea, M. J., Driscoll, E. M., Romson, J. L., Pitt, B. and Lucchesi, B. R.**, Effects of OKY 1581, a thromboxane synthetase inhibitor, on coronary thrombosis in the conscious dog, *Eur. J. Pharmacol.*, 105, 285, 1984.

418. **Hook, B. G., Schumacher, W. A., Lee, D. L., Jolly, S. R., and Lucchesi, B. R.**, Experimental coronary artery thrombosis in the absence of thromboxane A$_2$ synthesis: evidence for alternate pathways for coronary thrombosis, *J. Cardiovasc. Pharmacol.*, 7, 174, 1985.

419. **Randall, M. J. and Wilding, R. I. R.**, Acute arterial thrombosis in rabbits: reduced platelet accumulation after treatment with thromboxane synthetase inhibitor dazoxiben hydrochloride (UK 37,248-01), *Thromb. Res.*, 28, 607, 1982.

420. **Randall, M. J. and Wilding, R. I. R.**, Acute arterial thrombosis in rabbits: reduced platelet accumulation after treatment with dazoxiben hydrochloride UK 37,248-01, *Br. J. Pharmacol.*, 15, 49 S, 1983.

421. **Van Dergiessen, W. J. and Zijlstra, F. J.**, The thromboxane antagonist BK 13,177 inhibits experimentally induced coronary thrombosis, unlike aspirin, presented at Cardiovasc. Pharmacother. Int. Symp., Geneva, 140 (Abstr.), 1985.

422. **Lewis, G. P., Smith, J. R., and Williamson, I. H. M.**, Prostaglandin endoperoxides are more important than thromboxane A$_2$ in thrombus formation in vivo, presented at 9th Int. Congr. Thrombosis Haemostasis, Stockholm, 756 (Abstr.), 1983.

423. **Ambler, J., Butler, K. D., Ku, E. C., Maguire, E. D., Smith, J. R., and Wallis, R. B.**, CGS 12970: a novel long acting thromboxane synthetase inhibitor, *Br. J. Pharmacol.*, 86, 497, 1985.

424. **Van Reempts, J., Van Deuren, B., Borgers, M., and De Clerck, F.**, R 68070, a combined TXA$_2$-synthetase/TXA$_2$-prostaglandin endoperoxide receptor inhibitor reduces cerebral infarct size after photochemically initiated thrombosis in spontaneously hypertensive rats, presented at 11th Int. Congr. Thrombosis Haemostasis, Brussels, 671 (Abstr.), 1987.

425. **Zimmerman, R., Peter, J., Jung, G., Horsch, A., Mörl, H., and Harenberg, J.**, Antithrombotic and opposite effects of drugs influencing the prostaglandin system, *Thromb. Haemost.*, 46, 179, 1981.

426. **Heiss, M., Haas, S., and Blumel, G.**, The antithrombotic effect of a new thromboxane synthetase inhibitor (UK-37,248) in comparison with acetylsalicylic acid (ASA) in experimental thrombosis, *Haemostasis*, 12, 102, 1982.

427. **Bergqvist, D., Björck, C. G., Dougan, P., Exquivel, C. O., Lannerstad, O., Nilsson, B., Saldeen, P., and Saldeen, T.**, The effect of inhibition of thromboxane synthesis in experimental thrombosis and haemostasis, *Thromb. Res.*, 37, 435, 1985.

428. **Ogletree, M. L., Harris, D. N., Greenberg, R., Haslanger, M. F., and Nakane, M.**, Pharmacological actions of SQ 29 548, a novel selective thromboxane antagonist, *J. Pharmacol. Exp. Ther.*, 234, 435, 1985.

429. **Terres, W., Kupper, W., Hamm, C., and Bleifeld, W.,** Resting myocardial ischemia after intravenous infusion of BM 13 177, a thromboxane receptor antagonist, presented at 11th Int. Congr. Thrombosis Haemostasis, Brussels, 667 (Abstr.), 1987.

430. **Brezinski, M. E., Yanagisawa, A., and Lefer, A. M.,** Cardioprotective actions of specific thromboxane receptor antagonists in acute myocardial ischemia, *J. Cardiovasc. Pharmacol.,* 9, 65, 1987.

431. **De Gaetano, G., Cerletti, Ch., Dejana, E., Latini, R., and Villa, S.,** Thromboxane synthase inhibitor combined with thromboxane receptor blockade: a step forward in antithrombotic strategy?, *Thromb. Haemost.,* 52, 364, 1984.

432. **Gresele, P., Deckmyn, H., Arnout, J., Lemmen, J., Janssens, W., and Vermylen, J.,** BM 13.177, a selective blocker of platelet and vessel wall receptors, is active in man, *Lancet,* 1, 991, 1984.

433. **Stegmeir, K., Pill, J., Müller-Beckmann, B., Schmidt, F. M., Witte, E. C., Wolf, H. P., and Patscheke, H.,** The pharmacological profile of the thromboxane A_2 antagonist BM 13.177, a new antiplatelet and antithrombotic drug, *Thromb. Res.,* 35, 379, 1984.

434. **Ditter, H., Matthias, F. R., Voss, R., and Röttger, P.,** Prostacyclin improves survival and reduces microclot formation in rabbit endotoxemia, presented at 11th Int. Congr. Thrombosis Haemostasis, Brussels, 1892 (Abstr.), 1987.

435. **Romson, J. L., Haack, D. W., Abrams, G. D., and Lucchesi, B. R.,** Prevention of occlusive coronary artery thrombosis by prostacyclin infusion in the dog, *Circulation,* 64, 906, 1981.

436. **Schrör, K., Darius, H., Ohlendorf, R., Matzky, R., and Klaus, W.,** Dissociation of antiplatelet effects from myocardial cytoprotective activity during acute myocardial ischemia in cats by a new carbacyclin derivative (ZK 36 375), *J. Cardiovasc. Pharmacol.,* 4, 554, 1982.

437. **Maurin, N.,** Influence on platelet activity and red cell fluidity of epoprostenol and two stable prostacyclin analogues in vitro, *Arzneimittelforschung,* 36, 1180, 1986.

438. **Araki, H. and Lefer, A.,** Beneficial effect of prostacyclin (PGI_2) on the ischemic perfused rat heart, *Fed. Proc.,* 39, 1003, 1980.

439. **Jugdutt, B., Hutchins, G., Bulkley, B., and Becker, L.,** Infarct size reduction by prostacyclin after coronary occlusion in conscious dogs, *Clin. Res.,* 27, 117 A, 1979.

440. **Ogletree, M., Lefer, A., Smith, J., and Nicolau, K.,** Studies on the protective effect of prostacyclin in acute myocardial ischemia, *Eur. J. Pharmacol.,* 56, 95, 1979.

441. **Ubatuba, F. B., Moncada, S., and Vane, J. R.,** The effect of prostacyclin (PGI_2) on platelet behavior. Thrombus formation in vivo and bleeding time, *Thromb. Res.,* 41, 425, 1979.

442. **Bousser, M.-G. and Lecrubier, Ch.,** Effect of prostaglandin E_1 on experimental thrombosis and platelet aggregation in rabbits, *Haemostasis,* 1, 294, 1972/73.

443. **Sim, A. K., Mc Craw, A. P., Cleland, M. E., Aibara, H., Otomo, S., and Hosoda, K.,** The effect of prostaglandin E_1 incorporated in lipid microspheres on thrombus formation and thrombus disaggregation and its potential to target to the site of vascular lesions, *Arzneimittelforschung,* 36, 1206, 1986.

444. **Hladovec, J.,** Prostaglandins and endothelial stability, *Arzneimittelforschung,* 31, 46, 1981.

445. **Zawilska, K., Begent, N. A., and Born, G. V. R.,** Further evidence that haemostasis depends more on ADP than on thromboxane A_2, presented at 9th Int. Congr. Thrombosis Haemostasis, Stockholm, 1070 (Abstr.), 1983.

446. **Kloeze, J., Don, J. A., Haddeman, E., and Kivits, G. A. A.,** Are lipoxygenase products of more significance in arterial thrombosis than cyclooxygenase products?, presented at 9th Int. Congr. Thrombosis Haemostasis, Stockholm, 1090 (Abstr.), 1983.

447. **Hanson, S. R. and Harker, L. A.,** Effect of dazoxiben on arterial graft thrombosis in the baboon, *Br. J. Clin. Pharmacol.,* 15 (Suppl. 1—4), 57 S, 1983.

448. **Needleman, P., Minkes, M., and Raz, A.,** Thromboxanes: selective biosynthesis and distinct biological properties, *Science,* 193, 163, 1976.

449. **Butler, K. D., Maguire, E. D., Smith, J. R., Turnbull, A. A., Wallis, R. B., and White, A. M.,** Prolongation of rat tail bleeding time caused by oral doses of thromboxane synthetase inhibitors which have little effect on platelet aggregation, *Thromb. Haemost.,* 47, 46, 1982.

450. **Hook, B. G., Schumacher, W. A., Lee, D. L., Jolly, S. R., and Lucchesi, B. R.,** Experimental coronary artery thrombosis in the absence of thromboxane A_2 synthesis: evidence for alternate pathways for coronary thrombosis, *J. Cardiovasc. Pharmacol.,* 7, 174, 1985.

451. **Hallam, T. J., Scrutton, M. C., and Wallis, R. B.,** Responses of rabbit platelets to adrenaline induced by other agonists, *Thromb. Res.,* 20, 413, 1981.

452. **Rao, G. H. R., Gerrard, J. M., and White, J. G.,** Epinephrine induced potentiation of arachidonate aggregation in Quin 2 loaded platelets is not mediated by elevation of cytosolic calcium, presented at 11th Int. Congr. Thrombosis Haemostasis, Brussels, 962 (Abstr.), 1987.

453. **Swart, S. S., Wood, J. K., and Barnett, D. B.,** Differential labelling of platelet alpha$_2$adrenoceptors by 3 H-dihydroergocryptine and 3 H-yohimbine in patients with myeloproliferative disorders, *Thromb. Res.,* 40, 623, 1985.

454. **Smith, G. M.**, The influence of beta-adrenolytic blocking drugs on platelet aggregation, 6th Conference Microcirculation, Aalborg, 1970, 18.

455. **Salzman, E. W.**, Cyclic AMP and platelet function, *N. Engl. J. Med.*, 286, 358, 1972.

456. **Haslam, R. J., Davidson, M. M. L., and Lynham, J. A.**, Cyclic nucleotides in platelet function, *Thromb. Haemost.*, 40, 232, 1978.

457. **Owen, N. E. and Lebreton, G. C.**, The involvement of calcium in epinephrine and ADP potentiation of human platelet aggregation, *Thromb. Res.*, 17, 855, 1980.

458. **Koutouzov, S., Cothenet-Vernoux, L., Marche, P., and Dausse, J. P.**, Influence of alpha- and beta-adrenoceptors on thrombin-induced serotonin release in rat platelets, *Thromb. Res.*, 40, 147, 1985.

459. **Winther, K., Klysner, R., Geisler, A., and Andersen, P. H.**, Characterization of human platelet beta-adrenoceptors, *Thromb. Res.*, 40, 751, 1985.

460. **Hansen, K. W., Klysner, R., Geisler, A., Knudsen, J. B., Glaser, S., and Gormsen, J.**, Platelet aggregation and beta-blockers, *Lancet*, 1, 224, 1982.

461. **Greer, I. A., Walker, J. J., Calder, A. A., and Forbes, C. D.**, Inhibition of platelet aggregation in whole blood by adrenoceptor antagonists, *Thromb. Res.*, 40, 631, 1985.

462. **Campbell, W. B., Johnson, A. R., Callahan, K. S., and Graham, R. M.**, Anti-platelet activity of beta-adrenergic antagonists. Inhibition of thromboxane synthesis and platelet aggregation in patients receiving long-term propranolol treatment, *Lancet*, 2, 1382, 1981.

463. **Förster, W.**, Effect of various agents in prostaglandin biosynthesis and the anti-aggregatory effect, *Acta Med. Scand.*, 642, 35, 1980.

464. **Hawiger, J. and White, R. B.**, Propranolol and prostacyclin inhibit human platelet phospholipase A_2-induced release of arachidonic acid, *Circulation*, 57/58 (Suppl. 2), II.137, 1978.

465. **Vanderhoek, J. Y. and Feinstein, M. B.**, Local anesthetics, chlorpromazine and propranolol inhibit stimulus-activation of phospholipase A_2 in human platelets, *Mol. Pharmacol.*, 16, 171, 1979.

466. **Malta, E., Schini, V., and Miller, R. C.**, Effect of endothelium on basal and alfa-adrenoceptor stimulated calcium fluxes in rat aorta, *Naunyn Schmiedebergs Arch. Pharmacol.*, 334, 63, 1986.

467. **Levine, S. P., Towell, B. L., Suarez, A. M., Knieriem, L. K., Harris, M. M., and George, J. N.**, Platelet activation and secretion associated with emotional stress, *Circulation*, 71, 1129, 1985.

468. **Furberg, C. D. and May, G. S.**, Effect of long-term prophylactic treatment on survival after myocardial infarction, *Am. J. Med.*, 76 (Suppl. 6A), 76, 1984.

469. **Frishman, W. H., Weksler, B., Christodoulos, J. P., Smithen, C., and Killip, T.**, Reversal of abnormal platelet aggregation and change in exercise tolerance in patients with angina pectoris following oral propranolol, *Circulation*, 50, 887, 1974.

470. **Myers, A. K., Furman, G., Torres-Duarte, A. P., Penhos, J., and Ramwell, P.**, Comparison of verapamil and nifedipine in thrombosis models, *Proc. Soc. Exp. Biol. Med.*, 183, 86, 1986.

471. **Moriau, M., Noel, H., and Masure, R.**, Effects of alpha- and beta-receptor stimulating and blocking agents on experimental DIC, *Thromb. Diath. Haemorrh.*, 32, 157, 1974.

472. **McKay, D. G., Latour, J.-G., and Lopez, A. M.**, Production of the generalized Shwartzman reaction by activated Hageman factor and alpha-adrenergic stimulation, *Thromb. Diath. Haemorrh.*, 26, 71, 1971.

473. **Müller-Berghaus, G. and Lasch, H.-G.**, Microcirculatory disturbances induced by generalized intravascular coagulation, in *Handbook of Experimental Pharmacology*, Vol. 16 (Part III), Schmier, J. and Eichler, O., Eds., Springer-Verlag, 1975, 465.

474. **Berk, J. L., Hagen, J. F., Beyer, W. A., Gerber, M. J., and Dochat, G. R.**, The treatment of endotoxin shock by beta-adrenergic blockade, *Ann. Surg.*, 169, 74, 1969.

475. **Vick, J. A., Ciuchta, H. P., and Manthei, J. H.**, Use of isoproterenol and phenoxybenzamine in treatment of endotoxin shock, *J. Pharmacol. Exp. Ther.*, 150, 382, 1968.

476. **Halmagyi, D. F. J., Starzecki, B., and Horner, G. J.**, Mechanism and pharmacology of endotoxin shock in sheep, *J. Appl. Physiol.*, 18, 544, 1963.

477. **Swendenborg, J. and Olsson, P.**, Activation of plasma coagulation in vivo by epinephrine and platelet release reaction. An experimental study in the dog, *Thromb. Res.*, 13, 37, 1978.

478. **Nowak, G. and Markwardt, F.**, The influence of drugs on disseminated intravascular coagulation (DIC). V. Effects of alpha-adrenoceptor blocking agents on thrombin-induced DIC in rats, *Thromb. Res.*, 22, 417, 1981.

479. **Haft, J. I., Kranz, P. D., Albert, F. J., and Fani, K.**, Intravascular platelet aggregation in the heart induced by epinephrine, *Circulation*, 46, 698, 1972.

480. **Haft, J. I., Fani, K., Alcorta, C., and Toor, M.**, Effect of propranolol on stress-induced intravascular platelet aggregation in the heart, *Circulation*, 7—8 (Suppl. 4), 57, 1973.

481. **Haft, J. I. and Fani, K.**, Intravascular platelet aggregation in the heart induced by stress, *Circulation*, 47, 353, 1973.

482. **Folts, J. D. and Bonebrake, F. C.**, The effects of cigarette smoke and nicotine on platelet thrombus formation in stenosed dog coronary arteries: inhibition with phentolamine, *Circulation*, 65, 465, 1982.

483. **Hoak, J. C., Warner, E. D., and Connor, W. E.,** New concept of levarterenol-induced myocardial necrosis, *Arch. Pathol. Lab. Med.,* 87, 332, 1969.
484. **Bush, L. R., Buja, L. M., Tilton, G., Wathen, M., Apprill, P., Ashton, J., and Willerson, J. T.,** Effects of propranolol and dilthiazem alone and in combination on the recovery of left ventricular segmental function after temporary coronary occlusion and long-term reperfusion in conscious dogs, *Circulation,* 72, 413, 1985.
485. **Reimer, K. A., Rasmussen, M. M., and Jennings, R. B.,** Reduction by propranolol of myocardial necrosis following temporary coronary occlusion in dogs, *Circ. Res.,* 33, 353, 1973.
486. **Ozge, A. H., Mustard, J. F., Hegardt, B., Rowsell, H. C., and Downie, H. G.,** The effect of adrenaline on blood coagulation, platelet economy and thrombus formation, *Can. Med. Assoc. J.,* 88, 265, 1963.
487. **Rowsell, H. C., Hegardt, B., Downie, H. G., Mustard, J. F., and Murphy, E. A.,** Adrenaline and experimental thrombosis, *Br. J. Haematol.,* 12, 66, 1966.
488. **Van de Werf, F., Vanhaecke, J., Ik-Kyung Jang, Flameng, W., Collen, D., and De Geest, H.,** Reduction of infarct size and enhanced recovery of systolic function after coronary thrombolysis with tissue-type plasminogen activator combined with beta-adrenergic blockade with metoprolol, *Circulation,* 75, 830, 1987.
489. **Green, D., Rossi, E. C., and Haring, O.,** The beta-blocker heart attack trial: studies of platelets and factor VIII, *Thromb. Res.,* 28, 261, 1982.
490. **Pick, R. and Glick, G.,** Effects of propranolol, minoxidil, and clofibrate on cholesterol-induced atherosclerosis in stumptail macaques (Macaca arctoides), *Atherosclerosis,* 27, 71, 1977.
491. **Buonassisi, V. and Venter, J. C.,** Hormone and neurotransmitter receptors in an established endothelial cell line, *Proc. Natl. Acad. Sci. U.S.A.,* 73, 1612, 1976.
492. **Angus, J. A., Cocks, T. M., and Satoh, K.,** The alpha-adrenoceptors on endothelial cells, *Fed. Proc.,* 45, 2355, 1986.
493. **Freissmuth, M., Hausleithner, V., Nees, S., Böck, M., and Schütz, W.,** Cardiac ventricular beta$_2$-adrenoceptors in guinea-pigs and rats are localized on the coronary endothelium, *Naunyn Schmiedebergs Arch. Pharmacol.,* 334, 56, 1986.
494. **Baranczyk-Kuzma, A., Anders, K. L., and Borchardt, R. T.,** Catecholamine-metabolizing enzymes of bovine brain microvessel endothelial cell monolayers, *J. Neurochem.,* 46, 1956, 1986.
495. **Spatz, M. and Kaneda, N.,** The presence of catechol-o-methyltransferase activity in separately cultured cerebromicrovascular endothelial and smooth muscle cells, *Brain Res.,* 381, 363, 1986.
496. **Sunaga, T., Yamashita, Y., and Shimamoto, T.,** Epinephrine effect on arterial endothelial cells observed by scanning electron microscope, *Proc. Jpn. Acad.,* 45, 808, 1969.
497. **Mills, D. C. B. and Roberts, G. C. K.,** Membrane active drugs and the aggregation of human blood platelets, *Nature,* 213, 35, 1967.
498. **Dachary-Prigent, J., Dufourcq, J., Lussau, C., and Boisseau, M.,** Propranolol, chlorpromazine and platelet membrane: a fluorescence study of the drug-membrane interaction, *Thromb. Res.,* 14, 15, 1979.
499. **Hladovec, J.,** Circulating endothelial cells as a sign of vessel wall lesions, *Physiol. Bohemoslov.,* 27, 140, 1978.
500. **Hladovec, J. and Přerovský, I.,** Effects of hydroxyethylrutosides on circulating endothelial cells in experimental animals and man, in: hydroxyethylrutosides in vascular disease, Condensed Proceedings of an international symposium, Moretonhampstead, The Royal Society of Medicine, International Congress and Symposium Series, No. 42, 1981, 19.
501. **Detwiler, R. C., Charo, I. F., and Feinman, R. D.,** Evidence that calcium regulates platelet function, *Thromb. Haemost.,* 40, 207, 1978.
502. **Fleckenstein, A.,** Specific pharmacology of calcium in myocardium, cardiac pacemakers, and vascular smooth muscle, *Annu. Rev. Pharmacol. Toxicol.,* 17, 149, 1977.
503. **Fleckenstein, A.,** Calcium antagonists in heart and vascular smooth muscle, *Med. Res. Rev.,* 5, 395, 1985.
504. **Ahn, Y. S., Jy, W., Harrington, W. J., Shanbaky, N., Fernandez, L. F., and Haynes, D. H.,** Increased platelet calcium in thrombosis and related disorders and its correction by nifedipine, *Thromb. Res.,* 45, 535, 1987.
505. **Nayler, W. G.,** Calcium antagonists and ischemic myocardium, *Int. J. Cardiol.,* 15, 267, 1987.
506. **Ware, J. A., Johnson, P. C., Smith, M., and Salzman, E. W.,** Inhibition of human platelet aggregation and cytoplasmic calcium response by calcium antagonists: studies with aequorin and Quin 2, *Circ. Res.,* 59, 39, 1986.
507. **Ardlie, N. G., Jarret, J. J., and Bell, L. K.,** Collagen increases cytoplasmic free calcium in human platelets, *Thromb. Res.,* 42, 115, 1986.
508. **Valone, F. H.,** Inhibition of platelet-activating factor binding to human platelets by calcium channel blockers, *Thromb. Res.,* 45, 427, 1987.
509. **Ono, H. and Kimura, M.,** Effect of Ca^{2+}-antagonistic vasodilators, dilthiazem, nifedipine and verapamil, on platelet aggregation in vitro, *Arzneimittelforschung,* 31, 1131, 1981.

510. **Johnsson, H.**, Effects by nifedipine (Adalat®) on platelet function in vitro and in vivo, *Thromb. Res.*, 21, 523, 1981.

511. **Westwick, J., Mark, G., Powling, M. J., and Kakkar, V. V.**, Dilthiazem, the cardiac slow channel calcium antagonist, is a potent selective and competitive inhibitor of platelet activating factor (PAF) on human platelets, *Thromb. Haemost.*, 50, 42, 1983.

512. **Horwitz, P. M., Grazer, J. M., Lippton, H. L., McNamara, D. B., Porter, M. K., and Kadowiz, P. J.**, Effects of dilthiazem and verapamil on platelet aggregation, *Fed. Proc.*, 43, 977, 1984.

513. **Cremer, K. F., Pieper, J. A., Joyal, M., and Mehta, J.**, Effects of dilthiazem, dipyridamole, and their combinations on hemostasis, *Clin. Pharmacol. Ther.*, 36, 641, 1984.

514. **Mehta, P., Mehta, J., Ostrowski, N., and Brigmon, L.**, Inhibitory effects of dilthiazem on platelet activation caused by ionophore A 23187 plus ADP or epinephrine in subthreshold concentrations, *J. Lab. Clin. Med.*, 102, 332, 1983.

515. **Barnathan, E. S., Addonizio, V. P., and Shattil, S. J.**, Interaction of verapamil with human platelet alfa-adrenergic receptors, *Am. J. Physiol.*, 242, H19, 1982.

516. **Carlsson, A. and Waldeck, B.**, On the mechanism of action of prenylamine on tissue monoamines, *Biochim. Appl.*, 14 (Suppl. 1), 41, 1968.

517. **Chierchia, S., Crea, F., Bernini, W., Gensini, G., Parodi, O., De Caterina, R., and Maseri, A.**, Antiplatelet effects of verapamil in man, *Am. J. Cardiol.*, 47, 399, 1981.

518. **Shea, M. J., Bush, L. R., Romson, J. L., Driscoll, E. M., and Lucchesi, B. R.**, The effect of dilthiazem on coronary thrombosis in the conscious canine, *Eur. J. Pharmacol.*, 77, 67, 1982.

519. **Henry, P. D., Schuchleib, R., Borda, L. J., Roberts, R., Williamson, J. R., and Sobel, B.**, Effects of nifedipine on myocardial perfusion and ischemic injury in dogs, *Circ. Res.*, 43, 372, 1978.

520. **Haft, J. I.**, Role of blood platelets in coronary artery diseases, *Am. J. Cardiol.*, 43, 1197, 1979.

521. **Okamatsu, S., Peck, R. C., and Lefer, A. M.**, Effects of calcium channel blockers on arachidonate-induced sudden death in rabbits, *Proc. Coc. Exp. Biol. Med.*, 166, 551, 1981.

522. **Ortega, M. P., Sunkel, C., Priego, J. G., and Statkow, P. R.**, The antithrombogenic in vivo effects of calcium channel blockers in experimental thrombosis in mice, *Thromb. Haemost.*, 57, 283, 1987.

523. **Kramsch, D. M., Aspen, A. J., and Apstein, C. S.**, Suppression of experimental atherosclerosis by the Ca^{2+}-antagonist lanthanum, *J. Clin. Invest.*, 65, 967, 1980.

524. **Henry, P. D. and Bentley, K. I.**, Suppression of atherogenesis in cholesterol-fed rabbits treated with nifedipine, *J. Clin. Invest.*, 68, 1366, 1981.

525. **Rouleau, J. L., Parmley, W. W., Stevens, J., Wikman-Coffelt, J., Sievers, R., Mahley, R. W., and Havel, R. J.**, Verapamil suppresses atherosclerosis in cholesterol-fed rabbits, *J. Am. Coll. Cardiol.*, 1, 1453, 1983.

526. **Willis, A. L., Nagel, B., Churchill, V., Whyte, A., Smith, D. L., Mahmud, I., and Puppione, D. L.**, Antiatherosclerotic effect of nicardipine and nifedipine in cholesterol-fed rabbits, *Arteriosclerosis*, 5, 250, 1985.

527. **Stender, S., Stender, I., Nordestgaard, B., and Kjeldsen, K.**, No effect of nifedipine on atherogenesis in cholesterol-fed rabbits, *Arteriosclerosis*, 4, 389, 1984.

528. **Van Nierkerk, J. L. M., Hendricks, T., De Boer, H. H. M., and Van't Larr, A.**, Does nifedipine suppress atherogenesis in WHHL rabbits?, *Atherosclerosis*, 53, 91, 1984.

529. **Hladovec, J.**, The influence of calcium antagonists on endothelium, *Arzneimittelforschung*, 29, 1101, 1979.

530. **Hladovec, J. and De Clerk, F.**, Protection by flunarizine against endothelial cell injury in vivo, *Angiology*, 32, 448, 1981.

531. **De Clerck, F., Xhonneux, B., Leysen, J., and Janssen, P. A. J.**, The involvement of 5-HT_2-receptor sites in the activation of cat platelets, *Thromb. Res.*, 33, 305, 1984.

532. **Vanhoutte, P. M., Ed.**, *Serotonin and the Cardiovascular System*, Raven Press, New York, 1985.

533. **Pletscher, A.**, The 5-hydroxytryptamine system of blood platelets: physiology and pathophysiology, *Int. J. Cardiol.*, 14, 177, 1987.

534. **Marwood, J. F. and Stokes, G. S.**, Serotonin(5-HT) and its cantagonists: involvement in the cardiovascular system, *Clin. Exp. Pharmacol. Physiol.*, 11, 439, 1984.

535. **De Clerck, F., Somers, Y., and Van Gorp, L.**, Platelet-vessel wall interactions in hemostasis: implication of 5-hydroxytryptamine, *Agents Actions*, 15, 627, 1984.

536. **De Clerck, F., Van Nueten, J. M., and Reneman, R. S.**, Platelet-vessel wall interactions: implication of 5-hydroxytryptamine. A review, *Agents Actions*, 15, 612, 1984.

537. **De Clerck, F., Xhonneux, B., and Van de Wiele, R.**, Biochemical mechanisms in 5-hydroxytryptamine-induced human platelet aggregation, *Agents Actions*, 17, 270, 1985.

538. **Oei, H. H. H., Hughes, W. E., Schaffer, S. W., Longenecker, G. L., and Glenn, T. M.**, Platelet serotonin uptake during myocardial ischemia, *Am. Heart J.*, 106, 1081, 1983.

539. **Vanhoutte, P. M. and Cohen, R. A.**, The elusory role of serotonin in vascular function and disease, *Biochem. Pharmacol.*, 32, 3671, 1983.

540. **Sullenberger, J. W., Anlyan, W. G., and Weawer, W. T.**, Serotonin in intravascular thrombosis, *Surgery,* 46, 22, 1959.

541. **Marschall, R.**, Serotonin and embolization by small blood clots in dogs, *Thorax,* 21, 266, 1966.

542. **Huval, V. W., Mathieson, M. A., Stemp, L. I., Dunham, B. M., Jones, A. G., Shepro, D., and Hechtman, H. B.**, Therapeutic benefits of 5-hydroxytryptamine inhibition following pulmonary embolism, *Ann. Surg.,* 197, 220, 1983.

543. **Benedict, C. R., Mathew, B., Rex, K. A., Cartwright, J., Jr., and Sordahl, L. A.**, Correlation of plasma serotonin changes with platelet aggregation in an in vivo dog model of spontaneous occlusive coronary thrombus formation, *Circ. Res.,* 58, 58, 1986.

544. **Aiken, J. W.**, Pharmacological analysis of factors influencing platelet aggregation in stenosed coronary arteries of dogs, *Ann. N.Y. Acad. Sci.,* 454, 131, 1985.

545. **Amery, A., Fagard, R., Fiocchi, R., Lijnen, P., Staessen, J., and Vermylen, J.**, Antihypertensive action and serotonin-induced platelet aggregation during long-term ketanserin treatment in hypertensive patients, *J. Cardiovasc. Pharmacol.,* 6, 182, 1984.

546. **De Clerck, F. and Xhonneaux, B.**, Continuous inhibition of platelet S_2-serotonergic receptors during chronic administration of ketanserin in humans, *J. Cardiovasc. Pharmacol.,* 7 (Suppl. 7), S 23, 1985.

547. **De Clerck, F., Xhonneaux, B., Tollenaere, J. P., and Janssen, P. A. J.**, Dependence of the antagonism at human platelet 5-HT_2 receptors by ketanserin on the reaction pH, *Thromb. Res.,* 40, 581, 1985.

548. **Vermylen, J., Arnout, J., Deckmyn, H., Xhonneaux, B., and De Clerk, F.**, Continuous inhibition of the platelet S_2-serotonergic receptors during the long term administration of ketanserin, *Thromb. Res.,* 42, 721, 1986.

549. **Buczko, W., Gambino, M. C., and de Gaetano, G.**, Prolongation of rat tail bleeding time by ketanserin: mechanism of action, *Eur. J. Pharm.,* 103, 261, 1984.

550. **Völkl, K.-P.**, The prolongation of the platelet survival times mediated by ketanserin in rats, *Thromb. Res.,* Suppl. 6, 61, 1986.

551. **Swank, R. L.**, Platelet aggregation: its role and cause in surgical shock, *J. Trauma,* 8, 872, 1968.

552. **Walker, R. T., Matrai, A., Bogar, L., and Dormandy, J. A.**, Serotonin and the flow properties of blood, *J. Cardiovasc. Pharmacol.,* 7 (Suppl. 7), S 35, 1985.

553. **Zannad, F., Voisin, Ph., Pointel, J. P., Schmitt, C., Frietag, B., and Stoltz, J. F.**, Effects of ketanserin on platelet function and red cell filterability in hypertension and peripheral vascular disease, *J. Cardiovasc. Pharmacol.,* 7 (Suppl. 7), S 32, 1985.

554. **Longstaff, J., Gush, R., Williams, E. H., and Jayson, M. I. V.**, Effects of ketanserin on peripheral blood flow, haemorheology, and platelet function in patients with Raynaud's phenomenon, *J. Cardiovasc. Pharmacol.,* 7 (Suppl. 7), S 99, 1985.

555. **Badyda, C., Bielski, J., and Chodera, A.**, The influence of some antiserotonin drugs on blood clotting, *Acta Physiol. Pol.,* 14, 645, 1963.

556. **Gautier, J.-C., Derouesne, T., Held, T., and Lhermitte, F.**, Thromboses plaquettaires expérimentales dans les artères cérébrales. Effets du dipyridamole, de dérivés de l'ergot de seigle et d'antisérotonines, *Presse Med.,* 78, 1775, 1970.

557. **Humphrey, W. R. and Aiken, J. W.**, Antithrombotic and hypotensive effects of the serotonin$_2$-receptor antagonist ketanserine in anesthetized dogs, *Pharmacologist,* 24, 196, 1982.

558. **Bush, L. R., Campbell, W. B., Kern, K., Tilton, G. D., Apprill, P., Ashton, J., Schmitz, J., Buja, L. M., and Willerson, J. T.**, The effects of alfa$_2$-adrenergic and serotonergic receptor antagonists on cyclic blood flow alterations in stenosed canine coronary arteries, *Circ. Res.,* 55, 642, 1984.

559. **Bush, L. R., Evans, R. M., Gaul, S. L., and Reitz, P. M.**, Effects of the serotonin antagonists, cyproheptadine, ketanserin and mianserin, on cyclic flow reductions in stenosed canine coronary arteries, *J. Pharmacol. Exp. Ther.,* 240, 674, 1986.

560. **Ashton, J. H., Benedict, C. R., Fitzgerald, Ch., Raheja, S., Taylor, A., Campbell, W. B., Buja, L. M., and Willerson, J. T.**, Serotonin as a mediator of cyclic flow variations in stenosed canine coronary arteries, *Circulation,* 73, 572, 1986.

561. **Ashton, J. H., Ogletree, M. L., Michel, I. M., Golino, P., McNatt, J. M., Taylor, A. L., Raheja, S., Schmitz, J., Buja, L. M., Campbell, W. B., and Willerson, J. T.**, Cooperative mediation by serotonin S_2 and thromboxane A_2/prostaglandin H_2 receptor activation of cyclic flow variation in dogs with severe coronary artery stenoses, *Circulation,* 76, 952, 1987.

562. **De Clerck, F., Loots, W., Jageneau, A., and Nevelsteen, A.**, Correction by ketanserin of the platelet-mediated inhibition of peripheral collateral circulation in the cat: measurement of blood flow with radioactive microspheres, *Drug Dev. Res.,* 8, 149, 1986.

563. **Kordenat, R. K. and Kezdi, P.**, Serotonin blockade during experimental coronary thrombosis, *Am. Heart J.,* 97, 329, 1979.

564. **Sandler, H. and Gerdin, B.**, Effect of methysergide pretreatment on thrombin-induced pulmonary oedema in the rat, *Upsala J. Med. Sci.,* 89, 221, 1984.

565. **Nowak, G. and Markwardt, F.**, Influence of cyproheptadine on endotoxin-induced disseminated intravascular coagulation (DIC) in weaned pigs, *Thromb. Haemost.*, 53, 252, 1985.

566. **Der Agopian, Rosa, A., Gautier, J.-C., and Lhermitte, F.**, Thromboses artérielles expérimentales. Effet d'un alpha-bloquant: La nicergoline, *Presse Med.*, 2, 2521, 1973.

567. **Bolli, R., Ware, J. A., Brandon, T. A., Weilbaecher, D. G., and Mace, M. L.**, Platelet-mediated thrombosis in stenosed canine coronary arteries. Inhibition by nicergoline, a platelet-active alpha-adrenergic antagonist, *J. Am. Coll. Cardiol.*, 3, 1417, 1984.

568. **Okuma, M., Tokuyama, T., Senoh, S., Hirata, F., and Hayaishi, O.**, Antagonism of 5-hydroxykynurenamine against serotonin action on platelet aggregation, *Proc. Natl. Acad. Sci. U.S.A.*, 73, 643, 1976.

569. **Michal, F. and Penglis, F.**, Inhibition of serotonin-induced platelet aggregation in relation to thrombus production, *J. Pharmacol. Exp. Then.*, 166, 276, 1969.

570. **Hladovec, J.**, The effect of some platelet aggregating and potential thrombosis-promoting substances on the development of experimental arterial thrombosis, *Thromb. Dieth. Haemorrh.*, 29, 196, 1973.

571. **Hladovec, J.**, A new model of arterial thrombosis, *Thromb. Res.*, 41, 659, 1986.

572. **Casley-Smith, J. R. and Casley-Smith, J. R.**, *High Protein Oedemas and the Benzo-pyrones*, J. B. Lippincott, Sydney, 1986.

573. **Földi, M.**, Vitamin P and lymphatics, in *Klinische Pharmakologie, Flavonoide und Gefässwand, Symposia Angiologica Santoriana*, 4th International Symposium, Fribourg, Nyon, 1972, Comèl, M., and Laszt, L., Eds., S. Karger, Basel, 1973, published simultaneously in *Angiologica*, 9, 375, 1972.

574. **Gábor, M.**, *Abriss der Pharmakologie von Flavonoiden unter besonderer Berücksichtigung der antiödematösen und antiphlogistischen Effekte*, Akadémiai Kiadó, Budapest, 1975.

575. **Gábor, M.**, Pharmacologic effects of flavonoids on blood vessels, *Angiologica*, 9, 355, 1972.

576. **Robbins, R. C.**, Antithrombogenic properties of a hexamethoxylated flavonoid, *Atherosclerosis*, 18, 73, 1973.

577. **Robbins, R. C.**, Effect of phenyl benzo-gamma-pyrone derivatives (flavonoids) on blood cell aggregation: basis for a concept of mode of action, *Clin. Chem.*, 17, 433, 1971.

578. **Robbins, R. C.**, In vitro effects of penta-, hexa-, and hepta-methoxylated flavones on aggregation of cells in blood of hospitalized patients, *J. Clin. Pharmacol.*, 13, 271, 1973.

579. **Robbins, R. C.**, Actions of flavonoids on blood cells: trimodal action of flavonoids elucidates their inconsistent physiologic effects, *Int. J. Vitam. Nutr. Res.*, 44, 203, 1974.

580. **Robbins, R. C., Hammer, R. H., and Simpson, C. F.**, Methoxylated phenyl benzo-gamma-pyrone derivatives(flavonoids) that highly inhibit erythrocyte aggregation, *Clin. Chem.*, 17, 1109, 1971.

581. **Mac Intyre, D. E. and Gordon, J. L.**, Semi-synthetic flavonoids as inhibitors of platelet aggregation and the release reaction, presented at 1st Am.-Eur. Symp. Venous Diseases, Montreux, 1974.

582. **Kahlé, L. H., Dannijs, G. J., and Ten Cate, J. W.**, Effects of some semisynthetic rutoside derivatives on human platelets, *Bibl. Anat.*, 13, 263, 1975.

583. **van Haeringen, N. J., Glasius, E., Ten Cate, J. W., Gerritsen, J., and van Geet, J.**, Effect of O-(beta-hydroxyethyl)-rutoside on red cell and platelet functions in man, presented at 7th Eur. Conf. Microcirculation, Aberdeen, 1972, Part II, *Bibl. Anat.*, 12, 459, 1973.

584. **Ten Cate, I. W., Gerritsen, J., van Geet, J., van Haeringen, N. J., and Glasius, E.**, In vitro inhibition of erythrocyte and platelet functions by O-(beta-hydroxyethyl)-rutoside (HR), in *Erythrocytes, Thrombocytes, Leukocytes*, Gerlach, E., Moses, K., Deutsch, E., and Wilmanns, W., Eds., Thieme Verlag, Stuttgart, 1973.

585. **Ten Cate, J. W., van Haeringen, N. J., Gerritsen, J., and Glasius, E.**, Biological activity of a semisynthetic flavonoids, O-(beta-hydroxyethyl)rutoside: light scattering and metabolic studies of human red cells and platelets, *Clin. Chem.*, 19, 31, 1973.

586. **Pollock, J. and Heath, H.**, Studies on the effects of beta beta' iminodi-propionitrile and O-(beta-hydroxyethyl)-rutoside on ADP-activated aggregation on rat platelets in relation to the development of diabetic microangiopathy, *Biochem. Pharmacol.*, 24, 397, 1975.

587. **Heidrich, H., Höfner, J., Schneider, D., and Wollensak, J.**, Calcium dobesilate (Dexium®) and platelet aggregation, in *Microcirculation und Blutrheologie*, Müller-Wiefel, H., Ed., G. Witzstrock, New York, 1980, 259.

588. **Thomas, J., Dorme, N., Sergant, M., Raynaud, G., and Bouvet, P.**, Action du dobesilate de calcium sur la résistance et la perméabilité capillaires et sur le temps de saignement et l'adhésivité plaquettaire modifiés par le dextran, *Ann. Pharm. Fr.*, 30, 415, 1972.

589. **Vinazzer, H.**, Clinical and experimental studies on the action of ethamsylate on haemostasis and platelet functions, *Thromb. Res.*, 19, 783, 1980.

590. **Hoogendijk, E. M. G. and Ten Cate, J. W.**, The effects of intravenous hydroxyethylrutosides on platelet function in normal volunteers. The Royal Society of Medicine, International Congress and Symposium Series, No. 42, 1980, 49.

591. **van Haeringen, H. N. J.**, Effect of tri- and tetra-O-(beta-hydroxyethyl)-rutoside on red blood cell aggregation of human blood, 8th Eur. Conf. Microcirculation, Le Touquet, 1974, *Bibl. Anat.*, 13, 197, 1975.

592. **Schmid-Schönbein, H., Volger, E., Weiss, J., and Brandhuber, M.,** Effect of O-(beta-hydroxyethyl)-rutosides on the microrheology of human blood under defined flow conditions, *Vasa,* 4, 263, 1975.

593. **Oughton, J. W. and Barnes, A.,** An assessment of the effects of hydroxyethylrutosides given intravenously in high doses on blood viscosity and red-cell deformability in normal and diabetic patients, The Royal Society of Medicine, International Congress and Symposium Series, No. 42, 1980, 61.

594. **Beretz, A., Lanza, F., Stierlé, A., and Cazenave, J.-P.,** Cyclic nucleotide phosphodiesterase inhibitors prevent aggregation and secretion of human platelets by raising cyclic AMP and reducing cytoplasmic free calcium mobilization, presented at 11th Int. Congr. Thrombosis Haemostasis, Brussels, 787 (Abstr.), 1987.

595. **Arturson, G. and Johnsson, C.-E.,** Stimulation and inhibition of biosynthesis of prostaglandins in human skin by some hydroxyethylated rutosides, *Prostaglandins,* 10, 941, 1975.

596. **Gryglewski, R. J., Korbut, R., Robak, J., and Swies, J.,** On the mechanism of antithrombotic action of flavonoids, *Biochem. Pharmacol.,* 36, 317, 1987.

597. **Hennings, G.,** Zum molekularen Wirkungsmechanismus von (+)-cyanidanol-3, *Arzneimittelforschung,* 29, 720, 1979.

598. **Kimura, Y., Okuda, H., Arichi, S., Baba, K., and Kozawa, M.,** Inhibition of the formation of 5-hydroxy-6,8,11,14-eicosatetraenoic acid from arachidonic acid in polymorphonuclear leukocytes by various coumarins, *Biochim. Biophys. Acta,* 834, 224, 1985.

599. **Kappus, H.,** (+)-cyanidanol-3 inhibition of lipid peroxidation induced by hepatotoxic chemicals in the rat, in international workshop on (+)-cyanidanol-3 in diseases of the liver, The Royal Society of Medicine, International Congress Series, No. 47, 1981, 17.

600. **Slater, T. F. and Eakins, M. N.,** Interactions of (+)-cyanidanol-3 with free radical generating systems, in *New Trends in the Therapy of Liver Diseases,* Int. Symp. Tirrenia, 1974, S. Karger, Basel, 1975, 84.

601. **van Wauwe, J. and Goossens, J.,** Effects of antioxidants on cyclo-oxygenase activities in intact human platelets, *Prostaglandins,* 26, 725, 1984.

602. **Rodney, G., Swanson, A., Wheeler, L. M., Smith, G., and Worrel, C.,** The effect of a series of flavonoids on hyaluronidase and some related enzymes, *J. Biol. Chem.,* 183, 739, 1950.

603. **Niebes, P.,** Influence des flavonoides sur le métabolisme des mucopolysaccharides dans la paroi veineuse, *Angiologica,* 9, 226, 1972.

604. **Grochal, M., Sempinska-Edelberg, E., and Plewinski, J.,** Effect of Venoruton on the factor XIII activity in rat plasma, *Polish J. Pharmacol. Pharm.,* 30, 659, 1979.

605. **Naegeli, T. and Matis, P.,** Significance of several vitamins for the theory of thromboembolism, *Int. Z. Vitam. Ernaehrungsforsch.,* 27, 324, 1957.

606. **Földi, M. and Zoltan, O. T.,** Experimentelle Thrombophlebitis and und deren therapeutische Beeinflussung, *Arzneimittelforschung,* 15, 901, 1965.

607. **Földi, M., Zoltan, O. T., and Piukovich, I.,** Die Wirkung von Rutin und Cumarin auf den Verlauf einer experimentellen Thrombophlebitis, *Arzneimittelforschung,* 11, 1629, 1970.

608. **Piukovich, I., Zoltan, O. T., Traub, A., and Földi, M.,** Weitere Untersuchungen über die therapeutische Beeinflussung der experimentellen Thrombophlebitis, *Arzneimittelforschung,* 16, 94, 1966.

609. **Mirkovitch, V., Borgeaud, J., Meyer, S., and Niebes, P.,** Prévention de thrombose expérimentale par O-(beta-hydroxyéthyl)-rutosides, *Helv. Chir. Acta,* 39, 379, 1972.

610. **Casley-Smith, J. R., Gaffney, R. M.,** Excess plasma protein as a cause of chronic inflammation and lymphoedema. Quantitative electron microscopy, *J. Pathol.,* 133, 243, 1981.

611. **Bergqvist, D., Svensjö, E., and Arfors, K. E.,** The effect of O-(beta-hydroxyethyl)-rutoside (HR) on macromolecular leakage, thrombosis and haemostasis in experimental animals, *Upsala J. Med. Sci.,* 83, 123, 1978.

612. **Srinivasan, S., Lucas, T., Burrowes, C. B., Wanderman, N. A., Redner, A., Bernstein, S., and Sawyer, P. N.,** Effects of some flavonoids on the surface charge characteristics of the vascular system and their antithrombogenic characteristics, presented at 6th Eur. Conf. Microcirculation, Aalborg, 1971, 394.

613. **Klemm, J.,** Ionisierende Strahlen und terminale Strombahn. Eine mikrocolor-phasenkontrast-kinematographische Untersuchung an der Kaninchenohrkammer, *Fortschr. Med.,* 86, 154, 1968.

614. **Zalewski, A. and Maroko, P. R.,** Protective effect of rutosides on ischemic myocardium, *J. Am. Coll. Cardiol.,* 1, 677, 1983.

615. A cooperative trial in the primary prevention of ischaemic heart diseae using clofibrate. Report from the Committee of Principal Investigators, *Br. Heart. J.,* 40, 1069, 1978.

616. **Symons, C., de Toszeghi, A., and Cook, I. J. Y.,** Effect of ethyl chlorophenoxy isobutyrate with or without androsterone on platelet stickiness, *Lancet,* 2, 233, 1964.

617. **O'Brien, J. R. and Heywood, J. B.,** A comparison of platelet stickiness tests during an atromid-S trial, *Thromb. Diath. Haemorrh.,* 16, 768, 1966.

618. **Carson, P., McDonald, L., Pickard, S., Pilkington, T., Davies, B., and Love, F.,** Effect of clofibrate with androsterone (Atromid) and without androsterone (Atromid-S) on blood platelets and lipids in ischemic heart disease, *Br. Heart J.,* 28, 400, 1966.

619. **Carvalho, A. C. A., Colman, R. W., and Lees, R. S.**, Platelet function in hyperlipoproteinemia, *N. Engl. J. Med.*, 290, 434, 1974.

620. **Packham, M. A. and Mustard, J. F.**, Pharmacology of platelet-affecting drugs, *Circulation*, 62 (Suppl. 5), 26, 1980.

621. **Robinson, R. W.**, Platelet adhesiveness and aggregation with chlorophenoxyisobutyric ester, *Am. J. Med. Sci.*, 253, 76, 1967.

622. **Liu, C. Y. and Smith, S.**, The effect of halofenate and clofibrate on aggregation and release of serotonin by human platelets, *Life Sci.*, 18, 563, 1976.

623. **Steele, P. and Rainwater, J.**, Effects of dietary and pharmacologic alterations of serum lipids on platelet survival time, *Circulation*, 58, 365, 1978.

624. **Harker, L. A. and Hazzard, W.**, Platelet kinetic studies in patients with hyperlipoproteinemia: effects of clofibrate therapy, *Circulation*, 60, 492, 1979.

625. **Glynn, M. F., Murphy, E. A., and Mustard, J. F.**, Effect of clofibrate on platelet economy, *Lancet*, 2, 447, 1967.

626. **Gilbert, J. B. and Mustard, J. F.**, Some effects of Atromid on platelet economy and blood coagulation in man, *J. Atheroscler. Res.*, 3, 623, 1963.

627. **Colman, R. W., Bennett, J. S., Sheridan, J. F., Cooper, R. A., and Shattil, S. J.**, Halofenate, a potent inhibitor of normal and hypersensitive platelets, *J. Lab. Clin. Med.*, 88, 282, 1976.

628. **Favis, G. R. and Colman, R. W.**, The action of halofenate on platelet shape change and prostaglandin synthesis, *J. Lab. Clin. Med.*, 92, 45, 1978.

629. **Enger, S. Ch., Johnsen, V., Samuelsen, A., and Laws, E. A.**, The effect of clofibrate on glucose tolerance, insulin secretion, triglycerides and fibrinogen in patients with coronary heart disease, *Acta Med. Scand.*, 201, 563, 1977.

630. **Nakagawa, M., Ishibara, N., Shimokawa, T., and Kojima, S.**, Effect of clofibrate on lipid peroxidation in rats treated with aspirin and 4-pentenoic acid, *J. Biochem. (Tokyo)*, 101, 81, 1987.

631. **Sim, A. K., Davies, M. E., McCraw, A. P., and Metz, G.**, Effect of etofylline clofibrate on experimental thrombosis and platelet function, *Arzneimittelforschung*, 30, 2042, 1980.

632. **Metz, G., Sim, A. K., McCraw, A. P., and Cleland, M. E.**, Effect of etofylline clofibrate on experimental thrombus formation and prostacyclin activation, *Arzneimittelforschung*, 36, 1363, 1986.

633. **Chakrabarti, R., Fearnley, G. R., and Evans, J. F.**, Effects of clofibrate on fibrinolysis, platelet stickiness, plasma fibrinogen, and serum-cholesterol, *Lancet*, 2, 1007, 1968.

634. **Haft, J. I., Kranz, P. D., Albert, F., and Oestreicher, R.**, Protection against epinephrine induced myocardial necrosis with clofibrate, *Am. Heart J.*, 86, 805, 1973.

635. **Wexler, B. C. and Greenberg, B. P.**, Protective effects of clofibrate on isoproterenol-induced myocardial infarction in arteriosclerotic and non-arteriosclerotic rats, *Atherosclerosis*, 29, 373, 1978.

636. **Fleming, J. S., Buyniski, J. P., Cavanagh, R. L., and Bierwagen, M. E.**, Pharmacology of a potent, new antithrombotic agents, 6-methyl-1,2,3,5-tetrahydroimidazo (2,1-b) quinazolin-2-one hydrochloride monohydrate (BL-3459), *J. Pharmacol. Exp. Ther.*, 194, 435, 1975.

637. **Fleming, J. S. and Buyniski, J. P.**, Anagrelide, in *Cardiovascular Drugs*, Scriabine, E., Ed., Raven Press, New York, 1983, 277.

638. **Clark, W. F., Reid, B. D., and Tevaarwerk, G. J. M.**, Anagrelide: inhibitor of collagen- and forming immune complex-induced platelet aggregation and release, *Thromb. Res.*, 21, 215, 1981.

639. **Andes, W. A., Noveck, R. J., and Fleming, J. S.**, Inhibition of platelet production induced by an antiplatelet drug, Anagrelide, in normal volunteers, *Thromb. Haemost.*, 52, 325, 1984.

640. **Dhall, D. P., Bennett, P., McKenzie, F. N., and Matheson, N. A.**, Effects of dextran on human platelets, *Bibl. Anat.*, 9, 295, 1967.

641. **Ts'ao, C. H. and Krajewski, D. V.**, Effect of dextran on platelet activation by polymerizing fibrin, *Am. J. Pathol.*, 106, 1, 1982.

642. **Muzaffar, T. Z., Stalker, A. L., Bryce, W. A. J., Dhall, D. P., and Smith, G.**, Quantitative studies on fibrin formation and effects of dextran, presented at 7th Eur. Conf. Microcirculation, Aberdeen, 1972, *Bibl. Anat.*, 12 (Part II), 340, 1973.

643. **Tangen, O., Wik, K. O., Almqvist, I. A. M., Arfors, K.-E., and Hint, H. C.**, Effects of dextran on the structure and plasmin-induced lysis of human fibrin, *Thromb. Res.*, 1, 487, 1972.

644. **Aberg, M., Hedner, U., and Bergentz, S. E.**, The antithrombotic effect of dextran, *Scand. J. Haematol.*, 22 (Suppl. 34), 61, 1979.

645. **Battle, J., del Rio, F., Lopez, C., Borrasca, A. L., and Lopez Fernandez, M. F.**, Effect of dextran on factor VIII/von Willebrand factor structure and function, *Thromb. Haemost.*, 54, P 450, 1985.

646. **Arendt, K. A., Berman, H. J., and Fulton, G. P.**, Effect of dextran on bleeding time, vascular fragility and platelet thrombus formation in the hamster, *Fed. Proc.*, 16, 4, 1957.

647. **Ashwin, J. G. and Jaques, L. B.**, The effect of phosphorus 32, dextran, reserpine and stypturon on thrombus formation in rats, *Thromb. Diath. Haemorrh.*, 5, 543, 1961.

648. **Józsa, L., Perneczky, J., Pataky, J., and Luszting, G.,** Untersuchungen der Dextran- und Heparinwirkung am Mesoappendix von Kaninchen, *Z. Gesamte Inn. Med.,* 17, 203, 1962.

649. **Ernst, C. B., Fry, W. J., Kraft, R. O., and De Weese, M. S.,** The role of low molecular weight dextran in the management of venous thrombosis, *Surg. Gynecol. Obstet.,* 119, 1243, 1964.

650. **Sawyer, R. B. and Moncrieff, J. A.,** Dextran specificity in thrombosis inhibition, *Arch. Surg.,* 90, 562, 1965.

651. **Bryant, M. F., Bloom, W. L., and Brewer, S. S.,** Study of the anti-thrombotic properties of dextran of large molecular weight, *J. Cardiovasc. Surg.,* 5, 48, 1964.

652. **Aubert, N., Mauzac, M., and Jozefonvicz, J.,** Anticoagulant hydrogels derived from crosslinked dextran, Part I. Synthesis, characterization and antithrombotic activity, *Biomaterials,* 8, 24, 1987.

653. **Gruber, U. F., Saldeen, T., Brokop, T., Eklöf, B., Eriksson, I., Goldee, I., Gran, L., Hohl, M., Johnsson, T., Kristersson, S., Ljungström, K. G., Lund, T., Maartman, M. H., Svensjö, E., Thomson, D., Torhorst, J., Trippestad, A., and Ulstein, M.,** Incidence of fatal postoperative pulmonary embolism after prophylaxis with dextran 70 and low dose heparin; an international multicentre study, *Br. Med. J.,* 280, 69, 1980.

654. **Williams, R. D. and Elliot, D. W.,** The effects of heparin and coumarin derivatives on a standardized intravenous thrombosis, *Surg. Forum,* 9, 138, 1958.

655. **Reber, K.,** Versuche zur Beeinflussung der Thrombozytenadhäsivität in vivo, *Thromb. Diath. Haemorrh.,* Suppl. 24, 35, 1967.

656. **Richards, R. K. and Cortell, R.,** Studies on the anticoagulant 3,3′-methylenebis-(4-hydroxycoumarin), *Proc. Soc. Exp. Biol. Med.,* 50, 237, 1942.

657. **Thill, C. J., Stafford, W. T., Spooner, M., and Meyer, O. O.,** Hemorrhagic agent 3,3′-methylenebis-(4-hydroxycoumarin). V. Its effects in prevention of experimental thrombosis, *Proc. Soc. Exp. Biol. Med.,* 54, 333, 1941.

658. **Janssen, K. F. and Tage-Hansen, E.,** Dicoumarol in experimental thrombosis, *Acta Chir. Scand.,* 98, 152, 1949.

659. **Kubik, M. and Wright, H.-P.,** Coumarin treatment of experimental thrombosis, Proc. 3rd Congr. Int. Soc. Haematology, 477, 1950.

660. **Wright, H.-P., Kubik, M. M., and Hayden, M.,** Influence of anticoagulant administration on the rate of recanalization of experimentally thrombosed veins, *Br. J. Surg.,* 40, 163, 1952.

661. **Jewell, P., Pilkington, T., and Robinson, B.,** Heparin and ethylbiscoumacetate in prevention of experimental venous thrombosis, *Br. Med. J.,* 1, 1013, 1954.

662. **Kamiya, K., Takeuchi, K., Hayashi, R., and Suzuki, K.,** The treatment of intravascular clots with blood anticoagulants and proteolytic enzymes, *Jpn. Circ. J.,* 23, 417, 1959.

663. **Dale, D. and Jaques, L. B.,** The prevention of experimental thrombosis by dicoumarin, *Can. Med. Assoc. J.,* 46, 546, 1942.

664. **Rogers, F., Barrett, R. J., and Lam, C. R.,** The effect of moderate degree of dicumarol-induced hypoprothrombinemia on experimental intravascular thrombosis, *Surg. Gynecol. Obstet.,* 89, 339, 1949.

665. **Holden, W. D., Cameron, D. B., Shea, P. C., Jr., and Shaw, B. W.,** Trypsin and thrombin induced venous thrombosis and its prevention with 3,3′-methylenebis (4-hydroxycoumarin), *Surg. Gynecol. Obstet.,* 88, 635, 1949.

666. **Wright, H.-P., Kubik, M. M., and Hayden, M.,** Recanalization of thrombosed arteries under anticoagulant therapy, *Br. Med. J.,* 1, 1021, 1953.

667. **Baeckeland, E.,** Etude de la recanalisation sous traitement anticoagulant des artères thrombosées expérimentalement, *Thromb. Diath. Haemorrh.,* 3, 386, 1959.

668. **Wessler, S., Ballon, J. D., and Katz, J. H.,** Studies in intravascular coagulation V. A distinction between the anticoagulant and antithrombotic effects of dicumarol, *N. Engl. J. Med.,* 256, 1223, 1957.

669. **Davidson, E., Howard, A. N., and Gresham, G. A.,** The effect of pheninindione on rats fed diets which produce thrombosis and epxerimental arteriosclerosis, *Br. J. Exp. Pathol.,* 43, 418, 1962.

670. **Murphy, E. A., Mustard, J. F., Rowsell, H. C., and Downie, H. G.,** Quantitative studies on the effect of dicumarol on experimental thrombosis, *J. Lab. Clin. Med.,* 61, 935, 1963.

671. **Kahn, R. A., Johnson, S. A., and de Graff, A. F.,** Effects of sodium warfarin on capillary ultrastructure, *Am. J. Pathol.,* 65, 149, 1971.

672. **Markwardt, F. and Landmann, H.,** Blutgerinnungshemmende Proteine, in *Handbuch der Experimentellen Pharmacokologie,* Vol. 27, Antikoagulantien, Markwardt, F., Ed., Springer-Verlag, Berlin, 1971, 76.

673. **Hauptmann, J. and Markwardt, F.,** Pharmakologie synthetischer Thrombin-Inhibitoren. Beiträge zur Wirkstofforschung, Oehme, P., Löwe, H., and Gores, E., Eds., Heft 26, Akademie-Industrie-Komplex, Dresden, 1986.

674. **Markwardt, F., Nowak, G., and Hoffmann, J.,** The influence of drugs on disseminated intravascular coagulation (DIC). II. Effect of naturally occurring and synthetic thrombin inhibitors, *Thromb. Res.,* 11, 275, 1977.

675. **Markwardt, F.,** Über den Einfluss des Hirudins auf die Thrombenbildung, *Naunyn Schmiedebergs Arch. Pharmacol.,* 236, 286, 1959.

676. **Nikonov, G. and Baskova, I.,** Protective antithrombotic action of the preparations from the leeches Hirudo officinalis, *Thromb. Haemost.,* 58 (Suppl. 1), 81, 1987.

677. **Freund, M., Cazenave, J.-P., Wiesel, M. L., Roitsch, C., Riehl-Bellon, N., Loison, G., Lemoine, Y., Brown, S., and Courtney, M.,** Recombinant hirudin inhibits experimental venous thrombosis induced by injection of tissue factor and stasis, presented at 11th Int. Congr. Thrombosis Haemotasis, Brussels, 1118 (Abstr.), 1987.

678. **Markwardt, F. and Klöcking, H.-P.,** The antithrombotic effect of synthetic thrombin inhibitors, *Thromb. Res.,* 1, 243, 1972.

679. **Hauptmann, J. and Markwardt, F.,** Studies on the anticoagulant and antithrombotic action of an irreversible thrombin inhibitor, *Thromb. Res.,* 20, 347, 1980.

680. **Hauptmann, J., Kaiser, B., Markwardt, F., and Nowak, G.,** Anticoagulant and antithrombotic action of novel specific inhibitors of thrombin, *Thromb. Haemost.,* 43, 118, 1980.

681. **Hauptmann, J., Barth, A., Schönberger, F.-P., and Markwardt, F.,** Comparative study on the antithrombotic effects of a synthetic thrombin inhibitor and of heparin in animal models, *Biomed. Biochim. Acta,* 42, 959, 1983.

682. **Kaiser, B., Hauptmann, J., Weiss, A., and Markwardt, F.,** Pharmacological characterization of a new highly effective synthetic thrombin inhibitor, *Biomed. Biochim. Acta,* 44, 1201, 1985.

683. **Mattson, Ch., Eriksson, E., and Nilsson, S.,** Anti-coagulant and antithrombotic effects of some protease inhibitors, *Folia Haematol.,* 109, 43, 1982.

684. **Tremoli, E., Morazzoni, G., Maderna, P., Colli, S., and Paoletti, R.,** Studies on the antithrombotic action of BOC-D-Phe-Pro-ARG H (GYKI 14,451) *Thromb. Res.,* 23, 549, 1981.

685. **Ikoma, H., Ohtsu, K., Tamao, Y., Kikumoto, R., and Okamoto, S.,** Effect of a potent thrombin inhibitor, MCI-9038, on novel experimental arterial thrombosis, *Blood Vessel (Tokyo),* 13, 72, 1982.

686. **Markwardt, F., Nowak, G., and Hoffmann, J.,** Comparative study on thrombin inhibitors in experimental microthrombosis, *Thromb. Haemost.,* 49, 235, 1983.

687. **Yoshikawa, T., Murakami, M., Furukawa, Y., Kato, H., Takemura, S., and Kondo, M.,** Effects of FUT-175, a new synthetic protease inhibitor on endotoxin-induced disseminated intravascular coagulation in rats, *Haemostasis,* 13, 374, 1983.

688. **Schaeffer, R. C., Chilton, S.-M., Hadden, T. J., and Carlson, R. W.,** Pulmonary fibrin microembolism with Echis carinatus venom in dogs: effects of a synthetic thrombin inhibitor, *J. Appl. Physiol.,* 57, 1824, 1984.

689. **Hara, H., Tamao, Y., Kikumoto, R., and Okamoto, S.,** Effect of a synthetic thrombin inhibitor MCI-9038 on experimental models of disseminated intravascular coagulation in rabbits, *Thromb. Haemost.,* 57, 165, 1987.

690. **Oedekoven, B., Bey, R., Mottaghy, K., and Schmid-Schönbein, H.,** Gabexate mesilate (Foy) as an anticoagulant in extracorporeal circulation in dogs and sheep, *Thromb. Haemost.,* 29, 329, 1984.

691. **García-Raffanell, J., Ramis, J., Gomez, L., and Forn, J.,** Effect of triflusal and other salicylic acid derivatives on cyclic AMP levels in rat platelets, *Arch. Int. Pharmacodyn. Ther.,* 284, 155, 1986.

692. **Rosenblum, W. I. and El-Sabban, F.,** Use of AHR-5850 and AHR-6293 to distinguish the effect of antiplatelet aggregating drug properties from the effect of anti-inflammatory properties on an in vivo model of platelet aggregation, *Microvasc. Res.,* 17, 309, 1979.

693. **Inwood, M. J.,** Experimental evidence in support of the hypothesis that intravascular bubbles activate the hemostatic process, Proc. Symp. Blood Bubbles, Interaction in Decompression Sickness, DCIEM 73, CP-960. 171, 1973.

694. **Culp, J. R., Erdös, E. G., Hinshaw, L. B., and Holmes, D. D.,** Effects of anti-inflammatory drugs in shock caused by injection of living *E. coli* cells, *Proc. Soc. Exp. Biol. Med.,* 137, 219, 1971.

695. **Butler, K. D., Pay, G. F., Roberts, J. M., and White, A. M.,** The effect of sulfinpyrazone and other drugs on the platelet response during the acute phase of the active Arthus reaction in guinea pigs, *Thromb. Res.,* 15, 319, 1979.

696. **Nishizawa, E. E. and Wynalda, D. J.,** Inhibitory effect of ibuprofen (Motrin®) on platelet function, *Thromb. Res.,* 21, 347, 1981.

697. **Perlman, M. B., Johnson, A., and Malik, A. B.,** Ibuprofen prevents thrombin-induced lung vascular injury: mechanism of effect, *Am. J. Physiol.,* 252, H 605, 1987.

698. **Gloviczki, P., Hollier, L. H., Dowanjee, M. K., Trastek, V. F., Kopesky, K. R., and Kaye, M. P.,** Quantitative evaluation of ibuprofen treatment on thrombogenicity of expanded polytetrafluoroethylene vascular grafts, *Surgery,* 95, 160, 1984.

699. **Romson, J. L., Hook, B. G., Rigot, V. H., Schork, M. A., Swanson, D. P., and Lucchesi, B. R.,** The effect of ibuprofen on accumulation of indium-111-labeled platelets and leukocytes in experimental myocardial infarction, *Circulation,* 66, 1002, 1982.

700. **Carrieri, P., Donzelli, R., Orefice, G., Cerillo, A., Volpentesta, G., and Tayana, G.,** Antithrombotic effect of indobufen in an experimental model of arterio-arterial microanastomosis in the rat, *Thromb. Res.,* 45, 195, 1987.

701. **Esquivel, C. O., Bergqvist, D., Björck, C.-G., and Carson, S. N.,** Assessment of antithrombotic properties of sodium ibuprofen, *Thromb. Haemost.,* 48, 87, 1982.

702. **Herrmann, R. G., Marshall, W. S., Crowe, V. G., Frank, J. D., Marlett, D. L., and Lacefield, W. B.,** Effect of a new anti-inflammatory drug, fenoprofen, on platelet aggregation and thrombus formation, *Proc. Soc. Exp. Biol. Med.,* 139, 548, 1972.

703. **Jansen, J. W. C. M.,** Antithrombotische Wirkung von Benzydamin, *Arzneimittelforschung,* 37, 626, 1987.

704. **Todd, P. A. and Heel, R. C.,** Suprofen. A review of its pharmacodynamic and pharmacokinetic properties, and analgesic efficacy, *Drugs,* 30, 514, 1985.

705. **Imai, H., Muramaku, Y., Niu, K., Nozaki, M., and Fujimura, H.,** Inhibitory effect of TN-762 (suprofen) on the platelet aggregation, *Folia Pharmacol. Jpn.,* 80, 61, 1982.

706. **Caprino, L., Borelli, F., and Falchetti, R.,** Effect of 4,5-diphenyl-2-bis(2-hydroxyethyl)aminoxazole (Ditazol) on platelet aggregation, adhesiveness and bleeding time, *Arzneimittelforschung,* 23, 1277, 1973.

707. **de Gaetano, G., Cavenaghi, A. E., and Stella, L.,** Ditazole and platelets. II. Effect of ditazole on in vivo platelet aggregation and bleeding time in rats, *Haemostasis,* 6, 190, 1977.

708. **de Gaetano, G., Tonolli, M. C., Bertoni, M. P., and Roncaglioni, M. C.,** Ditazole and platelets, I. Effect of ditazole on human platelet function in vivo, *Haemostasis,* 6, 127, 1977.

709. **Caprino, L., Borrelli, F., Falchetti, R., Cafiero, C., and Gandolfo, G. M.,** Ditazole activity and its interaction with urokinase on experimental thrombosis, *Haemostasis,* 6, 310, 1977.

710. **Mari, D., Cattaneo, M., Gattinoni, A., and Dioguardi, N.,** Thrombogenicity of an artificial surface is decreased by the antiplatelet agent ditazol, *Thromb. Res.,* 12, 59, 1977.

711. **Sim, A. K., McCraw, A. P., Caprino, L., Antonetti, F., Martelli, F., and Morelli, L.,** The vascular protection of ditazole and its effects on arachidonic acid metabolism, *Thromb. Res.,* 32, 479, 1983.

712. **Cox, C. P. and Wood, K. L.,** Selective antagonism of platelet-activating factor (PAF)-induced aggregation and secretion of washed rabbit platelets by CV-3988, L-652731, triazolam and alprazolam, *Thromb. Res.,* 47, 249, 1987.

713. **Simon, M. F., Chap, H., Braquet, P., and Douste-Blazy, L.,** Effect of BN 52021, a specific antagonist of platelet activating factor (PAF-acether), on calcium movements and phosphatidic acid production induced by PAF-acether in human platelets, *Thromb. Res.,* 45, 299, 1987.

714. **Montruccio, G., Alloatti, G., Mariano, F., Tetta, C., Emanuelli, G., and Camussi, G.,** Cardiovascular alteration in the rabbit infused with platelet activating factor (PAF): effect of kadsurenone, a PAF-receptor antagonist, *Int. J. Tissue React.,* 8, 497, 1986.

715. **Etienne, A., Barrogi, N., Andries, R., Clostre, F., Esanu, A., Bourgain, R., and Braquet, P.,** Antithrombotic activity of BN 50 341, a structurally new compound with anticalcic and PAF-antagonistic properties, *Thromb. Res.,* Suppl. 6, 148, 1986.

716. **Schaub, R. G., Ochoa, R., Simmons, C. A., and Lincoln, K. L.,** Renal microthrombosis following endotoxin infusion may be mediated by lipoxygenase products, *Circ. Shock,* 21, 261, 1987.

717. **Croset, M. and Lagarde, M.,** Inhibition of platelet aggregation by lipoxygenase derivatives of eicosaenoic acids, presented at 9th Int. Congr. Thrombosis Haemostasis, Stockholm, 297 (Abstr.), 1983.

718. **Schaub, R. G. and Yamashita, A.,** Leukocyte mediated vein injury and thrombosis is reduced by a lipoxygenase inhibitor, *Exp. Mol. Pathol.,* 45, 343, 1986.

719. **Beetens, J. R., Loots, W., Somers, Y., Coene, M. C., and de Clerck, F.,** Ketoconazole inhibits the biosynthesis of leukotriens in vitro and in vivo, *Biochem. Pharmacol.,* 35, 883, 1986.

720. **Brown, C. H., Bradshaw, M. W., Natelson, E. A., Alfrey, C. P., Jr., and Williams, T. W., Jr.,** Defective platelet function following the administration of penicillin compounds, *Blood,* 47, 949, 1976.

721. **Cazenave, J.-P., Guccione, M. A., Packham, M. A., and Mustard, J. F.,** Effects of cephalothin and penicillin G on platelet function in vitro, *Br. J. Haematol.,* 35, 135, 1977.

722. **Johnson, G. J., Heckel, R., Leis, L. A., and Franciosa, J.,** Effect of inhibition of platelet function with carbencillin or aspirin on experimental canine sudden death, *J. Lab. Clin. Med.,* 98, 660, 1981.

723. **Bruce, I. J. and Kerry, R.,** The effect of chloramphenicol and cycloheximide on platelet aggregation and protein synthesis, *Biochem. Pharmacol.,* 36, 1769, 1987.

724. **Gallus, A. S.,** Antiplatelet drugs, clinical pharmacology and therapeutic use, *Drugs,* 18, 439, 1979.

725. **Carter, A. E. and Eban, R.,** Prevention of postoperative deep venous thrombosis in legs by orally administered hydroxychloroquine sulphate, *Br. Med. J.,* 3, 94, 1974.

726. **Griffiths, M. V., Fredrickson, J. M., and Glynn, M. F.,** Effect of a new antithrombotic agent at microvenous anastomotic sites, *Arch. Otolaryngol.,* 103, 318, 1977.

727. **Ulutin, O. N., Tunali, H., Ugur, M. S., Aytis, S., Erbengi, T., and Balkuv-Ulutin, S.,** Effect of defibrotide in electrically induced thrombosis in dogs, *Haemostasis,* 16, Suppl. 1, 9, 1986.

728. **Niada, R., Pescador, R., Porta, R., Mantovani, M., and Prino, G.,** Defibrotide is antithrombotic and thrombolytic against rabbit venous thrombosis, *Haemostasis,* 16 (Suppl. 1), 3, 1986.

729. **Rosenblum, W. I. and El-Sabban, F.,** Iproniazid inhibits platelet aggregation in mesenteric microvessels, *Blood Vessels,* 17, 324, 1981.

730. **Duval, D. L., Didisheim, P., Spittell, J. A., Jr., and Owen, C. A., Jr.,** Effect of monoamine oxidase inhibitor, glyceryl guaiacolate and ethanol on experimental arterial thrombosis, *Mayo Clin. Proc.,* 45, 579, 1970.

731. **Just, M., Martorana, P. A., and Zoller, G.,** Inhibition of experimental arterial and venous thrombosis by the novel pyridazinone-derivative, C 85-3143, *Thromb. Res.,* Suppl. 6, 147, 1986.

732. **Nawroth, P. P., Kisiel, W., and Stern, D. M.,** Anticoagulant and antithrombotic properties of a gamma-carboxyglutamic acid-rich peptide derived from the light chain of blood coagulation factor X. *Thromb. Res.,* 44, 625, 1986.

733. **Breddin, H. K. and Weichert, W.,** Inhibition of platelet thrombus formation in rat mesenteric vessels by molsidomine and SIN-1, *Pathol. Biol. (Paris),* 35, 223, 1987.

734. **Grodzinska, L., Basista, M., and Koenig, E.,** SIN-1, the active metabolite of molsidomine, is a potent antithrombotic agent, *Pathol. Biol. (Paris),* 35, 211, 1987.

735. **Herrmann, K. S., Grosse-Heitmeyer, A., and Kreuzer, H.,** Antithrombotic efficacy and its time course after application of naftidrofuryl in vivo, *Arch. Int. Pharmacodyn. Ther.,* 284, 145, 1986.

736. **Lecker, D. and Kumar, A.,** Effects of 6-(p-(4-phenylacetylpiperazin-1-y1)-phenyl)- 4,5-dihydro-3(2H) pyridazinone (CCI 17810) and aspirin on experimental arterial thrombosis in rats, *Thromb. Haemost.,* 44, 9, 1980.

737. **Ott, H. and Smith, G. M.,** Anti-thrombotic activity of a benzo-(c)(1,6) naphthyridine, *Br. J. Pharmacol.,* 43, 461 P, 1971.

738. **Andriuli, G., Mastecchi, R., and Barbanti, M.,** Antithrombotic activity of a glycosaminoglycan (Sulodexide) in rats, *Thromb. Res.,* 34, 81, 1984.

Chapter 5

DRUG COMBINATIONS

I. INTRODUCTION

The hemostatic system is notoriously known as being very well ensured against all failures with most partial functions having several alternative ways of consummation and/ or at least duplicate checks. The pathogenesis of most existing symptomatic thrombotic defects is the result of coincident failures at various sites of the control system. Thus, it is not surprising that the attempts at treatment are often unsuccessful. Correspondingly, the after all successful interventions by drugs are probably based on their pluripotential character of action. Another way to favorably influence the process of thrombogenesis is by using combinations of several drugs with well-defined single or prevailing activities which would complement each other in an overall synergistic effect. This was stressed by some authors, e.g., O'Brien,[1] de Gaetano,[2] Ritter and Dollery.[3] The main difficulty is, however, the adjustment of a dose relation schedule in the most effective way. In fact, it might be expected that many combinations would have a strictly defined dose relation optimum. This adjustment is probably directly impossible in clinical treatment as it is difficult to prove that a single drug at one dose is clinically effective at all. Thus, to demonstrate a significant decrease by about 10% in secondary mortality from myocardial infarction by ASA, it was necessary to combine six trials involving a total of 10,703 patients.[4] Let us assume now that this percentage could be increased to about 14 to 15% by the use of a suitable combination. How many patients would be necessary to prove the superior effectiveness of the drug combination as compared with a single drug effect? Meanwhile, it is not possible to dismiss this difference as irrelevant as it may represent many thousands of human lives. In addition, the selected dose ratio would be arbitrary and probably not optimal. Such trials are also very expensive and not many drug companies are ready to support them unless their own drug figures on top of the list. Therefore, it is necessary to rely upon the only possible rational means to assess optimum doses, that is well designed or selected animal models. Such models can also be used for the prediction of particularly suitable indications and interactions of antithrombotics with other concomitantly administered drugs. This chapter presents an attempt at such drug combination screening.

II. COMBINATIONS OF ASA WITH DIPYRIDAMOLE

The most often clinically used combination is that of ASA with dipyridamole. However, not all clinical trials were positive and those which were are liable to doubts.[5-7] Some authors suppose that all favorable effects if any, were due to ASA alone. However, the difficulties with an objective assessment have already been discussed and most negative conclusions are laden with a beta error. On the other hand, many biomodel studies were positive and completely negative results were exceptional. This is surprising in view of the large differences in the type of models, the dose ration, and absolute dosage (Table 1).

In vitro studies are of little help in this respect, despite some positive results.[8,9] Even *ex vivo* studies using whole blood aggregation tests may be both positive and negative.[10] The attempts to explain the supposed synergism by pharmacokinetic interactions, by phosphodiesterase inhibition or by the effect on the eicosanoid control system are probably either too speculative or one-sided. The explanation is simply not known.[11]

Danese and Haimov[16] tested one combination of ASA with dipyridamole in dogs with a carotid artery intimectomy and counting of occluded vessels. Polterauer et al.[17] used rabbits

TABLE 1
ASA + Dipyridamole Experimental Combination Studies

Author	Dose-ratio ASA:Dipyridamole	ASA mg/kg	Route of administration	Relative effectiveness	Comment
		In Biomodels			
Polterauer et al.	20:1	100	p.o.	−	Excessive dose
Danese and Haimov	15:1	18	p.o.	±	Positive trend
Silver et al.	11:1	8	i.p.	+	
Dean and Sundt	10:1	30/d	p.o.	+	
Hanson and Harker	8:1	20/d	p.o.	+	
Honour et al.	6:1	12/d	p.o.	+	
Metke et al., Josa et al.	6:1	18/d	p.o.	+	
Oblath et al.	3:1	15/d	p.o.	+	
Moreno et al.	2:1	36/d	p.o.	+	
Moncada and Korbut	3:1 (1.5:1)	10	i.v.	+	
Faxon et al.	1.2:1	32/d	p.o.	+	
Folts and Smith	1:1	1—2	i.v.	−	
Rosenblum and El-Sab-ban	1:1	1 (10)	i.p.	−	
Louie and Gurewich	1:2	1	i.v.	+	
Weselcouch et al.	1:2 (1:6)	0.03—0.1	i.v.	+	
		Clinical platelet survival studies			
Harker[12]	10:1	15/d	p.o.		
Fuster et al.,[13] Ritchie and Harker[14] Steele et al.[15]	5:1	15/d	p.o.		
		Clinical treatment			
Average dosage	5:1	15/d	p.o.		
More recently	5:1	5/d	p.o.		

with jugular veins injured by a topical silver nitrate application and reported accumulation of radiolabeled red cells. Honour et al.[18,19] observed white body formation in cortical microcirculation of alloxan-diabetic rabbits after topical ADP. Beside dipyridamole, they used the related drug SH 1117. Rosenblum and El-Sabban[20] injured cortical microvessels in mice by UV irradiation. Oblath et al.[21] implanted artificial grafts in dogs and estimated the accumulation of radiolabeled platelets. Moncada and Korbut[22] in fact used an *ex vivo* method. The Achilles tendons of rabbits were superfused from an A/V-shunt and the weight of tendons was continuously registered. Metke et al.[23] and Josa et al.[24] used coronary bypass grafts in dogs. They were particularly interested in the chronic intimal thickening. Deen and Sundt[25] endarterectomized segments of dog carotid arteries. Louie and Gurewich[26] observed thrombus formation on a polyethylene cannula inserted into rabbit carotid arteries. Silver et al.[27] traumatized ear arteries in rabbits and using electron microscopy investigated platelet adhesion. Faxon et al.[28] carried out experimental angioplasty in cholesterol-fed rabbits. Hanson et al.[29] implanted an artificial A/V-shunt in baboons and observed platelet consumption. Weselcouch et al.[30] registered cyclic flow decreases in canine stenosed coronaries. A similar method was used by Folts and Smith.[31] Moreno et al.[32] used streptozotocine-diabetic rats and investigated retinal vessels.

It was not easy to compare the dosages and results in all these studies as the drugs were often administered for several days, dosages were not always expressed in weight per weight terms, routes of administration were different, just as the time intervals of administration and evaluation methods were different. Despite many differences some general conclusions are possible. It is evident that almost always a single dose ratio was only used and its choice was not clarified. The majority of models showed positive difference of combinations versus single drugs. The dose-relations were extremely variable, but in more recent studies a trend to a decrease of the ASA to dipyridamole ratio was observed. A similar decrease may be noted of the absolute dose level. For comparison, some data of platelet survival studies in man and the dosages used in the clinical treatment are shown. There is no question that the choice of clinical doses was arbitrary and was probably based on clinical tolerance rather than functional considerations.

In the author's laboratory combinations were investigated in the screening procedure including the arterial and venous model, while no interaction was observed in the earlier used electrical arterial thrombosis (Figure 3). The dose-to-effect relation studies in the new arterial model were based on using a just effective single dose of one drug combined with several doses of the other (Figures 1, 2). It is evident that the combinations are more effective than single drugs. These combinations allowed to decrease the necessary dose of ASA to about 2.5 mg/kg, but the combination of about 3:3 ratio mg/kg was probably the best one. Of course, the synergism disappeared when either drug was given at sufficient doses to obtain a full inhibitory effect and it is not necessary to look for complicated explanations. If the results are translated into a tentative prediction of the clinical effect, obviously the lately used "low-dose" ASA is sufficient and can possibly be decreased to about 200 to 250 mg pro dosi, whereas the dose of dipyridamole should be increased to about 200 mg of a single dose. Naturally, other considerations such as possible side-effects should be respected as well.

In the venous model, no mutual interaction was observed (Figure 3).

III. OTHER DRUG COMBINATIONS

Combinations of ASA with heparin were often tested clinically, but experimental studies are scarce. If carefully controlled at the start, the risk is probably acceptable and the effectiveness increases. It is true, that on the basis of clinical experience, Yett et al.[33] warned against the use of this combination. Their doses were 10 mg/kg ASA plus 800 U/kg of

ARTERIAL THROMBOSIS

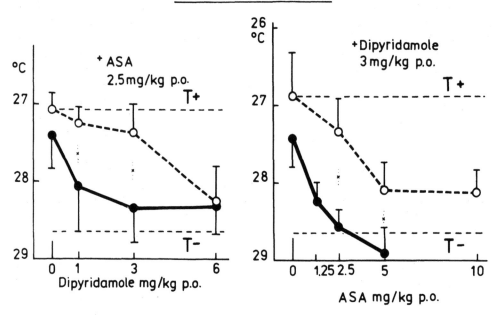

FIGURE 1. Effect of ASA-dipyridamole combination in the arterial model. Broken line: drugs separately, full line: drugs combined, asterisks: significant differences, T+: control with thrombosis, T−: control without thrombosis.

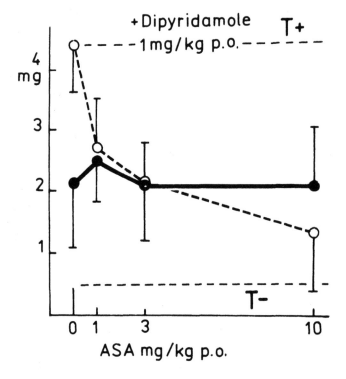

FIGURE 2. Effect of ASA-dipyridamole combination in the venous model.

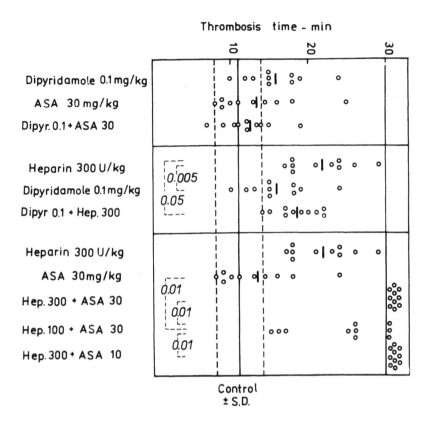

FIGURE 3.   Effect of ASA combination with heparin and dipyridamole, as well as heparin with dipyridamole in the electrically induced arterial thrombosis.

heparin. However, encouraging results were obtained by Donaldson et al.[34] after a combination of three agents, ASA, warfarin, and dipyridamole (75 mg). ASA plus heparin and ASA plus dicoumarole were not more effective than heparin alone in the hands of Benis et al.[35] using a canine extracorporeal model, and Piepgras et al.[36] in endarterectomized cats. The properties of the heparin-ASA complex were studied by Kudrjashov and Liapina.[37]

The combination of ASA with sulfinpyrazone was effective in the study performed by Hanson et al.[29] in baboons (platelet consumption in a chronic A/V-shunt). The combination was more effective than sulfinpyrazone alone, while ASA alone was almost without effect. According to Buchanan et al.,[38] ASA increased the rate of clearance of plasmatic sulfinpyrazone probably by displacing it from plasma protein binding. When free, the drug is more effectively metabolized to active compounds in the liver. Sulfinpyrazone was reported to interfere with the ASA effects on cyclo-oxygenase activity *ex vivo* in rats probably by the competition with the binding site.[39] Needless to say, it is difficult to draw any conclusions for the clinical use of drug combinations on the basis of such studies.

An interesting observation was described by Seiffge and Weithmann[40] who used a laser-induced thrombosis in the rat mesenteric microcirculation. ASA strongly potentiated the antithrombotic effect of pentoxifylline with an optimum ratio of 1:1 (10 mg/kg p.o.), but only if ASA was administered first followed by pentoxifylline 30 to 90 min later. Similar potentiation of antithrombotic activity was observed in adjuvant arthritic rats and hypercholesterolemic rabbits. The study introduced another factor which may be of importance for drug combinations: the sequential principle.

The combination of ASA with dilthiazem was investigated *ex vivo* on platelet aggregation by Ring et al.[41]

ASA was successfully combined with calcium dobesilate in the model of microcirculation thrombosis in the hamster cheek pouch by Michal and Giessinger[42] and with PGE_1 in the rabbit cortical microcirculation (method of Honour and Ross-Russell) by Bousser.[43]

The problem of interaction of ASA with oral anticoagulants is an old one. It is generally considered unfavorable and explained as displacement of anticoagulants from protein binding and a direct effect on liver metabolism. On the other hand, little attention is paid to the possibility of a well-controlled combination which could be more effective. Thus ASA with warfarin in rabbit jugular autografts was superior to the effect of either drug alone in preserving graft patency.[44] Some authors reported no effect of combined clinical administration of ASA 1500 mg together with phenprocoumon on Quick's time, bleeding tests, and the occurrence of complications.[45]

Combinations of ASA with other NSAID were studied quite often, particularly the combination of ASA with its metabolic product, salicylic acid. According to some authors, mostly on the basis of *in vitro* studies, salicylic acid interferes with acetylation protecting cyclo-oxygenase in the endothelium. Many NSAID should exert an effect similar to that of competitive and relatively weak cyclo-oxygenase inhibitors with the notable exception of indomethacine.[46-48] This protective effect was suggested as a solution to the much disputed "aspirin dilemma" of both favorable (inhibition of thromboxane production in platelets) and unfavorable (inhibition of prostacyclin production in the endothelium) effects of ASA. On the other hand, the existence of such relations *in vivo* may be questioned,[49] particularly if salicylic acid alone has a marked antithrombotic activity (see Chapter 4 on ASA).

According to Bertelé et al.,[50] and on the basis of *in vitro* studies, the combination of low doses of ASA with thromboxane synthetase inhibitor might offer a greater antithrombotic potential than either drug alone.

Combinations of heparin with other antithrombotics involve mainly oral anticoagulants. This combination did not prevent the formation of small thrombi in the microcirculation of the rabbit ear chamber, but both agents alone were just as ineffective.[51] Of course, this may serve as an example of inadequate model selection for answering a particular question. Heparin has been very often clinically combined with dihydroergotamine (DHE) which contributes to the antithrombotic effect probably by its venoconstricting activity. Experimentally, LMW-heparin with DHE was administered in a chemically induced rabbit venous thrombosis by Bergquist and Nilsson.[52] The danger of serious side-effects, e.g., gangrene of extremities or coronary spasm is well known.[53,54] Even more intriguing is the effect of combinations of heparin with adrenolytics. The clinical study of heparin combined with atenolol, i.e., a relatively pure $beta_1$-adrenolytic, in the intermediary coronary syndrome has shown no advantage in comparison with heparin alone.[55] The study was criticized for an unsuitable manner of atenolol administration and other technical flaws.[56] Another combination tested this time in an animal model (canine sodium morrhuate-induced thrombosis of the saphenous vein) was heparin with cortisone. The effects of the combination were inferior in comparison with heparin alone.[57] Harker and Fuster[58] pointed out the possibility of using heparin combined with prostacyclin which might be useful if coagulation prevails in thrombogenesis and less useful if platelets have a dominant role.

The effectiveness of dipyridamole in combination with adenosine or its derivatives has been suggested on the basis of the supposed mechanism of dipyridamole action, i.e., inhibition of adenosine accumulation in cells. Thus, the inhibitory adenosine effects on white body formation in the rabbit and rat cerebral cortex microcirculation were particularly potentiated by dipyridamole[59] and potentiation was likewise observed *in vitro* by Dawicki et al.,[60] who also used some drugs related to dipyridamole (dilazep and RA 233). Other studies have shown a potentiation by dipyridamole of prostacyclin effects on platelet adhesion to collagen-coated glass.[61] The inhibitory effects of the combination of eterylate (derivative of ASA) with dipyridamole were demonstrated in collagen and epinephrine-induced DIC in mice by Ortega.[62] Harker[63] stated, on the basis of his experience with the cannula platelet consumption rate in baboons, that the combination of dipyridamole and sulfinpyrazone has only additive inhibitory effects. *In vitro* potentiation of aggregation inhibition by dipyridamole was systematically investigated by Praga et al.[64] Particularly effective were ergoline derivatives, metergoline, and nimergoline. Clinical *ex vivo* platelet studies have shown positive effects of the combination nifedipine-dipyridamole in ischemic heart disease.[65] Vermylen et al.[66] observed *ex vivo* potentiation of the dipyridamole antiaggregatory effect by nafazatrom probably due to a complementary effect on the prostacylin level.

Mutual combination studies with other potential antithrombotics were rare. Thus the combination of the beta-adrenolytic propranolol with the calcium channel blocker dilthiazem seemed to improve the recovery of the myocardial function after occlusion and reperfusion of canine coronary.[67] The extent to which the antithrombotic activity participated was not established. Onoda et al.[68] observed *in vitro* with aggregation tests a synergistic effect of calcium channel blockers with prostacyclin and thromboxane synthetase inhibitors.

The effect of ketanserin on bleeding time was potentiated by the alpha-blocking adrenergic agent prozosin supposedly due to the interference with the synergism of serotonin and catecholamines in hemostasis.[69]

Marked potentiation, as reflected by several *ex vivo* platelet function parameters, was observed after a combination of metoprolol (a beta adrenolytic agent) with sulfinpyrazone.[70]

Hanson et al.[71] found no potentiation of dipyridamole or sulfinpyrazone effects by dazoxiben in their baboon A/V-shunt model as reflected by platelet consumption. Smith and Egan[72] observed some inhibition of thrombin-induced DIC in rabbits by the combination of a phosphodiesterase inhibitor with a thromboxane synthetase inhibitor or with ASA.[73] The combination with prostacyclin was also effective. According to de Gaetano et al.[2] thromboxane synthesis inhibitors could be used with advantage in combination with ASA whereas the combination with dipyridamole affords no benefit.[74] On the other hand, the combination with thromboxane receptor blocking agents looks particularly logical.[75] Heparin may be successfully combined with prostacyclin to inhibit the coagulation pathway e.g., in venous thrombosis but not in arterial thrombosis.[58]

Clofibrate was originally combined with androsterone (Atromid), but the effect of the androsterone component on platelet functions was questioned. Carson et al.[76] suggested a synergistic effect on platelet stickiness. Some warnings have been issued against the combination of clofibrate with oral anticoagulants, but O'Reilly et al.[77] did not find any increased bleeding tendency and no change in platelet and clotting system functions *ex vivo*.

Ticlopidine was successfully combined with cyclosporin to delay hyperacute xenograft rejection of rabbit kidney in rats.[78]

The author investigated the effect of the combination of ASA with heparin, ASA with dipyridamole, and heparin with dipyridamole in electrically induced arterial thrombosis in rats.[79] ASA 30 mg/kg with heparin 100 U/kg was more effective than heparin 300 U/kg or ASA 30 mg/kg alone (both administered intravenously), and heparin 300 U/kg with ASA 10 mg/kg was just as fully effective as with ASA 30 mg/kg (Figure 3). However, the dosage was still relatively high due to the low sensitivity of the model. Negative results with other combinations could be explained in the same way. With the new multifactorial arterial thrombosis model included into the routine battery of tests, combination ASA plus heparin was tested with a resulting additive effect at effective ASA doses of 5 mg/kg p.o. and heparin doses of 10 U/kg (Figure 4). Evidently the strong antithrombotic effect of the combination was only present in the former electrically induced thrombosis with relatively high and risky doses particularly of heparin, while in the new model the effect of the combination as compared with single drugs and using more adequate doses was much less prominent. In the venous model, on the contrary, a trend was observed to an unfavorable interaction with effects of higher doses of heparin inhibited by a constant dose of ASA (1 mg/kg p.o.).

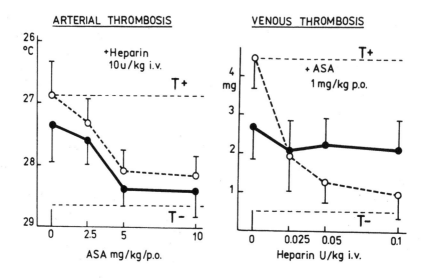

FIGURE 4.   Effect of ASA-heparin combination in the arterial and venous models.

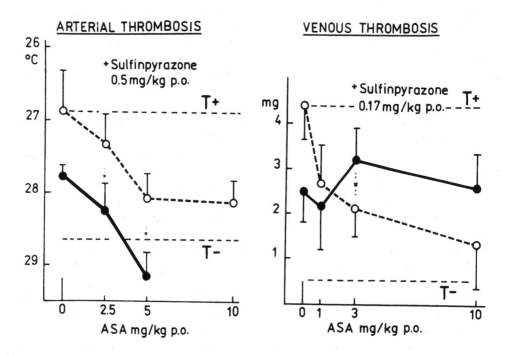

FIGURE 5.   Effect of ASA-sulfinpyrazone combination in the arterial and venous models.

The combination of ASA with dipyridamole was dealt with in a previous chapter. The combination with a constant dose of sulfinpyrazone in the arterial model was about two times more effective than ASA alone (Figure 5). In the venous model, higher doses of ASA were unfavorably influenced by a constant dose of sulfinpyrazone.

The combination of ASA with prenylamine was particularly effective at the dose of 0.25 mg/kg p.o. of prenylamine with 2.5 mg/kg p.o. ASA, but with higher doses of both ASA and prenylamine the synergistic effect was absent (Figure 6). No interaction was observed in the venous model (Figure 7). If, instead of prenylamine, nifedipine and verapamil were used in combination with ASA, a marked synergism was recorded with verapamil (Figures 8, 9).

ARTERIAL THROMBOSIS

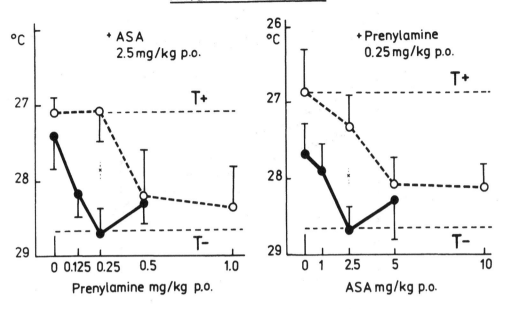

FIGURE 6.   Effect of ASA-prenylamine combination in the arterial model.

VENOUS THROMBOSIS

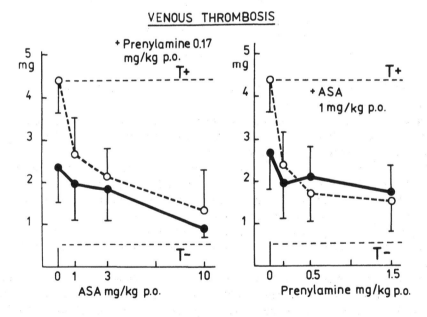

FIGURE 7.   Effect of ASA-prenylamine in the venous model.

The combination of ASA with a constant dose of troxerutin (10 mg/kg p.o.) in the arterial model was particularly advantageous showing not only about a fivefold increase in effect at a low dose of ASA which was not significantly effective alone (2.5 mg/kg p.o.), but also attaining full suppression of thrombus formation (Figure 10). In the venous model a significant effect was seen after a constant dose of troxerutin with rather low doses of ASA.

The combination of a constant dose of ASA with ketanserin was evidently unfavorable

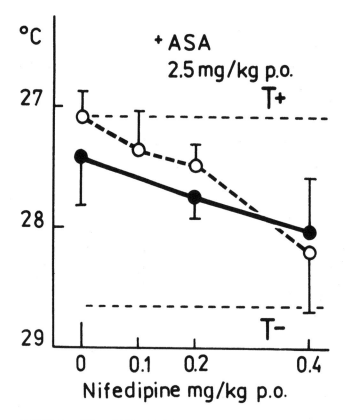

FIGURE 8.   Effect of ASA-nifedipine combination in the arterial model.

in the arterial model (Figure 11) and also tended to be unfavorable with higher doses of ASA in the venous model.

The combination of ASA with pentoxifylline revealed a narrow dose optimum of 2.5 mg/kg p.o. of ASA with 4 mg/kg p.o. of pentoxifylline (Figure 12). A marked antagonism of both drugs was observed in the venous model.

Pronounced synergism of ASA was recorded with the beta-adrenolytic metipranolol which was marked more with a constant dose of ASA 2.5 mg/kg p.o. than with the constant dose of metipranolol 1 mg/kg p.o. However, full inhibition was obtained with both (Figure 13). No synergism was observed in the venous model (Figure 14).

In general, ASA represents in comparison with other tested drugs, an arterial-type antithrombotic best suitable for most combinations but it cannot be combined as effectively in the venous model.

Heparin was, with some exceptions, not particularly suitable for combinations in both the arterial and venous models. Heparin administered intravenously 5 min before thrombus induction was combined with orally administered drugs 60 min in advance. Besides the combination with ASA already mentioned in the preceding section, heparin was combined also with dipyridamole. With a dose of 25 U/kg and higher a significant antagonism was observed (Figure 15). On the contrary, in the venous model a one dose combination had probably an additive effect (0.025 U/kg of heparin and 1 mg/kg p.o. of dipyridamole) which was significantly better than heparin alone in the one-tailed t-test. A pronounced antagonism was noted in the arterial model with heparin plus sulfinpyrazone starting with the dose of 10 mg/kg p.o. sulfinpyrazone (Figure 16), while no interference was recorded in the venous model. Similar antagonism as with sulfinpyrazone was seen in the arterial model with prenylamine (Figure 17) with almost no interaction in the venous model. A narrow zone of

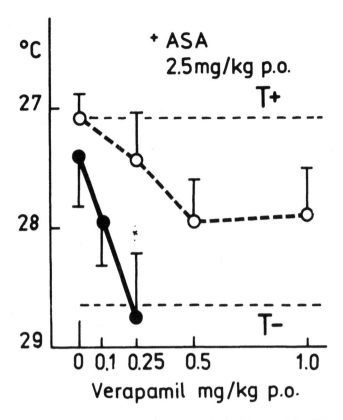

FIGURE 9. Effect of ASA-verapamil combination in the arterial model.

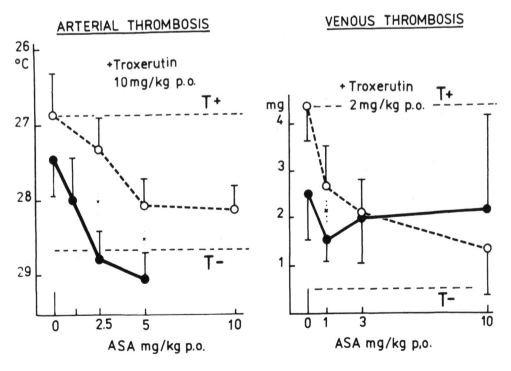

FIGURE 10. Effect of ASA-troxerutin combination in the arterial and venous models.

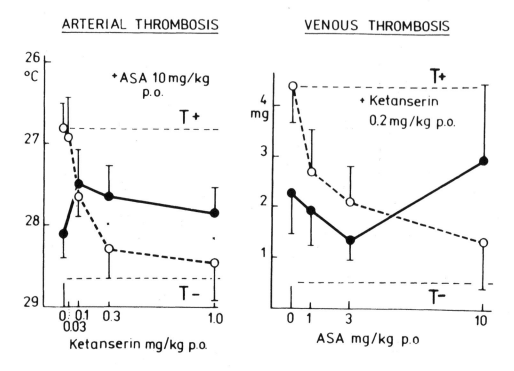

FIGURE 11.   Effect of ASA-ketanserin combination in the arterial and venous models.

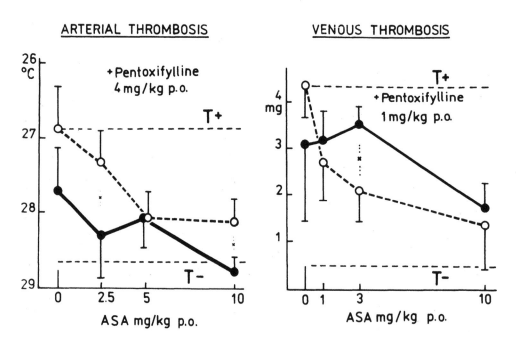

FIGURE 12.   Effect of ASA-pentoxifylline combination in the arterial and venous models.

ARTERIAL THROMBOSIS

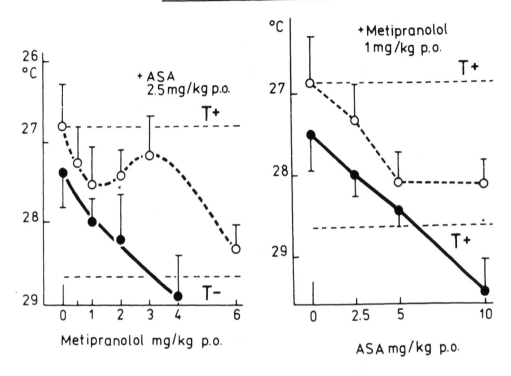

FIGURE 13. Effect of ASA metipranolol combination in the arterial model.

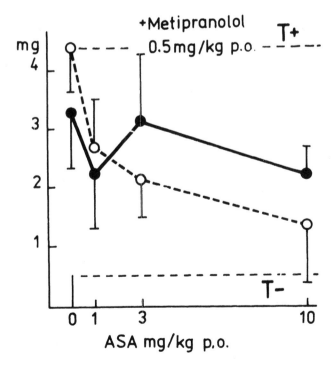

FIGURE 14. Effect of ASA-metipranolol combination in the venous model.

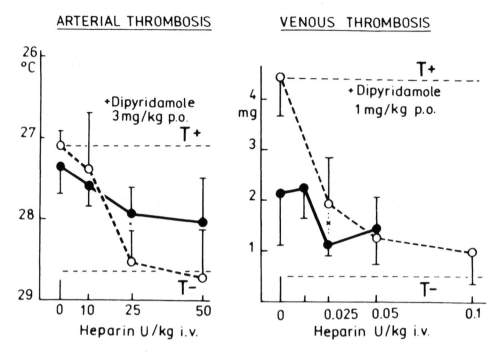

FIGURE 15. Effect of heparin-dipyridamole combination in the arterial and venous models.

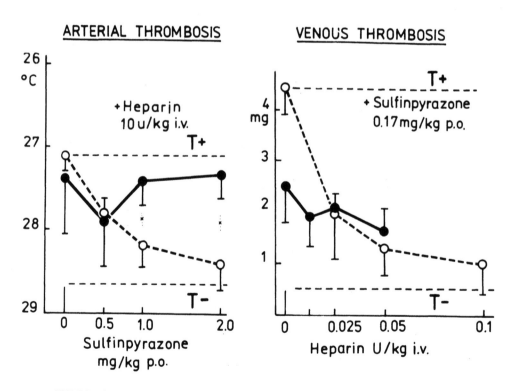

FIGURE 16. Effect of heparin-sulfinpyrazone combination in the arterial and venous models.

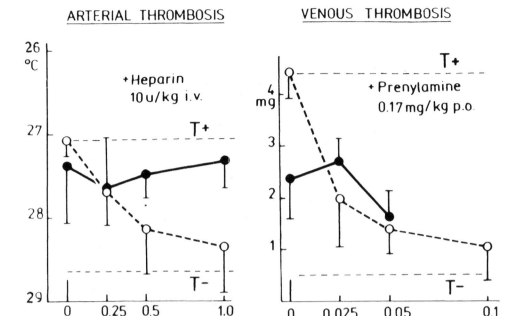

FIGURE 17. Effect of heparin-prenylamine combination in the arterial and venous models.

synergism was noted between heparin and troxerutin (5 mg/kg p.o. troxerutin and 10 U/kg i.v. heparin) (Figure 18). With higher doses of troxerutin a negative trend prevailed. In the venous model an antagonism also prevailed. An antagonistic interaction was noted between heparin and ketanserin in both the arterial and venous models (Figure 19). Pentoxyfylline entered practically no interaction with heparin in both the arterial and venous models (Figure 20).

The most surprising finding was the high degree of synergism in the arterial model between heparin and metipranolol (Figure 21). This synergism was not noted in the endothelemia test and some antagonism was seen instead (Figure 22). No interaction was revealed in the venous model (Figure 23). The synergism in the arterial thrombosis model was also seen with propranolol using only one dose in the screening procedure (Figure 36 in Chapter 4). Propranolol was also effective alone while prazosine had no effect alone, but was synergistic with heparin (Figure 37 in Chapter 4). Practolol was not effective alone or in combination with heparin (Figure 38 in Chapter 4). Yohimbine was partially effective alone but synergism was not noted with heparin (Figure 39 in Chapter 4). It may be concluded that the effect of the combinations is not related in a simple way to adrenergic receptors in terms of their classical concept. The effect may be directed more to endothelium than to platelet and other activities of adrenolytics may contribute to the total effect.

Among combinations of dipyridamole in the arterial model those with sulfinpyrazone can be mentioned. Significant antagonism was noted with higher sulfinpyrazone doses, while in the venous model some synergism with low doses was observed (Figure 24). A particularly marked antagonism in the arterial model was noted with pentoxifylline (Figure 25), which however, was not seen in the venous model. A somewhat less marked antagonism was seen with troxerutin in the arterial model (Figure 26) with no interaction in the venous model. Rather unfavorable interaction was observed with prenylamine in the arterial model that was less prominent in the venous model (Figure 27). Some trend to synergism with ketanserin was observed in the arterial model and no interaction in the venous model (Figures 28, 29). A similar lack of interaction was recorded with metipranolol in both models (Figure 30).

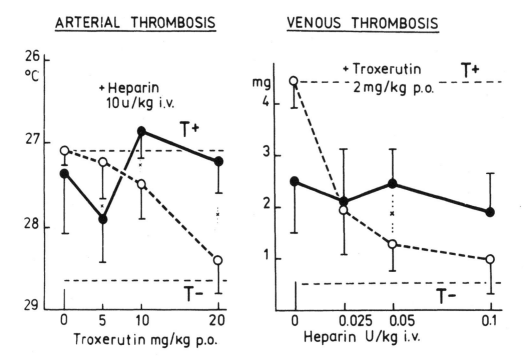

FIGURE 18.   Effect of heparin-troxerutin combination in the arterial and venous models.

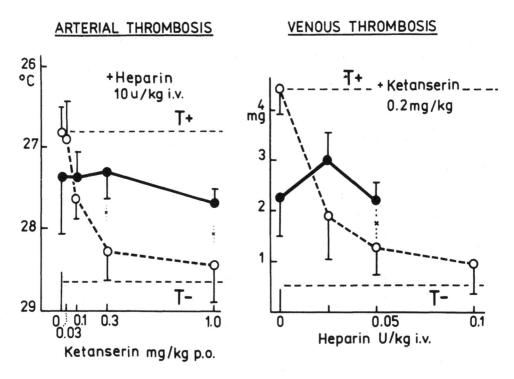

FIGURE 19.   Effect of heparin-ketanserin combination in the arterial and venous models.

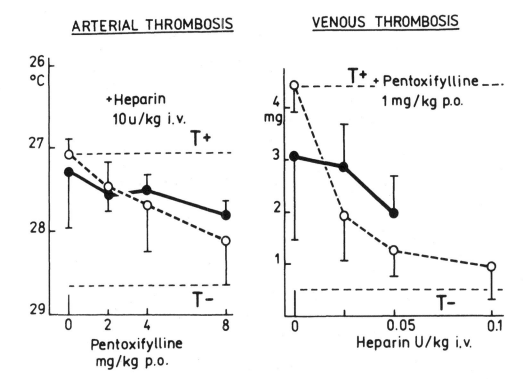

FIGURE 20.   Effect of heparin-pentoxifylline combination in the arterial and venous models.

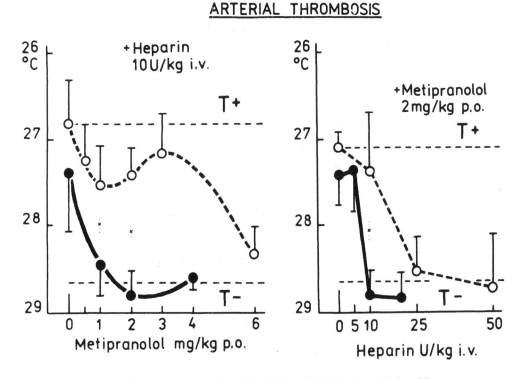

FIGURE 21.   Effect of heparin-metipranolol combination in the arterial model.

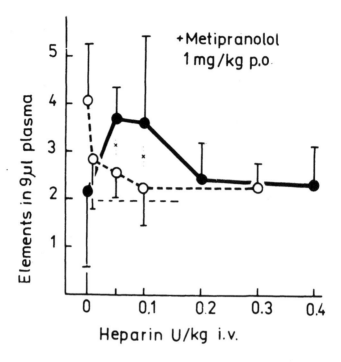

FIGURE 22.   Effect of heparin-metipranolol combination in endothelemia model after the hypotonic saline challenge.

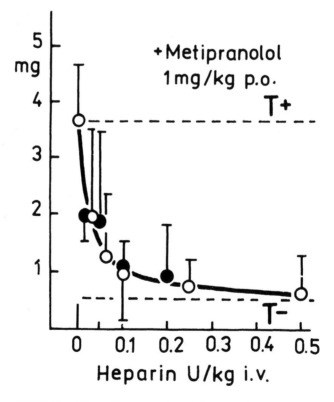

FIGURE 23.   Effect of heparin-metipranolol combination in the venous model (open circles: heparin alone).

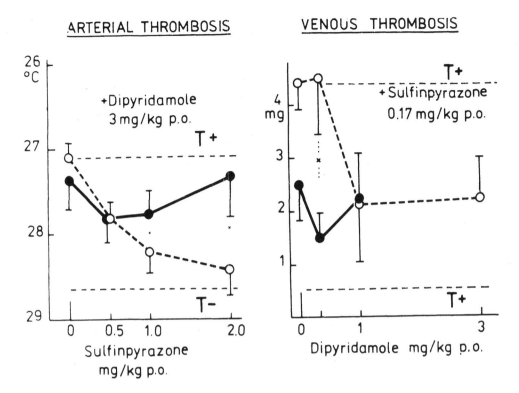

FIGURE 24. Effect of dipyridamole-sulfinpyrazone combination in the arterial and venous models.

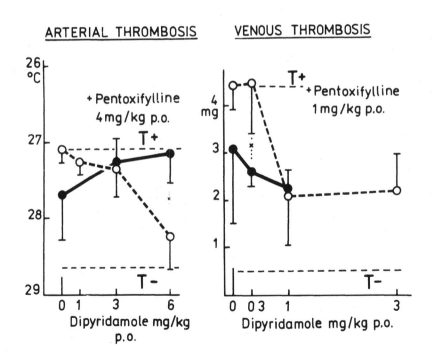

FIGURE 25. Effect of dipyridamole-pentoxifylline combination in the arterial and venous models.

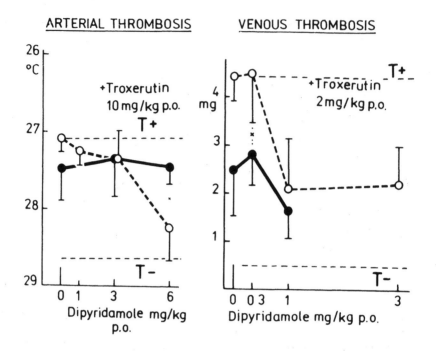

FIGURE 26.   Effect of dipyridamole-troxerutin combination in the arterial and venous models.

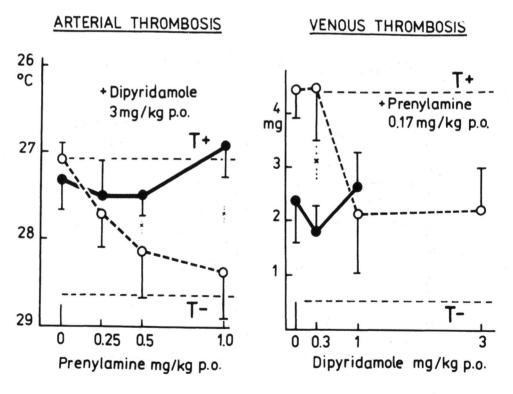

FIGURE 27.   Effect of dipyridamole-prenylamine combination in the arterial and venous models.

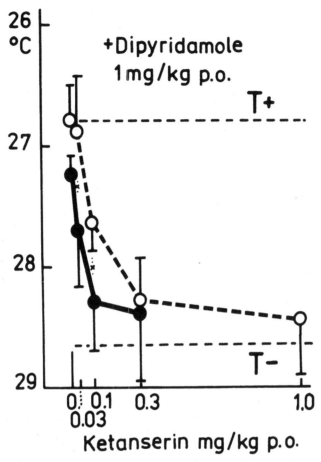

FIGURE 28.   Effect of dipyridamole-ketanserin combination in the arterial model.

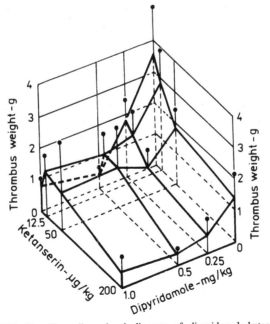

FIGURE 29.   Three-dimensional diagram of dipyridamole-ketanserin combination effect in the venous thrombosis.

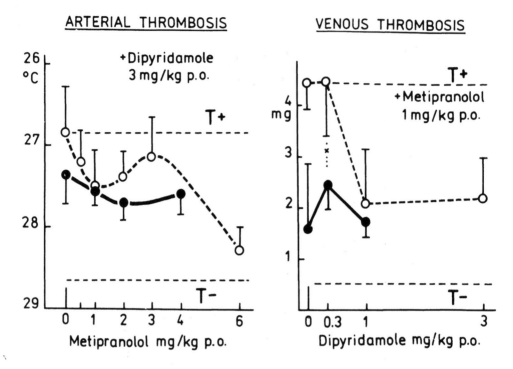

FIGURE 30. Effect of dipyridamole-metipranolol combination in the arterial and venous models.

An antagonistic interaction of sulfinpyrazone was seen in both the arterial and venous models with prenylamine (Figure 31), while a combination with troxerutin yielded opposite results in the arterial and venous models: a marked antagonism in the former and a similarly marked synergism in the latter (Figure 32). No interaction was noted with ketanserin in both the arterial and venous models (Figure 33), while with pentoxifylline similar marked opposite results were obtained as with troxerutin (Figure 34). The synergism in the venous model was probably the most prominent of all combinations. No interaction was registered in the arterial model and some synergism in the venous model with metipranolol (Figure 35).

Prenylamine combinations (minus the interactions with heparin, ASA, dipyridamole, and sulfinpyrazone which were mentioned previously) showed no marked interaction with troxerutin, at least with lower doses (Figure 36) in the arterial model and some synergism in the venous model. No interaction was recorded in the arterial model and a marked synergism in the venous model with pentoxifylline (Figure 37). A tendency to an antagonistic interaction was seen with metipranolol in both the arterial and venous models (Figure 38). An antagonism predominated with ketanserin, particularly with high doses, in the arterial model and a pronounced synergism in the venous model (Figure 39).

Troxerutin was antagonized by higher doses of ketanserin in the arterial model (Figure 40) and showed some synergism with lower doses of troxerutin in the venous model. It was particularly antagonized strongly in the arterial model by pentoxifylline, while in the venous model a tendency to synergistic effect was noted with lower doses of troxerutin (Figure 41). However, troxerutin did not interact with metipranolol in both the arterial and venous models (Figure 42).

Ketanserin showed a significant synergism with pentoxifylline in the arterial model at a narrow dose range and a tendency to antagonism in the venous model (Figure 43). It was antagonized by metipranolol in the arterial model and some similar tendency was also noted in the venous model (Figure 44).

No interaction was observed between pentoxifylline and metipranolol in the arterial

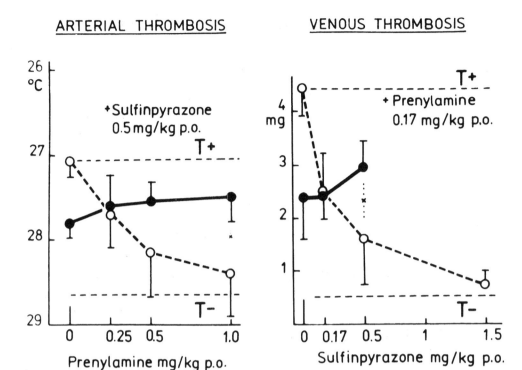

FIGURE 31. Effect of sulfinpyrazone-prenylamine combination in the arterial and venous thrombosis models.

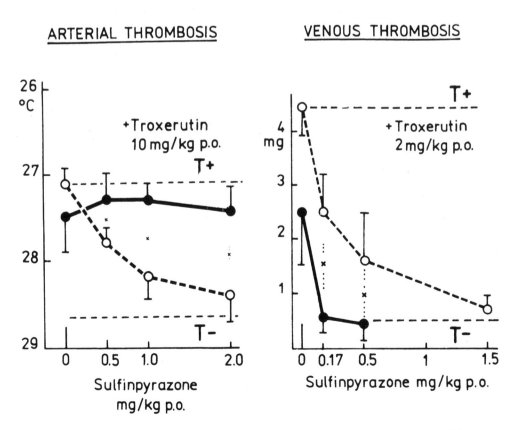

FIGURE 32. Effect of sulfinpyrazone-troxerutin combination in the arterial and venous models.

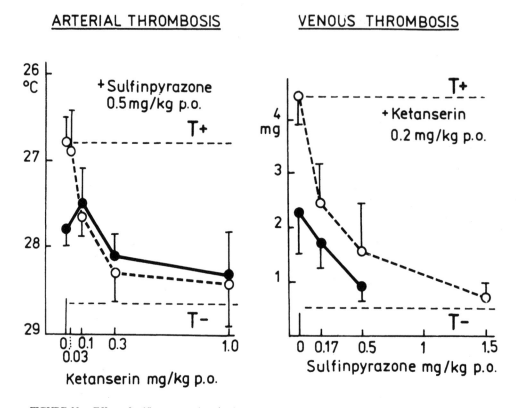

FIGURE 33.   Effect of sulfinpyrazone-ketanserin combination in the arterial and venous thrombosis models.

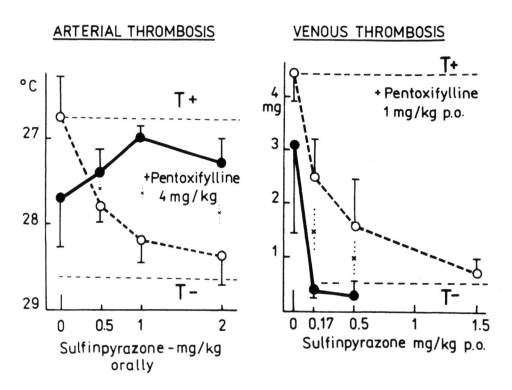

FIGURE 34.   Effect of sulfinpyrazone-pentoxifylline combination in the arterial and venous thrombosis models.

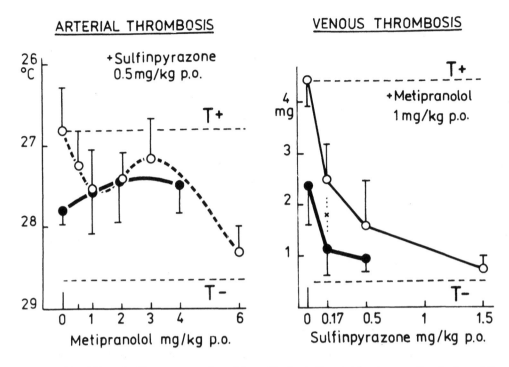

FIGURE 35. Effect of sulfinpyrazone-metipranolol combination in the arterial and venous thrombosis models.

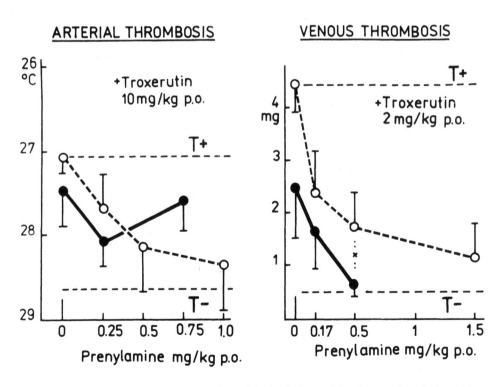

FIGURE 36. Effect of prenylamine-troxerutin combination in the arterial and venous thrombosis models.

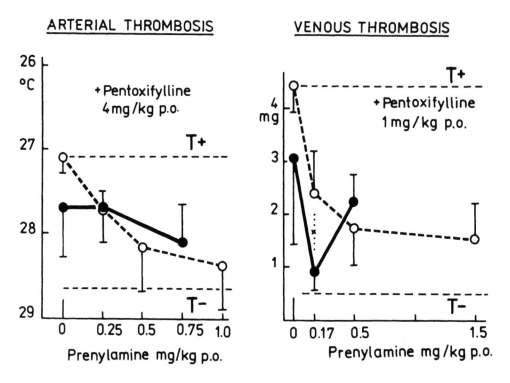

FIGURE 37.   Effect of prenylamine-pentoxifylline combination in the arterial and venous thrombosis models.

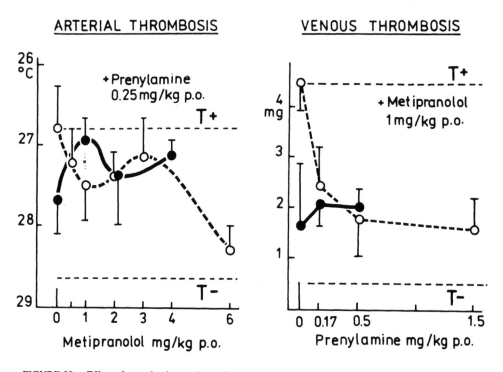

FIGURE 38.   Effect of prenylamine-metipranolol combination in the arterial and venous thrombosis models.

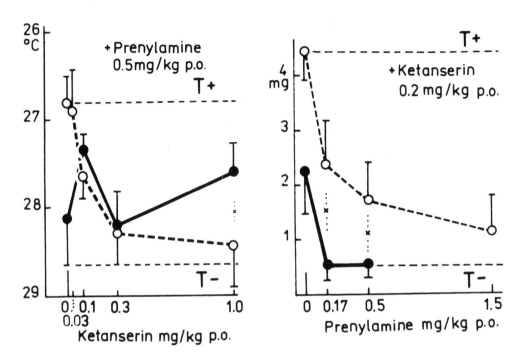

FIGURE 39.   Effect of prenylamine-ketanserin combination in the arterial and venous thrombosis models.

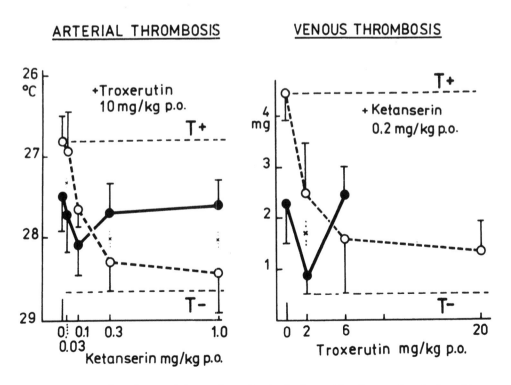

FIGURE 40.   Effect of troxerutin-ketanserin combination in the arterial and venous thrombosis models.

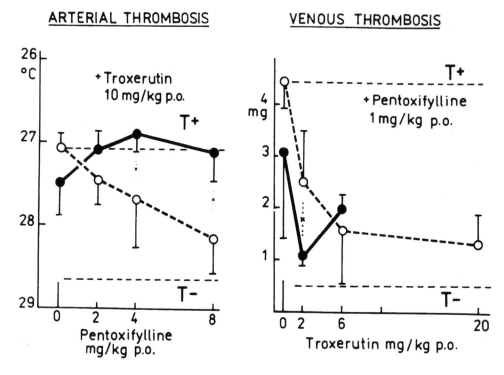

FIGURE 41. Effect of troxerutin-pentoxifylline combination in the arterial and venous thrombosis models.

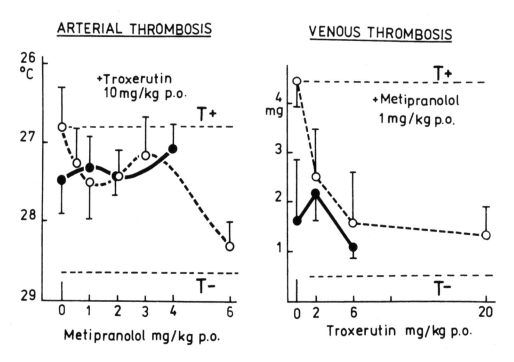

FIGURE 42. Effect of troxerutin-metipranolol combination in the arterial and venous thrombosis models.

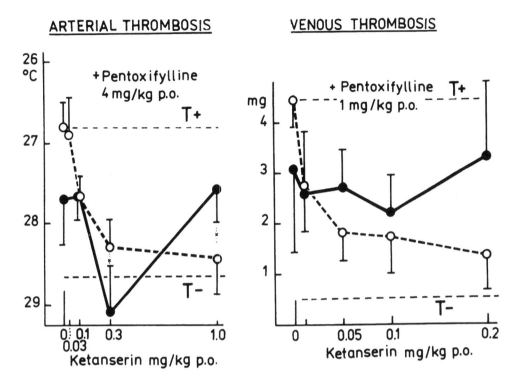

FIGURE 43. Effect of ketanserin-pentoxifylline combination in the arterial and venous thrombosis models.

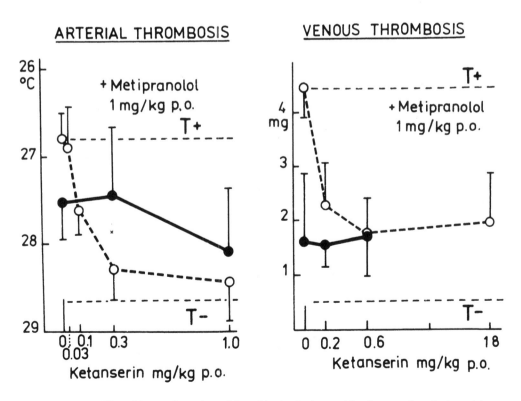

FIGURE 44. Effect of ketanserin-metipranolol combination in the arterial and venous thrombosis models.

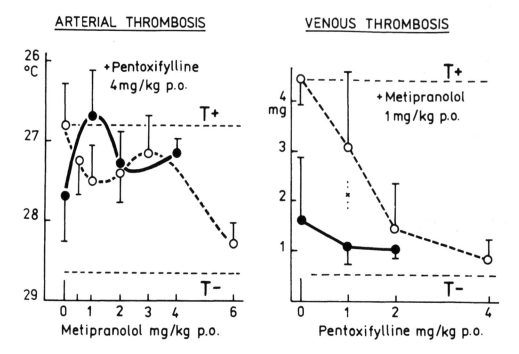

FIGURE 45.   Effect of metipranolol-pentoxifylline combination in the arterial and venous thrombosis models.

model, while on the contrary, a marked synergism was recorded in the venous model (Figure 45).

IV. CONCLUSIONS OF THE COMBINATION SECTION

Use of biomodels in the study of drug combinations is essential. Nevertheless, until now the studies carried out in this field have been virtually nonexistent or very fragmentary. An attempt has been made here to perform a systematic study with at least a portion of the drugs of interest.

After selecting the lowest, yet partially effective dose of each drug on the basis of preliminary dose-to-effect studies, it was possible to investigate the combinations of antithrombotics (and potential antithrombotics) in both the arterial and venous thrombosis models (Figures 46, 47). In the arterial model ASA was particularly suitable for combinations except with ketanserin. Some interesting observations were also recorded with other agents such as the potentiation of heparin effect by some adrenergic blocking agents, potentiation of ketanserin by dipyridamole, and possibly by troxerutin and pentoxifylline. On the other hand some unfavorable effects of combinations were noted as well. Thus heparin was not compatible with dipyridamole in arterial thrombosis even though the opposite was true in venous thrombosis, sulfinpyrazone was not compatible in the arterial model with troxerutin, dipyridamole with sulfinpyrazone, prenylamine, and particularly with pentoxifylline. Sulfinpyrazone effects were inhibited by prenylamine and especially by pentoxifylline, which evidently was not very suitable for most combinations. Prenylamine was not compatible with ketanserin and metipranolol, troxerutin with both ketanserin and metipranolol. In general, the possibility of both favorable and unfavorable effects of combinations should be kept in mind.

The venous model was somewhat less sensitive than the arterial one in combination studies and minor advantages or disadvantages of combinations might escape attention. Nevertheless, some observations can be pointed out. No correlation was found between results in the arterial and venous model and quite often they were of opposite character.

	Heparin	ASA	Dipyri-damole	Sulfin-pyrazone	Prenyl-amine	Troxerutin	Ketanserin	Pentoxi-fylline	Metipra-nolol
Heparin	✕	O	−	−	−	±	−	O	+
ASA	O	✕	+	+	+	+	−	O	+
Dipyri-damole	−	+	✕	−	−	−	+	−	O
Sulfin-pyrazone	−	+	−	✕	−	−	O	−	O
Prenyl-amine	−	+	−	−	✕	O	−	O	−
Troxerutin	±	+	−	−	O	✕	±	−	O
Ketanserin	−	−	+	O	−	±	✕	±	−
Pentoxi-fylline	O	O	−	−	O	−	±	✕	O
Metipra-nolol	+	+	O	O	−	O	−	O	✕

+ increased antithromb. effect
− decreased "
O no effect
± mixed effect

FIGURE 46.   Table of mutual combinations of nine antithrombotics and potential antithrombotics in the arterial model.

Both clear-cut synergism and antagonism were observed in the venous model. ASA did not yield good combinations, while sulfinpyrazone and prenylamine were good "mixers", showing some particularly effective combinations with troxerutin, ketanserin, pentoxifylline, and metipranolol. In general, the study of combinations in both the arterial and venous models can supply interesting and stimulating results both from the practical (better prevention, avoiding adverse interactions) and theoretical point of view.

	Heparin	ASA	Dipyri-damole	Sulfin-pyrazone	Prenyl-amine	Troxerutin	Ketanserin	Pentoxi-fylline	Metipra-nolol
Heparin	X	−	o	o	o	−	−	o	o
ASA	−	X	o	−	o	+−	o	−	o
Dipyri-damole	o	o	X	+	o	o	o	o	o
Sulfin-pyrazone	o	−	+	X	−	+	o	+	+
Prenyl-amine	o	o	o	−	X	+	+	+o	o
Troxerutin	−	+−	o	+	+	X	+o	+o	o
Ketanserin	−	o	o	o	+	+o	X	−	o
Pentoxi-fylline	o	−	o	+	+o	+o	−	X	o
Metipra-nolol	o	o	o	+	o	o	o	o	X

+ increased antithrombotic effect
− decreased   "   "
o no effect
+− two-phase effect

FIGURE 47. Table of mutual combinations of nine antithrombotics and potential antithrombotics in the venous model.

REFERENCES

1. **O'Brien, J. R.**, Multiple therapy for multifactorial thrombosis, *Thromb. Haemost.*, 57, 232, 1987.
2. **de Gaetano, G., Cerletti, Ch., Dejana, E., and Vermylen, J.**, Current issues in thrombosis prevention with antiplatelet drugs, *Drugs*, 31, 512, 1986.
3. **Ritter, J. M. and Dollery, C. T.**, Therapeutic opportunities in vasoocclusive disease, *Circulation*, 73, 240, 1986.
4. **Canner, P. L.**, Aspirin in coronary heart disease, *Isr. J. Med. Sci.*, 19, 413, 1983.
5. **Loeliger, E. A.**, Does dipyridamole have antithrombotic potential?, *Thromb. Haemost.*, 53, 437, 1985.
6. **Fitzgerald, G. A.**, Dipyridamole, *N. Engl. J. Med.*, 316, 1247, 1987.
7. **Harker, L. A.**, Clinical trials evaluating platelet-modifying drugs in patients with atherosclerotic cardiovascular disease and thrombosis, *Circulation*, 73, 206, 1986.
8. **Greer, I. A., Walker, J. J., Calder, A. A., and Forbes, C. D.**, Aspirin with an adrenergic and calcium-channel-blocking agent as a new combination therapy for arterial thrombosis, *Lancet*, 1, 351, 1985.
9. **Gresele, P., Arnout, J., Deckmyn, H., and Vermylen, J.**, Combining antiplatelet agents: potentiation between aspirin and dipyridamole, *Lancet*, 1, 937, 1985.
10. **Heptinstall, S., Fox, S., Crawford, J., and Hawkins, M.**, Inhibition of platelet aggregation in whole blood by dipyridamole and aspirin, *Thromb. Res.*, 42, 215, 1986.
11. **Rosenfeld, J., Buchanan, M. R., Reilly, P. A., and Turpie, A. G. G.**, Dipyridamole disposition after chronic administration: effect of aspirin, *Thromb. Res.*, Suppl. 4, 137, 1983.
12. **Harker, L. A.**, In vivo evaluation of antithrombotic therapy in man, *Thromb. Diath. Haemorrh.*, 60, 481, 1974.
13. **Fuster, V., Chesebro, J. H., Frye, R. L., and Elveback, L. R.**, Platelet survival and the development of coronary heart disease in the young: the effects of cigarette smoking, strong family history, and medical therapy, *Circulation*, 63, 546, 1981.

14. **Ritchie, J. L. and Harker, L. A.,** Platelet and fibrinogen survival in coronary atherosclerosis: response to medical and surgical therapy, *Am. J. Cardiol.,* 39, 595, 1977.

15. **Steele, P., Rainwater, J., Vogel, R., and Genton, E.,** Platelet-suppressant therapy in patients with coronary artery disease, *JAMA,* 240, 228, 1978.

16. **Danese, C. A. and Haimov, M.,** Inhibition of experimental arterial thrombosis in dogs with platelet-deaggregating agents, *Surgery,* 70, 927, 1971.

17. **Polterauer, P., Zekert, F., and Gottlob, R.,** Azetylsalizylsäure und Dipyridamol: Aggregationshemmung im Experiment am Kaninchen, *Vasa,* 4, 397, 1975.

18. **Honour, A. J., Hockaday, T. D. R., and Mann, J. I.,** The reversibility by dipyridamole of the increased sensitivity of in vivo platelet aggregation in rabbits after alloxane, *Br. J. Exp. Pathol.,* 57, 11, 1976.

19. **Honour, A. J., Hockaday, T. D. R., and Mann, J. I.,** The synergistic effect of aspirin and dipyridamole upon platelet thrombi in living blood vessels, *Br. J. Exp. Pathol.,* 58, 268, 1977.

20. **Rosenblum, W. J. and El-Sabban, F.,** Effect of dipyridamole on platelet aggregation in cerebral microcirculation of the mouse, *Thromb. Res.,* 12, 181, 1977.

21. **Oblath, R. W., Buckley, F. O., Green, R. M., Schwartz, S. I., and De Weese, J. A.,** Prevention of platelet aggregation and adherence to prosthetic vascular grafts by aspirin and dipyridamole, *Surgery,* 84, 37, 1978.

22. **Moncada, S. and Korbut, R.,** Dipyridamole and other phosphodiesterase inhibitors act as antithrombotic agents by potentiating endogenous prostacyclin, *Lancet,* 1, 1286, 1978.

23. **Metke, M. P., Lie, J. T., Fuster, V., Josa, M., and Kaye, M. P.,** Reduction of intimal thickening in canine coronary bypass vein grafts with dipyridamole and aspirin, *Am. J. Cardiol.,* 43, 1144, 1979.

24. **Josa, M., Lie, J. T., Bianco, R. L., and Kaye, M. P.,** Reduction of thrombosis in canine coronary bypass vein grafts with dipyridamole and aspirin, *Am. J. Cardiol.,* 47, 1248, 1981.

25. **Deen, H. G. and Sundt, T. M.,** The effect of combined aspirin and dipyridamole therapy on thrombus formation in an arterial thrombogenic lesion in the dog, *Stroke,* 13, 179, 1982.

26. **Louie, S. and Gurewich, V.,** The antithrombotic effect of aspirin and dipyridamole in relation to prostaglandin synthesis, *Thromb. Res.,* 30, 323, 1983.

27. **Thomas, D. P. and Wessler, S.,** Stasis thrombi induced by bacterial endotoxin, *Circ. Res.,* 14, 486, 1964.

28. **Faxon, D. P., Sanborn, T. A., Haudenschild, Ch. C., and Ryan, T. J.,** Effect of antiplatelet therapy on restenosis after experimental angioplasty, *Am. J. Cardiol.,* 53, 72 C, 1984.

29. **Hanson, S. R., Harker, L. A., and Bjornsson, T. D.,** Effects of platelet-modifying drugs on arterial thromboembolism in baboons. Aspirin potentiates the antithrombotic actions of dipyridamole and sulfinpyrazone by mechanism(s) independent of platelet cyclooxygenase inhibition, *J. Clin. Invest.,* 75, 1591, 1985.

30. **Weselcouch, E. O., Humphrey, W. R., and Aiken, J. W.,** Effects of low doses of aspirin and dipyridamole on platelet aggregation in the dog coronary artery, *J. Pharmacol. Exp. Ther.,* 240, 37, 1987.

31. **Folts, J. D. and Smith, S. R.,** Dipyridamole alone and with low dose aspirin does not prevent acute platelet thrombus formation in stenosed dog coronary arteries, presented at 11th Int. Congr. Thrombosis Haemostasis, Brussels, 778 (Abstr.), 1987.

32. **Moreno, A., de la Cruz, J. P., Campos, J. G., and de la Cuesta, F. S.,** Effect of dipyridamole plus ASA on the retinal vascular pattern of estreptozotocin-diabetic rats, presented at 11th Int. Congr. Thrombosis Haemostasis, Brussels, 299 (Abstr.), 1987.

33. **Yett, H. S., Skillman, J. J., and Salzman, E. W.,** The hazards of aspirin plus heparin, *N. Engl. J. Med.,* 298, 1092, 1978.

34. **Donaldson, D. R., Sreeharan, N., Crow, M. J., and Rajah, S. M.,** Assessment of the interaction of warfarin with aspirin and dipyridamole, *Thromb. Haemost.,* 47, 77, 1982.

35. **Benis, A. M., Nossel, H. L., Aledort, L. M., Koffsky, R. M., Stevenson, J. F., Leonard, E. F., Shiang, H., and Litwak, R. S.,** Extracorporeal model for study of factors affecting thrombus formation, *Thromb. Diath. Haemorrh.,* 34, 127, 1975.

36. **Piepgras, D. G., Sundt, T. M., and Didisheim, P.,** Effect of anticoagulants and inhibitors of platelet aggregation on thrombotic occlusion of endarterectomized cat carotid arteries, *Stroke,* 7, 248, 1976.

37. **Kudrjashov, B. A. and Liapina, L. A.,** Heparin-aspirin complex, its physicochemical and physiological properties, *Vopr. Med. Khim.,* 23, 44, 1977.

38. **Buchanan, M. R., Edrenyi, L., Giles, A. R., and Rosenfeld, J.,** The effect of aspirin on the pharmacokinetics of sulfinpyrazone in man, *Thromb. Res.,* Suppl. 4, 145, 1983.

39. **Rajtar, G., Cerletti, Ch., Livio, M., and de Gaetano, G.,** Sulphinpyrazone prevents in vivo the inhibitory effect of aspirin on rat platelet cyclo-oxygenase activity, *Biochem. Pharmacol.,* 30, 2773, 1981.

40. **Seiffge, D. and Weithmann, K. U.,** Surprising effects of the sequential administration of pentoxifylline and low dose acetylsalicylic acid on thrombus formation, *Thromb. Res.,* 46, 371, 1987.

41. **Ring, M. E., Corrigan, J. J., and Fenster, P. E.,** Effects of oral dilthiazem on platelet function: alone and in combinations with "low dose" aspirin, *Thromb. Res.,* 44, 391, 1986.

42. **Michal, M. and Giessinger, N.,** Effect of calcium dobesilate and its interaction with aspirin on thrombus formation in vivo, *Thromb. Res.,* 40, 215, 1985.

43. **Bousser, M.-G.,** Effects of combined prostaglandin E₁ and aspirin on experimental arterial thrombosis in rabbits, *Biomedicine,* 19, 90, 1973.

44. **Friedman, E. W., Frank, H. A., and Ponn, R.,** Patency of venous grafts in small veins- influence of aspirin and warfarin sodium, *Arch. Surg.,* 112, 1072, 1977.

45. **Barth, P., Walter, E., Zimmermann, R., and Weber, E.,** Über die Anwendung von Acetylsalicylsäure bei Antikoagulantientherapie, *Dtsch. Med. Wochenschr.,* 97, 1854, 1972.

46. **Vargaftig, B. B.,** The inhibition of cyclo-oxygenase of rabbit platelets by aspirin is prevented by salicylic acid and by phenanthroline, *Eur. J. Pharmacol.,* 50, 231, 1978.

47. **Brantmark, B., Hedner, U., Melander, A., and Wahlin-Boll, E.,** Salicylate inhibition of antiplatelet effect of aspirin, *Lancet,* 2, 1349, 1981.

48. **Dejana, E., Cerletti, Ch., and de Gaetano, G.,** Interaction of salicylate and other non-steroidal anti-inflammatory drugs with aspirin on platelet and vascular cyclo-oxygenase activity, *Thromb. Res.,* Suppl. 4, 153, 1983.

49. **Philp, R. B. and Paul, M. L.,** Non-interference by salicylate with aspirin inhibition of arterial thrombosis, *Prostaglandins Leukotrienes Med.,* 7, 91, 1981.

50. **Bertelé, V., Falanga, A., Tomasiak, M., Dejana, E., Cerletti, Ch., and de Gaetano, G.,** Platelet thromboxane synthetase inhibition and low doses of aspirin: Possible resolution of the "aspirin dilemma", *Science,* 220, 577, 1983.

51. **Allison, F., Jr. and Lancaster, M. G.,** Studies on the pathogenesis of acute inflammation. III. The failure of anticoagulants to prevent the leucocytic sticking reaction and the formation of small thrombi in rabbit ear chambers damaged by heat, *J. Exp. Med.,* 114, 535, 1961.

52. **Bergqvist, D.,** The influence on experimental thrombosis and haemostasis by low molecular weight heparin in combination with dihydroergotamine, presented at 11th Int. Congr. Thrombosis Haemostasis Brussels, 2054 (Abstr.), 1987.

53. **Rem, J. A., Gratzl, O., Follath, F., and Pult, I.,** Ergotism as complication of thromboembolic prophylaxis with heparin-dihydroergotamine, *Lancet,* 1, 219, 1987.

54. **Gatterer, R.,** Ergotism as complication of thromboembolic prophylaxis with heparin and dihydroergotamine, *Lancet,* 2, 638, 1986.

55. **Telford, A. M. and Wilson, Ch.,** Trial of heparin versus atenolol in prevention of myocardial infarction in intermediate coronary syndrome, *Lancet,* 1, 1225, 1981.

56. **Yusuf, S. and Sleight, P.,** Atenolol, heparin, and the intermediate coronary syndrome, *Lancet,* 2, 46, 1981.

57. **Zambouras, D. A., Anezyris, P., and Kalakonas, P.,** La cortisone et l'héparine dans les thrombophlébites expérimentales, *Presse Med.,* 69, 1134, 1961.

58. **Harker, L. A. and Fuster, V.,** Pharmacology of platelet inhibitors, *J. Am. Coll. Cardiol.,* 8, 21 B, 1986.

59. **Philp, R. B. and Lemieux, V.,** Comparison of some effects of dipyridamole and adenosine on thrombus formation, platelet adhesiveness and blood pressure in rabbits and rats, *Nature,* 218, 1072, 1968.

60. **Dawicki, D. D., Agarwal, K. C., and Parks, R. E., Jr.,** Potentiation of the antiplatelet action of adenosine in whole blood by dipyridamole or dilazep and the cAMP phosphodiesterase inhibitor, RA 233, *Thromb. Res.,* 43, 161, 1986.

61. **Groves, H. M., Kinlough-Rathbone, R. L., Cazenave, J.-P., Dejana, E., Richardson, M., and Mustard, J. F.,** Effect of dipyridamole and prostacyclin on rabbit platelet adherence in vitro and in vivo, *J. Lab. Clin. Med.,* 99, 548, 1982.

62. **Ortega, M. P.,** The antithrombotic in vivo effect of eterylate and dipyridamole in experimental thrombosis in mice, *Thromb. Res.,* 44, 555, 1986.

63. **Harker, L. A.,** Symposium discussion, *Thromb. Res.,* Suppl. 4, 151, 1983.

64. **Praga, C., Pogliani, E., Cortellaro, M., and Polli, E. E.,** Potentiating effect of various drugs on the inhibition of platelet aggregation by dipyridamole, in *Aggregazione Piastrinica,* Boehringer Ingelheim, Firenze, 1972, 97.

65. **Domingues, M. J., Aguirre, J. M., Iriarte, J. A., and Iriarte, M. M.,** Association nifedipine-dipyri-damole on platelets in ischemic heart disease, *Thromb. Res.,* Suppl. 6, 141, 1986.

66. **Vermylen, J., Chamone, D. A. F., and Verstraete, M.,** Stimulation of prostacyclin release from vessel wall by BAY g 6575, an antithrombotic compound, *Lancet,* 1, 518, 1979.

67. **Bush, L. R., Buja, L. M., Tilton, G., Wathen, M., Apprill, P., Ashton, J., and Willerson, J. T.,** Effects of propranolol and dilthiazem alone and in combination on the recovery of left ventricular segmental function after temporary coronary occlusion and long-term reperfusion in conscious dogs, *Circulation,* 72, 413, 1985.

68. **Onoda, J. M., Sloane, B. F., and Honn, K. V.,** Antithrombogenic effects of calcium channel blockers: Synergism with prostacyclin and thromboxane synthase inhibitors, *Thromb. Res.,* 34, 368, 1984.

69. **Buczko, W., Gambino, M. C., and de Gaetano, G.,** Prolongation of rat tail bleeding time by ketanserin: Mechanism of action, *Eur. J. Pharmacol.,* 103, 261, 1984.

70. **Cortellaro, M., Boschetti, C., Antoniazzi, V., Polli, E. E., de Gaetano, G., De Blasi, A., Gerua, M., Pezzi, L., and Garattini, S.,** A pharmacokinetic and platelet function study of the combined administration of metoprolol and sulfinpyrazone to healthy volunteers, *Thromb. Res., 34,* 65, 1984.

71. **Hanson, S. R. and Harker, L. A.,** Effect of dazoxiben on arterial graft thrombosis in the baboon, *Br. J. Clin. Pharmacol.,* Suppl. 1—4, 57 S, 1983.

72. **Smith, E. F. and Egan, J. W.,** Comparison of the effects of a thromboxane synthase inhibitor or prostacyclin in combination with a phosphodieterase inhibitor for prevention of experimental thrombosis and sudden death in rabbits, *J. Pharmacol. Exp. Ther., 241,* 855, 1987.

73. **Cerletti, C., Rajtar, G., Bertelé, V., and de Gaetano, G.,** Inhibition of arachidonate-induced human platelet aggregation by a single low oral dose of aspirin in combination with a thromboxane synthase inhibitor, *Thromb. Haemost., 52,* 215, 1984.

74. **Gresele, P., Deckmyn, H., Arnout, J., Zoja, C., and Vermylen, J.,** Lack of synergism between dazoxiben and dipyridamole following administration to man, *Thromb. Res., 37,* 231, 1985.

75. **Gresele, P., van Houtte, E., Arnout, J., Deckmyn, H., and Vermylen, J.,** Thromboxane synthase inhibition combined with thromboxane receptor blockade: a step forward in antithrombotic strategy?, *Thromb. Haemost., 52,* 364, 1984.

76. **Carson, P., McDonald, L., Pickard, S., Pilkington, T., Davies, B., and Love, F.,** Effect of clofibrate with androsterone (Atromid) and without androsterone (Atromid-S) on blood platelets and lipids in ischemic heart disease, *Br. Heart. J., 28,* 400, 1966.

77. **O'Reilly, R. A., Sahud, M. A., and Robinson, A. J.,** Studies on the interaction of warfarin and clofibrate in man, *Thromb. Diath. Haemorrh., 27,* 309, 1972.

78. **Green, C. J., Kemp, E., and Kemp, G.,** Effect of cyclosporin A, ticlopidine hydrochloride and cobra venom factor on the hyperacute rejection of discordant renal xenografts, *Invest. Cell. Pathol., 3,* 415, 1980.

79. **Hladovec, J.,** The effect of some antithrombotic drugs on experimental arterial thrombosis, *Cor. Vasa, 17,* 66, 1975.

Chapter 6

GENERAL CONCLUSIONS

After an attempt to look at thrombogenesis in a more integrated way taking into account particularly the still relatively neglected role of the vascular wall and emphasizing the multifactorial character of the process, the author introduced a novel system of biomodels constituting an integral battery of tests. The use of various tests as described in the literature in testing antithrombotic activity was surveyed including the results, if available, with the novel battery of tests used in the author's laboratory. The quantitative character of these tests and the ease with which the dose-to-effect relations can be investigated made it possible to study some acknowledged as well as potential antithrombotics and the results were presented against the background of previously published studies.

Throughout the text, the importance of animal models for the prediction of clinical use, dosages, and combinations of antithrombotics was emphasized. The *in vitro* tests and bio-chemical studies, however highly estimated as instruments of deeper knowledge, are not recommended for such prediction purposes and may be misleading without the necessary interface of biomodels. Even in the screening of new drugs they should be interpreted with due caution. The "holistic" approach stressing the response of the organism as a whole should be respected. Of course, this ideal is often not entirely fulfilled even in biomodels and it is necessary to look all the time for such models which would be approaching it as closely as possible.

INDEX

A

Acetylation, 85—86
Acetylsalicylic acid (ASA), 154
  acetylation capacity of, 85—86
  activation of, 76
  in aggregation tests, 77—78
  combinations of, 218
    with calcium dobesilate, 194
    with dihydroergotamine, 194
    with dilthiazem, 193—194
    with dipyridamole, 113, 189—193
    with heparin, 191, 193, 195, 196
    with ketanserin, 197—198, 200
    with metipranolol, 198, 201
    with nifedipine, 198
    with NSAID, 194
    with pentoxifylline, 198, 200
    with prenylamine, 196—197
    with sulfinpyrazone, 196
    with thromboxane synthetase inhibitor, 194
    with troxerutin, 197, 199
    with verapamil, 199
  dose range of, 51—52
  effectiveness of, 69, 75
  effects of, 75—76, 82—87
  interaction of with oral anticoagulants, 194
  introduction of, 75
  in microcirculation, 146
  optimum dose effect of, 56
  with phosphodiesterase inhibitor, 195
  platelet adhesivity and, 76—77
  release of, 78—87
  sensitivity to, 70
Activation, definition of, 76
Adenosine, 88
Adenosine-dipyridamole combination, 194—195
ADP, 25, 146, 158
  decreased platelet count with, 92
  in DIC model, 150
  iontophoretic administration of, 79
  platelet aggregation with, 113, 126
ADPase, 11
Adrenaline, 53
Adrenergic blocking agents, 128
Adrenolytics, 124—130
Aequorin, 131
Aggregating agents, 88
Aggregation tests, acetylsalicylic acid (ASA) in, 77—78
Aglycons, 142
Alkaline phosphatase, 46
Alpha-adrenergic blocking agents, 126
Alprazolam, 158
Aminoalcohol, sulfur-containing, 118
Aminopeptidase M, 45
Anagrelide, 151—152
Androsterone (Atromid), 149, 195
Angiostrongylosis, 25

Angiotensin II, 14
Angiotensin-converting enzyme, 11
Antiaggregating agents, 88
Anticoagulants, see also specific drugs
  interaction of with ASA, 194
  oral, effects of, 153—155
  testing of, 81, 101
Antifibrinolytics, 25
Antimalarics, 158
Antiplatelet agents, 70—71, 98, 151, see also specific drugs
Antiserotonin drugs, 135—141, see also specific drugs
Antiserotonin lisuride, 63
Antithrombin III deficiency, 4, 6
Antithrombotic drugs, see also specific drugs
  combination studies of, 195
  effective doses of, 160—161
  effectiveness of, 154, 156—159
  mutual combinations and potentials of, 218—220
  pitfalls of investigation of, 75
  testing of, 98
  in venous thrombosis prevention, 158
Antithrombotic factors, 12
Aorta
  ligation of, 63
  mechanical lesion of, 97
  occlusion of, 65
Aprotinin, 7
Arachidonic acid, 96
  DIC with, 133
  effects on citrate-induced endothelemia, 125
  metabolism of, 121
  pulmonary distress with, 97
Arenochrome-induced arrhythmias, 99
Arginine derivatives, 157
Arrhythmias, arenochrome-induced, 99
Arterial thrombosis, 20—21
  ASA effects on, 82—85
  dilthiazem effect in, 138
  dipyridamole therapy for, 92—93, 95
  electric current induction of, 62
  epinephrine in, 128
  heparin effects on, 107—108
  ketanserin for, 141
  methiotepine effects on, 144
  model of, 55—67
  nafazatrom effect in, 116
  oral yohimbine effect in, 135
  pipethiadene effects on, 145
  procedure to induce, 61—64
  prothrombotic agent effects on, 62
  sulfinpyrazone effect on, 102
  suloctidil effects on, 119, 120
Arteriolar thromboembolism, laser-induced, 145
Arthus reaction, 114
ASA, see Acetylsalicylic acid
Aspirin, 90, 101
AT III deficiency, see Antithrombin III deficiency

Atherosclerosis, modern theories of, 3
Atherosclerotic plaque, stenosis caused by, 57—58
ATPase, 11
Atrioventricular (AV) microshunt, 89
Atrioventricular (AV) shunts, 80, 81, 96, 191
  occlusive thrombi in, 141
  by sulfinpyrazone, 98

B

Benzamidine, 157
Benzopyrones, 142, 143, 146
Benzydamine, 158
Beta-adrenergic blocking agents, 126, 128
Bioflavonoids, 52, 141—149, 151
Biological inducing agents, 25
Biomodel, definition of, 19—20
BL-3459, 158
Blood
  fluidity regulation of, 11, 23
  infections of, 39
  rheological properties of, 9, 139
  viscosity of, 9
Blood-clotting activation, 15, 16, see also Coagula-
    tion system
Blood clotting factor, hereditary defect of, 4
Blood flow factors, 8—9, 19
BN 50341, 158
BN 52021, 158
Bürkers's chamber, 41—43

C

C 85-3143, 159
Calcium antagonists, 118
Calcium channel blockers
  clinical and experimental effective doses of, 137
  effects of, 130—135
  synergistic effect of with prostacyclin and
      thromboxane synthetase inhibitors, 195
Calcium chelating agents, protective and desqua-
    mating effects of, 55
Calcium dobesilate, 146, 147, 194
Calcium ion influx, 130—131
Calmodulin antagonists, 133
cAMP, see Cyclic adenosine-monophosphate
Capacitance vessels, 68
Carbencillin, 158
Carboanhydrase, 11
Carboxylation, vitamin K-dependent, 153—154
Cardiopulmonary bypass, retinal embolism with, 92
Carotid artery deendothelialization, 113
Catechin A, 146
Catecholamines, 126—128, 195
Challenging agents, 48—51, 71, see also specific
    agents
Chan's method, 159
Chemical challenges, 154
Chemical provocation, 24—25
2-Chloroadenosine, 88
Chlorophenoxy-isobutyrate, 149

Cinnarizine, 135, 139
Citrate
  effects of, 53
  potentiation of, 142
Citrate challenge, 84, 100, 107
Citrate-epinephrine synergism, 130
Clofibrate
  with androsterone, 195
  effects of, 149—151
Clot retraction, 69
Coagulation, 22, see also Disseminated intravascular
    coagulation (DIC)
Coagulation factor precursors, carboxylation of,
    153—154
Coagulation system, 3—6
Coagulation time, prolongation of, 104
Coagulopathy, consumption, 22
Collagen-induced aggregation, 77
Complement system, 19
Contraceptives, endothelial stability and, 61
Coronary artery thrombosis, 21, 132
Coumarin, 142, 145, 154
Curcuma longa, 159
Cyanidanole, 148
Cyclic adenosine-monophosphate, 88—89
Cyclo-oxygenase, 85, 96
Cyclosporin, with ticlopidine, 195
Cyproheptadine, 141
Cytoplasma, 39
Cytoprotective agents, 52

D

Dazoxiben, 121, 123—125
Deep vein thrombosis, 4, 24, 68
Defibrotide, 158—159
Desquamation, 39
  inhibition of, 129
  in ischemia, 45
  mechanisms of, 44
  of mesothelial cells, 53
Destabilizing agents, 52
Dextran, 152—153
DIC, see Disseminated intravascular coagulation
Dicoumarol, 105
Diferuloyl methane (curcumin), 159
Dihydroergotamine-Acetylsalicylic acid (ASA)
    combination, 194
Dilthiazem, 131—132, 134
  with ASA, 193
  effects of, 136, 138
  with propranolol, 195
Dipeptidyl peptidase, 45
Dipyridamole, 87, 95
  with adenosine, 194—195
  with ASA, 189—193
  combinations of, 203, 207—210
  effects of, 81, 88—94, 113
  with heparin, 202
  with nifedipine, 195
  testing of, 87—88

Direct mechanical trauma, 23—24
Dirofilariasis, 25
Disseminated intravascular coagulation (DIC), 3, 22,
    25, 79, 91
  endotoxin, 97
  heparin effectiveness in, 105
  lactic acid-induced, 114
  provocation of, 127
  suloctidil effects in, 118
  verapamil and nifedipine effects on, 133
Ditazole, 158
Drug combinations, 189—220, see also specific
    drugs
Drug screening, thrombotic models in, 71—72
Duncan's test, 72
Dysfibrinogenemias, 4

E

EACA, 7
EDTA, 53
Eicosanoids, role of, 85
Eicosanoid system, drugs interacting with, 121—124
Electrical thrombosis model, 92, 154
Electrochemical lesions, 24
Endarterectomy, 79, 90
Endocarditis, ulcerative, 39
Endothelemia, 148
  ASA effect in, 83
  challenges to, 151
  citrate-induced, 125
  differences with, 160
  hydroxychlorquine for, 158
  inhibition of, 130
  pentoxifylline effectiveness in, 112
  warfarin effect on, 154, 156
Endothelemia test, 71, 124, 161
Endothelial cells
  appearance of, 44
  carcasses of, 47
  characteristics of elements of, 48—49
  circulating elements of, 40—41, 52
  desquamation of, 39, 44, 45, 129
  elements of in microcirculation, 48
  factors inhibiting synthesis of, 4
  loss of coherence of, 44
  low density anuclear carcasses of, 40
  method of counting carcasses of, 40—44
  stabilizing drug effects on, 58
Endothelial cement, 44
Endothelial defensive functions, 118
Endothelial element count
  ASA effect on, 84
  diagnostic value of, 54
  ischemia and stasis effects on, 52
  methionine and, 54
  time course in, 49
Endothelial lesions, 10
  drugs inducing, 54
  homocysteine-induced, 92
  morphological changes of, 10
  noxious influences leading to, 14

Endothelial stability, 56—57
  ASA effects on, 85
  bioflavinoid effects on, 148
  calcium dobesilate effect on, 147
  catecholamine effects on, 128
  cinnarizine and lidoflazine effect on, 139
  contraceptive effects on, 61
  dilthiazem effects on, 136
  flunarizine effect on, 138, 139
  heparin effects on, 110
  mental stress effects on, 60
  physical exertion effects on, 59
  smoking effects on stability of, 58
  suloctidil effects on, 119
  test, sulfinpyrazone effect on, 99—100
  troxerutin effect on, 147
Endothelial vulnerability test, 51
Endotheliomas, 39
Endothelium, 11—12, 14—15
Endothelium-derived relaxing factor (EDRF),
    11, 13
Endotoxin, 25
Endotoxin thrombus model, 105
Epinephrine, 108, 126—129
Epsilonaminocaproic acid (EACA), 7
Erythrocyte aggregation, 143, 152
Esculetin, 143
Eterylate, inhibitory effects of, 194—195
Euglobulin lysis test, 45, 47
Experimental animals, 25—26

F

Factor VIIR:AG, 44
Factor VIII, 14
Factor VIIIR:AG immunoreaction, 43
Factor Xa absorption, 103
Factor XII deficiency, 4
Factor XIIa, antithrombotic activity of, 12
Factor C defect, 4
Femoral vein thrombosis, morrhuate-induced, 145—
    146
Fenoprofen, 158
Fernthrombose, 10
Fibrin, 12—13, 18—19, 70
Fibrin degradation products, prothrombotic activity
    of, 12
Fibrinogen
  coagulation of, 22
  decreased levels of, 50, 150
  detection of levels of, 47
  prothrombotic activity of, 12
  split products from, 12—13, 18—19
Fibrinogen uptake test, 16
Fibrinolytic system, 4, 6—7, 19
Fibrinopeptide B, 13
Fibronectin, 113
Flavonoids, 142—143, 145, 147, 149
Flavonols, 143
Flunarizine, 135, 138—140
Formalin, rebound thrombosis and, 104
FP-A test, 5

G

Giemsa's staining, 39, 40
Glomerular fibrin deposits, 91
Glucuronidation, 142
Glycocalyx, 11, 45, 149
Glycoproteins, 11, 114
Glycosaminoglycans, synthesis of, 11
Glycosaminoglycan sulodexide, 159
Gravimetric method, 47

H

Halofenate, 150
Hemostatic system, 189
Heparan monosulfate, 11
Heparin
    anticlotting effect of, 70
    with ASA, 191, 193, 195—196
    binding of to vascular endothelium and reticuloen-
        dothelial system, 103
    combinations of, 198, 202—206, 218
    discrepancy of effects of, 103
    effectiveness of, 194
    effects of, 69, 101—111
    low molecular weight, 102—103, 106—107
    sensitivity to, 108
    subcutaneous, 108
    testing of, 101
Heparin cofactor II, 103
Heparinoid SP 54, 107
Heparinoid thrombocid, 104
Hirudin, 157
HLA antigens, 4
Hodgkin's disease, 39
Homocysteine, 49, 53
Homocysteinemia, 4
5-HT, 63—64, 67
    as mediator and potentiating agent, 140—141
    release of from platelets, 136
Humoral factors, 4—8, 18, 19
Hyaluronidase inhibition, 143
Hydrogen peroxide
    as challenge agent, 147
    endothelemia-increasing activity of, 148
    endothelial stability and, 57
Hydroxychloroquine, 158—159
4-Hydroxycoumarin derivatives, 154
Hydroxyethylated rutosides (HR), 146, 148—149
5-Hydroxykynurenamide, 141
Hypercoagulability, 4—6, 29
Hypercoagulability tests, 6
Hyperfibrinolysis, 22
Hyperlipemia, 154
Hypotension, deep, 89
Hypotonic saline, 63—64
    as challenging agent, 107, 160
    effects of, 65, 67
    endothelial stability and, 110
    systemic administration of, 68

I

Ibuprofen, 158
Imidazoquinazoline, 151
Indalitan, 154, 155
Indandione derivatives, 154
Indication, method of, 26
Indobufen, 158
Interendothelial gaps, widening of, 44
Interleukin-1, 12
Intravenous citrate challenge, 46
    ASA effect on stability of, 56
    decreased euglobulin lysis time after, 47
    effects of, 50
Iproniazide, 159
Iron deficiency thrombocytosis, 7
Ischemia, 45, 52
Isoprenaline, 128

K

Kadsurenone, 158
Kallikrein system, 19
Kaolin, 70
Ketanserin
    with ASA, 197—198, 200
    bleeding time and, 195
    combinations of, 210, 217, 219
    with dipyridamole, 203, 209
    effects of, 135—141, 143
    with heparin, 204
    with prenylamine, 210, 215
    with sulfinpyrazone, 210, 212
    with troxerutin, 210, 215
6-Ketoprostaglandin F_{1a} formation, 117

L

L-652731, 158
Lanthanum, 133
Laser-induced lesions, 81—82
Laser-induced thrombi, 105, 116
Legalon, 148
Leukocytes, 7, 8
Lidoflazine, 135, 139
Lipid peroxidation, 150
Lipoperoxidase system, 143
Lipoprotein lipase, 11
Lipoxygenase inhibitors, 143, 158
Lipoxygenases, 117
Lisuride, 142
Localization, 20—23

M

Mechanical trauma, 23—24
Membrane-stabilizing agents, 52
Mental stress, endothelial stability and, 60
Mesenteric microcirculation, 89—90
Mesenteric vessel thrombosis, 68—69, 109, 121

Mesothelial cells, desquamation of, 53
Methionine
  desquamating activity of, 49
  effects of, 53
  endothelial element count and, 54
  as oral challenge, 51
Methiotepine, 141, 144
Metipranolol, 128—130
  with ASA, 198, 201
  combinations of, 219
  with dipyridamole, 203, 210
  effects of, 131
  with heparin, 203, 205, 206
  with ketanserin, 217
  with pentoxifylline, 210—218
  with prenylamine, 214
  with sulfinpyrazone, 210, 213
  with troxerutin, 210, 216
Metoprolol, 127
Metoprolol-sulfinpyrazone combination, 195
Microcirculation thrombosis, 78, 79, 104
Microembolism syndrome, 22
Mono-7-hydroxyethylrutoside, 146, 148
Monoaminooxidase
  inhibitors, 159
  metabolism of biogenic amines by, 13
Multifactorial pathogenesis, 15—19
Myocardial infarction, 99, 126, 189
Myocardial microcirculation, 90
Myocardial necrosis, 79, 99, 127

N

Nafazatrom, 115—118, 124
Naftidrofuryl, 159
Naphthyridine derivative, 159
Nicardipine, 133
Nifedipine, 131—134
Nifedipine-ASA combination, 198
Nifedipine-dipyridamole combination, 195
Nonsteroidal anti-inflammatory drugs (NSAIDs)
  with ASA, 194
  cyclo-oxygenase inhibitory action of, 96
  effectiveness of, 157
  membrane-stabilizing effects of, 86
  new type of, 158
5-Nucleotidase, 11

O

Oxygen burst, 8
Oxygen scavenger effect, free, 143

P

PAF, see Platelet-activating factor
PAI, see Plasminogen activator inhibitor
Penicillin, 158
Pentaerythritol tetranitrate (PETN), 64, 67
Pentoxifylline

  with ASA, 198, 200
  combinations of, 219
  with dipyridamole, 203, 207
  effects of, 111—112
  with heparin, 205
  with ketanserin, 210, 217
  with metipranolol, 210—218
  with prenylamine, 210, 214
  with sulfinpyrazone, 210, 212
  with troxerutin, 210, 216
Peripheral arterial disease, sulfinpyrazone effects on, 96
Peripheral circulation, 135
PGI_1, 123
PGI_2, 14, 81
Pharmacokinetics, 27
Phenoxybenzamine, 126
Phentolamine, 126, 127, 128
Phenylbutazone, 157
Phosphodiesterase, 89, 111, 143
Phosphodiesterase inhibitor, with thromboxane synthetase inhibitor or ASA, 195
Phospholipase A_2 inhibition, 158
Piette's method, 47
Pipethiadene, 141, 145
Pizotifen, 141, 144
Plasminogen activator inhibitor (PAI), 4—7, 12
Plasminogen, deficient or defective, 4
Platelet-activating factor (PAF), 131, 132, 158
Platelet activation tests, 8
Platelet aggregation, 146
  benzopyrone effects on, 143
  with epinephrine, 126
  inhibition of, 103, 152
  ketanserin effect on, 137
  serotonin-induced, 141
Platelet function tests, 150
Platelet microthrombi, 90
Platelets
  adhesivity of, 76—77
  constituents, release of, 70
  decreased count of, 92
  derangements, 7
  distribution after citrate challenge, 50
  drugs interacting with, 121
  in early thrombosis stages, 7—8
  inhibited adhesion of, 80
  interacting, 70—71
  interaction with vessel wall, 96, 101
  loss of local reactivity of, 89
  membrane reorganization in, 112
  radiolabeled, accumulation of, 114
  redistribution of, 131
  serotonin accumulation in, 60—61
  tests for early activation of, 15
Platelet sequestration, 47
  ASA inhibited, 82—83
  changes in, 48
  citrate-epinephrine synergism in, 130
  epinephrine effects on, 129

flunarizine effects on, 140
heparin effects on, 109
HR and mono-7-hydroxyethylrutoside effects on, 146
in vivo method of, 77
increased, 45
potentiation of citrate effect on, 142
pulmonary, 114
sulfinpyrazone effect on, after citrate challenge, 100
suloctidil effects on, 119, 120
Platelet sequestration test, 93, 94, 128
Platelet thrombus formation, transient, 140
Polytetrafluoroethylene grafts, 91
Postheparin thrombocytopenias, 7
Practolol, 130, 133
Practolol-heparin combination, 203
Prazosine, 130, 134
Prazosine-heparin combination, 203
Prenylamine, 134, 154
  with ASA, 196—197
  combinations of, 210, 213—215, 218
  with dipyridamole, 203, 208
  effects of, 137, 156, 157
  with heparin, 203
  with sulfinpyrazone, 210—211
Prethrombosis models, 57, 71, 78
Propranolol, 126, 127, 128, 130
  effects of, 132
Propranolol-dilthiazem combination, 195
Propranolol heart attack, 127
Propranolol-heparin combination, 203
Prostacyclin, 11
  availability of, 116
  combinations of, 195
  deficiency of, 7
  effects of, 123, 124
  synthesis of, 81, 88, 122
Prostaglandin, 123, 143
Prostanoids, 52
Prostheses, thrombosis on, 23
Proteases, 25
Protein C, 12, 13
Protein S deficiency, 4
Prothrombin, one stage, 154
Prothrombotic agents, 25, 62
Prothrombotic factors, 12
Provocation, type of, 23—25
Provoking factors, number of, 27
Prozosin, 195
Pulmonary vascular resistance, increased, 98
Pyridazinone derivative, 159
Pyridinolcarbamate, 151
Pyridoxine, 49, 53

Q

Quercetin, 143

R

RA 233, 89
RA 433, 89
Radiofibrinogen, 68, 106—107
Retinal embolism, 92
Reyers' method, 69—70
Rheological factors, 8
Rokitanski, C., 3
Rotation viscosimeters, 9
Russel's viper venom, 25
Rutin, 141, 142, 145

S

Sclerosing agents, 25
Serotonin, 136
  with catecholamines, 195
  effects of, 63, 140
  intravenous, 29
  in platelets, 60—61
  prothrombotic activity of, 12
  release of, 13
  thrombosis-stimulating effect of, 59—60
SH 1117, 90
Sickle cell anemia, 4, 8
Silymarine, 148
Smoking, effect of on endothelial stability, 58
Sodium salicylate, effects of, 80, 86
Stabilizing agents, 51—52, 58
Stenosis, mechanical occlusion stimulating, 57—58
Sulfinpyrazone
  activity of, 94
  with ASA, 196
  combinations of, 210—213, 218
  with dipyridamole, 203, 207
  effectiveness of, 69, 193
  effects of, 94—102
  with heparin, 198, 202
  with metoprolol, 195
  with prenylamine, 210, 211
  testing of, 98
  with troxerutin, 210—211
Suloctidil, effects of, 118—121

T

Thrombin, 25
  adsorption of in endothelium, 103
  intravascular, 154
  intravenous, 22
  prothrombotic activity of, 12
  release of, 13
Thrombin-induced thrombus, 106
Thrombin inhibitors, 156—157
Thrombocytopenia, heparin-induced, 6
Thrombocytosis, 7
Thrombogenesis, process of, 14—15

Thrombolysis, 3
Thrombophilia, 5, 29
Thrombophlebitis, 68, 145
Thromboplastin, 25
Thrombosis
  arterial, 20—21, 55—67, 82—85, 92—95, 102, 107—108, 116—120, 135, 138, 141, 144—145
  on artificial surfaces, 23
  deep vein, 4, 24, 68
  definition of, 3—4
  in experimental animals, 25—26
  freeze-induced, 115, 116
  laser-induced, 81—82, 105, 116
  localization of, 20—23
  methods of indication in, 26
  model of, 19—20
    classification of, 20—28
    comprehensiveness of viewpoint on, 27
    number of provoking factors in, 27
    research objectives for, 28
    time span of experiment in, 26—27
  multifactorial character of, 15—19, 55, 69—70
  new system of models of, 30
  pathogenetic role of, 1
  spontaneous, 25
  survey conclusions on, 28—30
  tendency to, 5
  type of provocation of, 23—25
  venous, 17—18, 21, 67—71, 97, 116, 121, 128, 141
Thrombosis factors, 27
  blood flow, 8—9
  humoral, 4—8
  interaction of, 15—19, 29
  vascular lesion, 9—15
Thrombosis triad, 3—4
Thrombotic ischemic accidents, study of, 71
Thrombotic microangiopathy, 22
Thrombotic thrombocytopenic purpura, 7
Thromboxane
  production of, in platelets, 117
  sources of, 122
Thromboxane A_2, 12, 121—122
Thromboxane-prostacyclin balance, 77, 85, 87
Thromboxane receptors, 123
Thromboxane synthetase inhibitor-acetylsalicylic acid (ASA) combination, 194
Thromboxane synthetase inhibitors, combinations of, 194—195
Thrombus
  cyclic formation, 107
  factors for induction of, 57—60
  mechanism of formation of, 55, 71
TIAs, see Transient ischemic accidents
Ticlopidine
  effects of, 113—115
  with cyclosporin, 195

Tissue cell system, drugs interacting with, 121
Tissue plasminogen activator (tPA)
  in blood fluidity regulation, 11
  defects in synthesis of, 6
  deficient, 4
  in testing for endothelial lesions, 14
Tissue thromboplastin, intravenous, 105
Transient ischemic accidents (TIAs), 21, 57
Triazolam, 158
Trihydroxyethylrutoside, 141
Troxerutin, 141, 146—147
  antithrombotic activity of, 149
  ASA combination, 197, 199
  combinations of, 210, 215—216, 218, 219
  dipyridamole combination, 208
  effects of, 150—151
  heparin combination, 203—204
  inhibitory effect of, 148
  prenylamine combination, 210, 213
  sulfinpyrazone combination, 210—211
Trypsin, 105
Turpentine oil, 145
TXSI, 122, 123

U

U-66,855, 158

V

Vascular factors, neglect of, 160
Vascular lesion
  categories of, 9—10
  definition of, 9
  etiological aspect of, 13
  generalized low-intensity, 58—59
  hypercoagulability and, 5—6
  model of, 39—54
  physical effects producing, 24
  in thrombosis, 9—15
  types of, 67—68
Venous occlusion, decreased endothelial element counts with, 48
Venous thrombosis
  epinephrine in, 128
  frequency of, 18
  idiopathic, 17—18, 21
  ketanserin for, 141
  model of, 67—71
  nafazatrom effect in, 116
  prevention of, 97
  suloctidil effects on, 121
Verapamil, 131—134, 196, 199
Virchow, R., 3
VK 744, 89—90
von Willebrand's disease, 152

W

Warfarin
  anticoagulant effect of, 52
  cumulative effect of, 156
  optimum dose effect of, 56
  therapeutic dose of, 154
Weibel-Pallade bodies, 45
Wessler's principle, 67
White bodies
  formation of
    electric current-induced, 118
    prevention of, 97, 105

shortened period of, 88—89
  reduction of, 127
Wu-Hoak method, 47

X

Xenograft rejection, hyperacute, 114

Y

Yohimbine
  effects of, 135
  with heparin, 203

9 780367 450984